Vitamins, Supplements, and Herbs for Health and Longevity

Boost Your Immunity, Increase Energy, and Feel Younger in Minutes a Day

HEALTH AND LONGEVITY MASTERY SERIES
VOLUME TWO

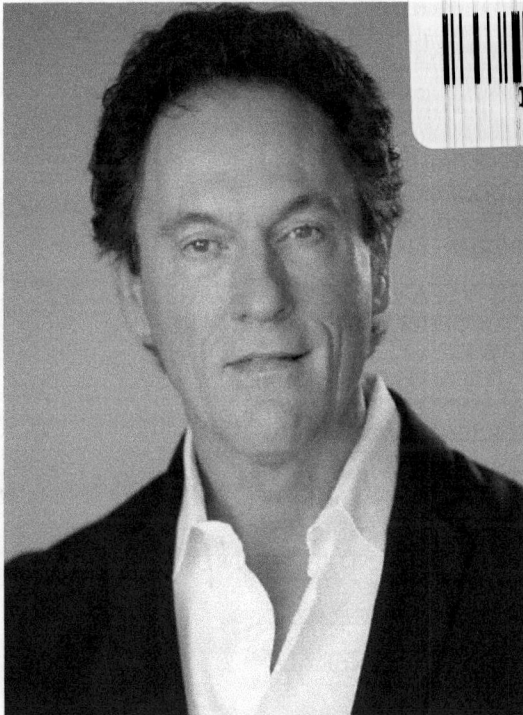

By Tad Sisler

TABLE OF CONTENTS

SECTION ONE: WHY SUPPLEMENTS MATTER
I.I.I: BRIDGING NUTRIENT GAPS
I.I.2: PERSONALIZED NUTRITION
I.I.3: COMMON MYTHS/MISCONCEPTIONS

SECTION TWO: THE BUILDING BLOCKS OF LIFE
I.2.I: MACRONUTRIENTS VS. MICRONUTRIENTS
I.2.2: THE ROLE OF ENZYMES AND COENZYMES
I.2.3: OXIDATIVE STRESS AND ANTIOXIDANTS

SECTION THREE: SAFETY, REGULATION, AND QUALITY
I.3.I: UNDERSTANDING LABELS AND CLAIMS
I.3.2: THIRD-PARTY TESTING AND GMP STANDARDS
I.3.3: KEY REGULATORY BODIES
I.3.4: CONSULTING HEALTHCARE PROFESSIONALS

SECTION ONE: VITAMIN A AND THE B-COMPLEX
2.I.I: VITAMIN A (RETINOL, BETA-CAROTENE)
2.I.2: THE B-COMPLEX OVERVIEW
2.I.3: INDIVIDUAL B-VITAMINS

SECTION TWO: VITAMINS C AND D
2.2.I: VITAMIN C (ASCORBIC ACID)
2.2.2: VITAMIN D2 (Ergocalciferol) vs. D3 (Cholecalciferol)
2.2.3: EMERGING RESEARCH ON VITAMIN D

SECTION THREE: VITAMINS E AND K, AMINO ACIDS
2.3.I: VITAMIN E (TOCOPHEROLS & TOCOTRIENOLS)
2.3.2: VITAMIN KI VS. K2
2.3.3: SYNERGY IN THE ALPHABET VITAMINS
2.3.4: THE ROLE OF AMINO ACIDS
2.3.5: VITAMIN DEFICIENCIES AND SYMPTOMS

SECTION ONE: MACRO MINERALS
3.I.I: CALCIUM, MAGNESIUM, AND PHOSPHORUS
3.I.2: POTASSIUM AND SODIUM
3.I.3: BIOAVAILABILITY AND INTERACTIONS

SECTION TWO: TRACE MINERALS
3.2.I: IRON, ZINC, COPPER
3.2.2: SELENIUM, IODINE, CHROMIUM
3.2.3: MANGANESE, MOLYBDENUM, BORON

SECTION TWO: PEPTIDES, GENE THERAPIES, AND PLASMA
APPROACHES
8.2.1: PEPTIDE THERAPIES (e.g. EPITHALON, THYMOSIN) AND POLYAMINES
(SPERMIDINE)
8.2.2: GENE EDITING (CRISPR) AND SiRNA
8.2.3: PLASMA EXCHANGE / APHERESIS
8.2.4: ETHICAL CONSIDERATIONS IN GENE THERAPIES

SECTION THREE: PRACTICAL CONSIDERATIONS AND RESPONSIBLE
USE
8.3.1: REGULATORY AND ETHICAL DIMENSIONS
8.3.2: LIFESTYLE INTEGRATION WITH EMERGING SCIENCE
8.3.3: MONITORING AND FOLLOW-UP

SECTION ONE: TRADITIONAL CHINESE MEDICINE (TCM) INSIGHTS
9.1.1: TCM HERBS (DANG GUI, HUANG QIN, DAN SHEN)
9.1.2: QI, YIN, AND YANG EXPLAINED BRIEFLY
9.1.3: KEY TCM FORMULAS (XAIO YAO SAN, LIU WEI DI HUANG WAN) AND
LONGEVITY HERBS (JIAOGULAN)

SECTION TWO: AYURVEDA AND OTHER GLOBAL TRADITIONS
9.2.1: AYURVEDIC STAPLES (AMLA, NEEM, GUDUCHI, GOTU KOLA)
9.2.2: LATIN AMERICAN AND INDIGENOUS REMEDIES (GRAVIOLA, YERBA MATE)
9.2.3: AFRICAN AND MIDDLE EASTERN HERBS (CINNAMON, FENUGREEK,
FRANKINCENSE)
9.2.4: AFRICAN AND NATIVE AMERICAN TRADITIONS

SECTION THREE: INTEGRATING HISTORICAL WISDOM WITH
MODERN SCIENCE
9.3.1: RESEARCH CHALLENGES
9.3.2: RESPECTING AND PRESERVING CULTURAL KNOWLEDGE
9.3.3: PERSONALIZED, HOLISTIC APPROACHES
9.3.4: VALIDATION OF HISTORICAL USES

SECTION FOUR: NUTRITION FROM LIVING ORGANISMS
9.4.1: COMMON STAPLES
9.4.2: ORGANIC DETOX AND CLEANSING AGENTS

SECTION ONE: MAJOR DISEASES
10.1.1: THE GREATEST KILLERS
10.1.2: MINOR ILLNESSES
10.1.3: LIFESTYLE FACTORS BEYOND SUPPLEMENTS
10.1.4: PERSONALIZED MEDICINE AND GENETICS

SECTION TWO: MODERN CHALLENGES
10.2.1: MODERN CHRONIC CONDITIONS
10.2.2: NEURODEVELOPMENTAL AND BEHAVIORAL CONDITIONS
10.2.3: AUTOIMMUNE CONDITIONS

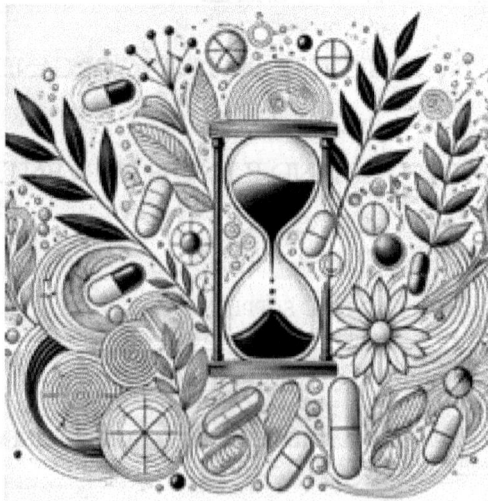

FOREWORD

My mother, **Elaine Witt Sisler**, was a child prodigy. She became a renowned concert pianist, performing as a soloist for the Chicago Symphony at 17. When she met my father, **Maynard Lee Sisler**, during World War II, he was a pharmacist's mate on a Navy ship, deployed to the South Pacific shortly after they met. Although my father didn't attend medical school until after the war, he had to learn quickly during battle, as he was sometimes the only medic on an entire ship. These were the early days of life-saving antibiotics; the ships would get small supplies.

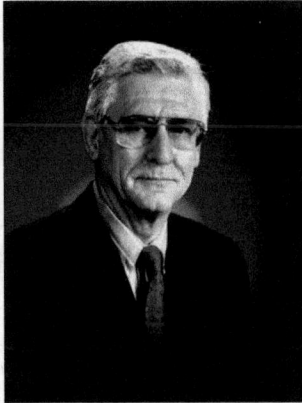

Tad Sisler's Father Maynard Lee Sisler, M.D., F.A.C.P
Source – Sisler Private collection

My father would dispense them to the sickest sailors, and others who also needed antibiotics were forced to drink urine from the sailors who initially received the antibiotics to stretch out the efficacy as far as they could to heal as many as possible. He learned surgical techniques on the fly, relying upon the fast advice of a handful of doctors and available medical books. Later, he became a *Fellow* in the **American College of Physicians** and a member of London's **Royal Society of Medicine.** My father instilled a love of medicine into me, and I probably would have become a doctor if my first love were not music. As my mother had done, I took the road less traveled and became a performing musician.

My parents divorced when I was 12, and my mother suffered a nervous breakdown. Although I have five older sisters, at that point, they were grown and gone, and I was alone with my mother, trying to help her through her grief. For a short period, she turned to alcohol and depressants, but she came out of it eventually and started searching for health and wellness without medication. Sometimes, when searching to save ourselves, we go out on a limb and might take our recovery to the limit. This probably explains why she filled every available cabinet in our house with vitamins and supplements.

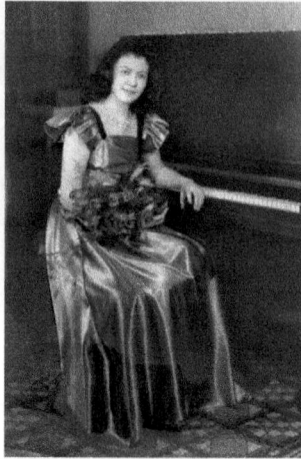

Tad Sisler's Mother Elaine Witt Sisler at Age 16
Source: Tad Sisler's personal collection

I became my mother's guinea pig! She would give me handfuls of vitamins in the morning before school. Once, she gave me niacin, and by the time I got to school I had become beet red, flushing from the effects of the vitamin right in front of my friends. It was embarrassing and, frankly, scary! Another morning, she gave me a cayenne pepper pill, and I burped fire! On another day, I got a garlic pill, and none of the other students would come close to me! Even though it seemed like an ordeal at the time, she had good intentions, and I received an extensive early education on vitamins and supplements! She had a remedy for everything, and most of the time, her suggestions worked. And I was probably the healthiest eighth grader at my school.

My **Robin** is a nurse, and she rolls her eyes when I take out my big table every month, put an enormous number of supplements on it, and dole out my daily supply for the next month. She, like my niece **Lori** and many other medical professionals, was trained to believe that when you take so many supplements like I do, you're probably just creating expensive pee. But I honestly don't know many men my age who feel as vibrant and healthy as I do, and I hear all the time that I look much younger than my chronological age.

I was also delighted to see that many health gurus also take multiple amounts of supplements. I just saw an article yesterday where **Robert F. Kennedy, Jr.** mentioned taking handfuls of supplements daily.

I'm not suggesting that you or anyone else do this, but my goal is to help you find the most current information on what might be right for you. If I can help you become even a bit healthier, I've hopefully done a good thing.

I read a great article recently on a study by *Stanford Medicine* about "smart toilets", disease-detecting toilets that can sense multiple signs of illness through automated urine and stool analysis. I read somewhere else that scientists are working on the idea of a futuristic 'smart house' where your toilet analyses your urine and stool, and by the time you get to the kitchen, your refrigerator is ready to dispense a perfect concoction of supplements, nutraceuticals and pharmaceuticals to keep you in optimum health for the day. The future has endless possibilities!

No matter what you do, however, the Universe may have other plans for you. One of the most genuine expressions I've heard is, ***"If you want to make God laugh, tell him what you're doing tomorrow."*** My sister **Judy** was beautiful. She was a registered nurse with a master's degree and focused entirely on her health. She was vibrant and full of life at the age of 64 when a tick bit her and she quickly contracted *Rocky Mountain Spotted Fever.* She tragically lost her life in just two weeks. My other sister, **Betsy**, had overcome her addictions and had been clean and sober for almost 30 years when she passed suddenly in an automobile accident. Another sister, **Kathleen,** was the healthiest of all my sisters, eating natural foods and taking every vitamin and supplement you could imagine. She had a heart defect and had mitral valve surgery at the age of 45. After three other heart surgeries, I believe strongly that her healthy lifestyle has brought her this far, and I'm grateful for every day I still have with her. The main thing is to do the most you can with what you have. Remember what my friend, the great actor **Robert Wagner**, said:

"I've learned one important thing about God's gifts – what we do with them is our gift to him."

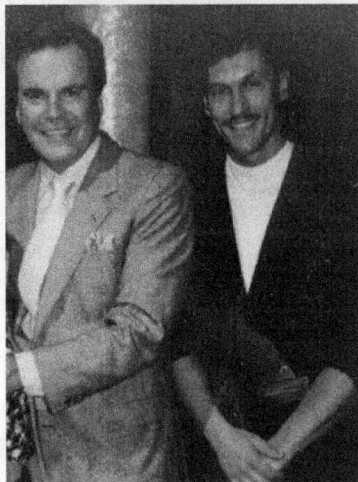

Robert Wagner and Tad Sisler
Source – Sisler Private Collection

Make it your mission to treat your body, the ultimate of God's gifts, with the utmost respect. We don't know if we will live until the end of the day or for another hundred years. All we can do is treat our body like a temple and do everything we can to stay healthy until new scientific advances increase our longevity even more. Remember the old saying, **"Trust in God, but keep your gunpowder dry."** Take care of yourself daily, and you'll do your part.

INTRODUCTION
UNLOCKING THE SECRETS OF LASTING VITALITY

When I began researching this book, I immediately understood why so many people feel information overload when trying to figure out what vitamins and supplements are necessary. It's challenging to differentiate between credible and misleading information about supplements and herbs. And there are so many to choose from! Which of these are essential for combating aging? Do some work against others in our bodies?

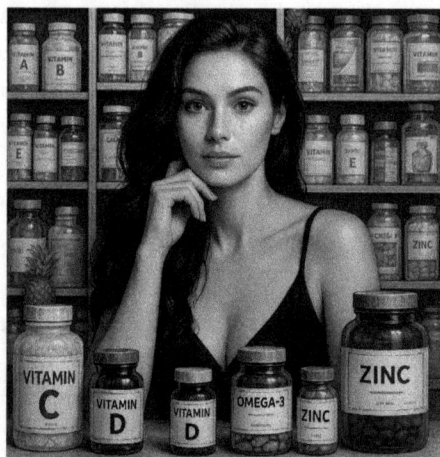

Like many people, I began to feel fatigue and low energy regularly despite trying various diets or routines. My stress levels were sometimes very high, leading to a desire for natural remedies to offset stress. When my beloved older sister **Suzanne** was diagnosed with Parkinson's Disease, I cried watching her struggle and at the same time I worried about how to prevent my own age-related diseases or how to "age well" in general. Finally, with my daily time constraints, how would I balance my busy schedule while still trying to incorporate health practices? How can I find the time and energy to apply this knowledge?

I could probably find all the information I need online for free, but what about unique or deeper insights that would help me better understand this new world I'm navigating? Is it too complicated? What if I don't understand scientific jargon or complex advice? And I always felt that the multivitamins I took when

I was younger didn't really do much for me. But not all vitamins are supposed to make you feel extra energy or really anything but normal. It's the absence of supplementation that our bodies notice. Just ask any old sailor who experienced scurvy from lack of Vitamin C! Still, imagine waking up each day brimming with energy without relying on endless cups of coffee. What if the key to feeling younger and more vibrant lies in some vitamins, supplements, and herbs we often overlook?

Embarking on my own personal journey of seeking better health and well-being, I boiled down my desires to a handful of significant things:

Improved Energy Levels: I wanted more energy to handle daily tasks and feel vibrant. Did nutritional deficiencies contribute to my low energy, or was it just aging? What vitamins and supplements could naturally boost my energy and help me feel like I could tackle anything?

Health Optimization: I wanted to find ways to boost my immunity, prevent illness, and promote longevity. Strengthening my immune system is a priority, especially when people with the flu surround me! What natural remedies could boost my immunity?

Clearer Skin and Appearance: I started looking for natural solutions to enhance the health of my skin and slow signs of aging. As a performer with people staring at me all night, I want to age gracefully, improving my external appearance while boosting my internal health.

Stress Management: What herbs and supplements could provide calm and focus? Like many people, my chronic stress levels made me search for natural ways to avoid the desire for anxiety medication.

Confidence in My Choices: I wanted trustworthy information to select the right vitamins and herbs. What supplements should I trust for safety, quality, and efficacy?

This book aims to highlight the growing popularity of dietary supplements, vitamins, and herbs. I strive to provide science-backed guidance on harnessing these compounds for immunity, energy, and longevity. Throughout the book, you'll see quotes from extraordinary individuals, enormous encouragement, and evidence-based information from peer-reviewed studies, regulatory considerations, and real-world use cases to help you in your own quest for health and long life.

My goal is to help you seamlessly incorporate vitamins, supplements, and herbs into your daily routine without becoming overwhelmed.

But before we discuss vitamins and herbs, let's first examine the fundamentals—how nutrition and supplementation actually work in the body. But, before that, here's the legal stuff:

EXTREMELY IMPORTANT – READ THIS BEFORE PROCEEDING

MEDICAL DISCLAIMER

The information provided in this book is for informational and educational purposes only and is not intended to replace or substitute professional advice, diagnosis, or treatment from a licensed medical practitioner, pharmacist, or other qualified healthcare provider. The author and publisher are not medical practitioners and do not claim to provide medical advice.

Readers are strongly advised to consult a qualified healthcare professional before starting any new health regimen, including but not limited to the use of vitamins, supplements, herbs, poultices, or dietary changes. Individual reactions to supplements and herbs can vary significantly based on personal health conditions, existing prescriptions, allergies, sensitivities, or dietary habits.

The methods, techniques, and practices described in this book may not be suitable for all individuals, and their safety and effectiveness depend on personal health factors. Some of the products, ideas, or techniques discussed may be experimental, not widely available, or still under development. No guarantees or warranties are made regarding their safety, efficacy, or suitability for any particular individual or circumstance.

Certain supplements, herbs, or poultices may interact negatively with prescription medications, over-the-counter drugs, foods, or other supplements. These interactions can result in adverse effects, reduced effectiveness of treatments, or unexpected health outcomes. Readers are solely responsible for verifying potential interactions with their healthcare providers prior to use.

The author and publisher expressly disclaim any liability for adverse reactions, harm, or damages that may arise from the use or misuse of the information in this book. The reader assumes full responsibility for any actions taken or decisions made based on the content of this book.

LEGAL DISCLAIMER

This book is presented for informational and educational purposes only and should not be considered a source of medical, legal, financial, or professional advice. The content is based on research, opinions, and sources believed to be reliable at the time of publication; however, the author and publisher make no representations or warranties regarding the accuracy, completeness, or timeliness of the information. Readers should consult qualified professionals for specific advice tailored to their individual needs and circumstances.

The use of any information contained in this book is at the reader's own risk. The reader agrees to indemnify and hold harmless the author, publisher, and affiliated parties from any and all claims, demands, damages, liabilities, or losses resulting from the use or misuse of the information provided. This includes, but is not limited to, adverse reactions, injuries, or complications related to the use of vitamins, supplements, herbs, poultices, or their interactions with prescription medications, over-the-counter drugs, foods, or other substances.

This book does not establish any form of professional relationship between the author, publisher, and reader. Any discussion of supplements, therapies, emerging scientific developments, or other practices is for informational purposes only and does not constitute an endorsement or guarantee.

The content of this book is subject to change as new research and evidence emerge. The author and publisher disclaim all responsibility for any errors or omissions, and they are not responsible for any consequences arising from the use of this book, including but not limited to misinterpretation of the content or failure to seek appropriate professional guidance.

By reading this book, the reader acknowledges and accepts these disclaimers, indemnifying the author, publisher, and affiliated parties from any liabilities or claims arising directly or indirectly from the use, misuse, or application of the content contained herein.

CHAPTER ONE
UNDERSTANDING THE FOUNDATIONS OF NUTRITION AND SUPPLEMENTATION

"Our body is the only one we've been given, so we need to maintain it; we need to give it the best nutrition." — Trudie Styler

Once upon a time, people believed that just 'eating well' was enough. But modern lifestyles, environmental factors, and personalized needs tell a different story — leading many of us to explore vitamins, supplements, and herbs more seriously. Also, new advances in longevity and age reversal research have identified supplements that could increase our lifespan and healthspan. These advances are particularly exciting for me. For a deep dive into the latest information on longevity and age reversal, please read my book **Stay Healthy, Stay Youthful: The Science of Living to 150.**

WHY DO I NEED SUPPLEMENTS?
So many of us find ourselves unhealthy, overweight, and generally unhappy with our overall well-being. And when you think about it, too much weight on you puts you in a position where you're more likely to get heart disease, diabetes, inflammation, and other maladies. While I'm plugging my books, I've done a deep dive into all the diets of the last century and their common denominators in my book **The Ultimate AI Diet - Consolidating the Best Diets Over the Last 100 Years.** It's packed with information on weight management.

Imagine a world where your body gets all the nutrition it needs to function at the highest level; a world where you can eat most anything in moderation and get away with it, if you follow a few guidelines such as burning more calories than you use. Supplements can be the key to a healthier life. My friend, legendary multi-platinum recording artist **Rod Stewart** said,

"I wish I knew what I know now before."

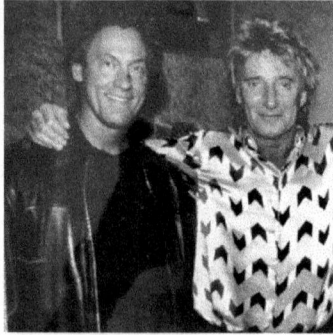

Tad Sisler with Rod Stewart
Source – Sisler Private Collection

Getting a head-start on your overall health as you age could add years on to your life. So, let's get started!

WHAT IS A DIETARY SUPPLEMENT?

Dietary supplements encompass a wide range of compounds that provide nutritional or therapeutic benefits. These supplements are typically consumed to enhance health, address specific deficiencies, or support physiological functions.

SECTION ONE: WHY SUPPLEMENTS MATTER
I.I.I: BRIDGING NUTRIENT GAPS

MANY DIETS LACK ESSENTIAL NUTRIENTS from processed foods and soil depletion. Regarding organic foods, one of my friends asked, *"Why is it that we have to pay more at the supermarket for foods that don't contain poison?"* Although that may not be entirely true, it's a sad reminder that we need to know what we're eating. It's difficult to count on the quality of our current food supply, although if you live in a first-world country like the United States, you have an outstanding advantage in abundance over third-world countries.

Modern farming practices, extended supply chains, and the widespread consumption of processed foods can significantly reduce the micronutrient content of our meals. Soil depletion means that fruits and vegetables may not contain the same levels of vitamins and minerals they once did, even if they look

14

the same in the grocery store. Consequently, even people who *think* they are eating a healthy, balanced diet may still miss vital nutrients. This makes supplementation an extremely important tool to make sure you have enough vitamins, minerals, and other key nutrients.

SUPPLEMENTS CAN FILL MICRONUTRIENT GAPS for busy or restrictive lifestyles. I performed almost exclusively at corporate and private events for over 15 years. During this time, I was always on the go, moving equipment, setting up, performing, breaking down, and moving on to the next event. I had to eat quickly and too many times I relied upon fast food because it was easy.

Many people struggle to maintain a perfectly balanced diet due to time constraints, food availability, or personal preferences. For instance, people who follow strict dietary protocols—like ketogenic, vegan, or low-FODMAP diets—can inadvertently eliminate entire food groups. Supplements act as substitutes for nutrition you may not be receiving by providing concentrated doses of the nutrients that may be lacking in day-to-day meals. For the busiest of us who may rely on convenience foods or have erratic eating schedules, supplements act as an important safety net to ensure consistent nutrient intake.

CASE STUDY: BRIAN

Meet my nephew **Brian,** a 32-year-old who switched to a vegan diet for ethical and environmental reasons. After a year, **Brian** began experiencing fatigue, weakness, and difficulty concentrating. Lab tests revealed low vitamin B12 levels. A B12 supplement quickly helped address his deficiency, providing the vital nutrients that weren't readily available through **Brian's** exclusively plant-based meals.

Supplementation becomes critical for specific diets—mainly vegan or vegetarian—where nutrients like vitamin B12 or iron may be scarce. It's important to recognize your unique nutritional context and adjust accordingly.

GOVERNMENT GUIDELINES SET MINIMUMS, NOT ALWAYS OPTIMAL LEVELS

Government agencies often provide Recommended Dietary Allowances (RDAs) and Dietary Reference Intakes (DRIs). These numbers are mostly aimed at stopping serious deficiencies, not making you feel your best. Unfortunately, lobbyists have influenced some of these guidelines over the years, so the numbers might not be perfect for everyone. If you're very active, under a lot of stress, or live in an environment that affects certain nutrients (like far from the equator where you get less Vitamin D), you might need more than the official minimums. Paying attention to "optimal" levels rather than just "enough to avoid disease" can help you stay energetic, support long-term health, and potentially live longer.

QUALITY SUPPLEMENTS CAN HELP

Not all supplements are the same. Some are cheaply made or might have contaminants. Others use forms of vitamins that your body can't absorb very well. Quality brands, on the other hand, tend to test their products to make sure you're getting what the label says. Their supplements usually use nutrients your body can actually use. By choosing reliable, well-tested supplements, you can fill nutritional gaps in your regular diet and give your body what it truly needs.

I.I.2: PERSONALIZED NUTRITION
IT'S NOT "ONE-SIZE-FITS-ALL"

Your genetics, your lab test results, what stage of life you're in, and advice from experts all matter when picking the right supplements.

Years ago, I heard **Dr. Dean Edell** on his radio show. He said that when you swallow a pill for back pain, it doesn't magically know to go straight to your back. It's really a marketing idea more than a scientific fact. The same goes for vitamins: for example, you might take Vitamin D to support your bones, but it can also help with your immune system, mood, and inflammation. So, you might start taking it just for strong bones and later notice it's also improving other parts of your health.

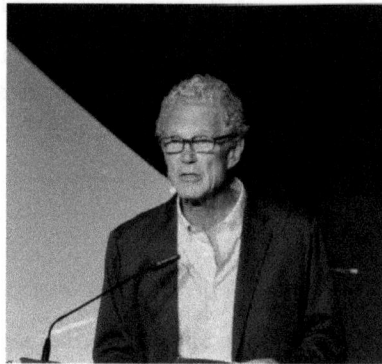

Dr. Dean Edell
Credit – Wikimedia Commons

GENETIC DIFFERENCES

How your body processes vitamins and minerals can vary, even among siblings. Your genes may mean you're faster or slower at breaking down certain nutrients, so you might need more (or sometimes less) than the usual guidelines suggest.

PERSONALIZED BLOODWORK

Regular blood tests can show if you're low in certain nutrients, even if you feel fine. For example, someone could discover they have low Vitamin D or iron by looking at their labs. Once you know your levels, you can adjust your diet or supplements to fix any issues. It's much smarter than just guessing. I've done this myself when I found out my white blood cell count was on the low side— I used supplements and foods that help boost white blood cells, and it really made a difference.

"I get a blood test every six months to narrow down what could be causing fatigue, exhaustion, dark thoughts, and obviously, eventually, how to be in my top shape. Blood doesn't lie. From vitamins that I'm lacking to natural foods, it's an educated guide to connect my physical internal and external look." – Eliza Gonzalez

CERTAIN LIFE STAGES

People at different stages of life have different nutritional needs. For instance, pregnant women need more folate and iron for the baby's health. Older adults can have trouble absorbing B12 or calcium, so they often need extra. By paying attention to these changing needs, you can adjust your supplements as you grow older or when big life events happen.

GWYNETH PALTROW

Gwyneth Paltrow is a very active actress who loves trying new health tips. One day, she kept yawning and felt drained, even though she was eating lots of veggies and doing yoga. After a check-up, her doctor said, "Your Vitamin D3 is really low." She wrote on her lifestyle website *GOOP* in 2010 about how she started taking a Vitamin D3 supplement. Before long, she felt more energetic and even noticed her bones seemed stronger.

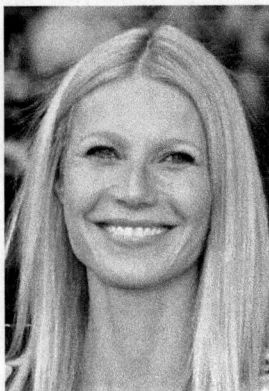

Gwyneth Paltrow
Credit – Wikimedia Commons

WORKING WITH HEALTHCARE PROVIDERS

It's great to do research on your own, but it's also wise to team up with experts—like nutritionists, naturopaths, or doctors who look at your whole lifestyle—to create a safe, personalized plan. They can review your genetic test results, bloodwork, and daily habits to suggest which supplements and doses make sense. They'll also check if there are any risks from mixing supplements with prescription medications. When you work together, you can enjoy the benefits of supplements while avoiding the pitfalls.

"Your genetics load the gun. Your lifestyle pulls the trigger."
– Dr. Mehmet Oz

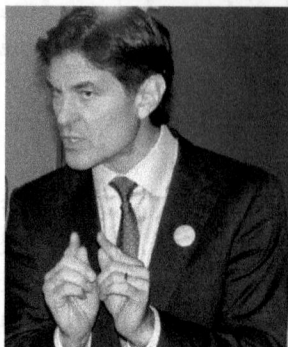

Dr. Mehmet Oz
Credit – Wikimedia Commons

I.I.3: COMMON MYTHS/MISCONCEPTIONS

I want you to know the truth behind these common myths about supplements. Used correctly, they can be powerful tools for good health. But it's important to use them wisely and keep potential risks in mind.

MYTH: "MORE IS ALWAYS BETTER."

This is the hardest myth for me personally! Sometimes you hear about huge doses of a certain vitamin changing someone's life. But often, those stories don't come from reliable, peer-reviewed research. People assume if a little is good, a lot must be better. The problem is, too much of certain vitamins can be toxic. Vitamins A, D, E, and K can build up in your tissues over time, potentially damaging your liver, bones, or kidneys if you overdo it. That's why it's important to follow recommended doses—or your doctor's guidance—and not go overboard.

MYTH: "SUPPLEMENTS ARE UNREGULATED."

It's true that rules for supplements can vary by country, and they aren't regulated as strictly as prescription drugs. But in many places—like the United States, Canada, and parts of Europe—manufacturers still have to follow certain standards, known as cGMP (current Good Manufacturing Practices). In the U.S., the FDA oversees supplements under the Dietary Supplement Health and Education Act (DSHEA). Many reputable companies also do voluntary tests on their products to ensure that what's on the label is really in the bottle. It's not perfect, but it's not a total free-for-all either. So, do a little homework on the brand before you buy.

MYTH: "ONE SUPPLEMENT CAN FIX EVERYTHING."

Our bodies are complex. Good health depends on a combination of a balanced diet, regular exercise, quality sleep, managing stress, and so on. No single "miracle pill" can tackle all health problems. Even if a nutrient is fantastic, it still only does a specific job. For example, a supplement alone can't fix the damage done by smoking, junk food, or chronic stress. The best results usually come from a balanced approach that includes healthy habits, plus targeted supplements for your unique needs.

MYTH: "ONLY OLDER ADULTS NEED SUPPLEMENTS."

It's true that older people often need extra Vitamin D, calcium, or B12. But younger folks can be low in nutrients too—maybe because they're busy, skip meals, eat a limited diet, or have specific eating styles like vegan or keto. Athletes can also need more of certain nutrients (like iron or magnesium) because their bodies work extra hard. Even your genes might mean you need more or less of a particular vitamin. In short, supplements aren't just for seniors.

MYTH: "'NATURAL' ALWAYS MEANS SAFE."

I have a friend named **John** who likes to point out that oil is "organic," but you definitely don't want to eat it! He's right. Many natural supplements come from plants or herbs, but that doesn't automatically make them harmless. A lot of "natural" substances—like caffeine—are powerful and can cause harm if you take too much. Plus, some herbal products can interact dangerously with prescription drugs. St. John's Wort can reduce how well some antidepressants and birth control pills work, and garlic supplements may thin the blood too much if you're on certain medications. So always ask your doctor, nurse, or pharmacist if your natural supplements might clash with any medications you take. "Natural" is great, but it's not a free pass to do whatever you want.

That covers the major points: understanding how government guidelines set minimum standards, the importance of quality and personalized supplements, and clearing up some big myths. Keep these ideas in mind as you explore vitamins and supplements to support your health!

SECTION TWO: THE BUILDING BLOCKS OF LIFE
1.2.1: MACRONUTRIENTS VS. MICRONUTRIENTS

"Getting all the nutrients you need simply cannot be done without supplements." – Dr. Steven Gundry

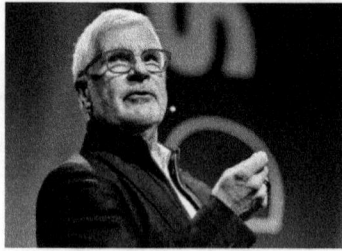

Dr. Steven Gundry
Credit- Wikimedia Commons

HOW OUR BODIES USE NUTRIENTS
From Cells to Energy
Good health starts at the tiniest level: our cells. When we eat, our digestive system breaks down food into amino acids (from proteins), simple sugars (from carbohydrates), and fatty acids (from fats). Vitamins and minerals also get absorbed during this process. After nutrients move through the small intestine and into the bloodstream, they travel to our cells to help create energy, build new tissues, and repair damage.

MACRONUTRIENTS VS. MICRONUTRIENTS
Macronutrients (Carbs, Proteins, Fats)
Macronutrients give us most of our energy and also help build and protect our bodies. Carbs offer quick energy, proteins help muscles and tissues grow and repair, and fats give us long-lasting energy, plus insulation and cushioning. People often focus on balancing these three when looking at calories or sports performance.

Micronutrients (Vitamins and Minerals)
Unlike macronutrients, vitamins and minerals don't have calories. However, they're absolutely crucial because they're like the spark plugs in your body's engine. They help with hundreds of processes, from making red blood cells to keeping your hormones balanced. If you only focus on carbs, protein, and fats—but ignore your vitamins and minerals—you could still end up feeling run-down or develop health issues later on.

THE IMPORTANCE OF SYNERGY
Why Vitamins Matter for Using Macros
It's not enough just to count carbs or protein. Vitamins and minerals unlock the energy from these macronutrients and keep your metabolism running well. For example, B vitamins (like B1, B2, B3, B6, and B12) are "helpers" in your body's energy production. If you don't get enough B vitamins, you might not fully benefit from all that healthy protein or the balanced carbs you eat.

Minerals also matter—a lot. Magnesium alone is involved in hundreds of body processes, including producing energy and controlling muscle movement. So even if you're great at balancing your macros, ignoring micronutrients could leave you tired or unable to perform at your best. Even something as simple as taking a daily multivitamin can make a difference.

MICRONUTRIENT DEFICIENCIES

When your body doesn't get enough vitamins or minerals, you might not notice big changes right away. Maybe you just feel more tired or catch colds more easily. But over time, these small warning signs can turn into bigger, long-term problems. For instance, low vitamin D can affect bone health and mood, and not getting enough B12 or folate may lead to anemia and nerve issues.

Because these problems often show up slowly, it's easy to miss them. That's why it's wise to check your diet and occasionally get blood tests. Spotting a deficiency early can save you a lot of trouble down the road.

ANNE HATHAWAY

Anne Hathaway once mentioned in an interview with *Harper's Bazaar* that she had switched to mostly vegan meals while filming a movie because she wanted a cleaner diet. Over time, she felt unusually weak, struggled to keep up with her fitness routine, and even had trouble concentrating on her lines. A blood test showed her ferritin levels were low. Under her doctor's advice, she introduced more iron into her diet—especially through leafy greens and certain iron supplements. Before long, Anne felt a noticeable boost in both energy and mental clarity.

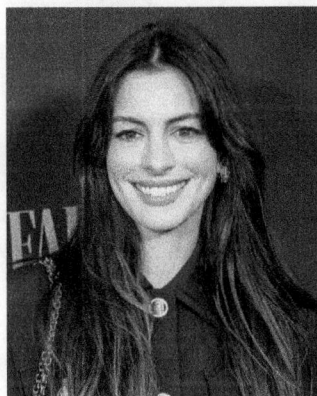

Anne Hathaway
Credit – Wikimedia Commons

FINDING BALANCE WITH FOOD AND SUPPLEMENTS

A balanced, nutrient-rich diet should be your first goal: include proteins, healthy fats, complex carbs, and a good variety of vitamins and minerals. If blood tests or diet reviews show specific gaps, supplements can step in to help. Think of supplements as a helpful add-on, not a replacement for real food. This combination gives you both quick wins (more energy) and long-term benefits (disease prevention and a better shot at aging well).

Remember, fundamentals don't change: eat right, move your body, get enough sleep, and use supplements to fill in the gaps. My good friend, *Major League Baseball Hall of Fame* Pitcher **Trevor Hoffman** had the most saves of any closer in history when he left the game. At a young age, he cultivated a work ethic and worked his way up to success. **Trevor** said:

"There is no shortcut to true success."

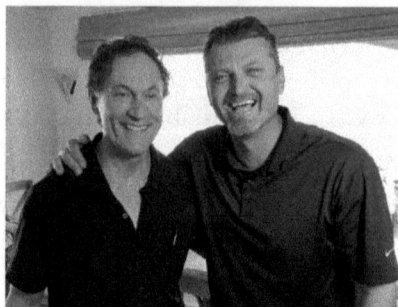

Tad Sisler with Trevor Hoffman
Source – Sisler Private Collection

1.2.2: THE ROLE OF ENZYMES AND COENZYMES
Enzymes—Your Body's Speed Boosters
Enzymes are little machines in your body that speed up chemical reactions so they happen fast enough to keep you alive. Coenzymes, which are often made from vitamins, are like the tools enzymes need to do their jobs. I personally use digestive enzymes every day to support my gut health.

"Enzymes are masters of chemistry. They evolved over billions of years to perform specific biological functions. They make complex materials with virtually no waste." – Frances Arnold

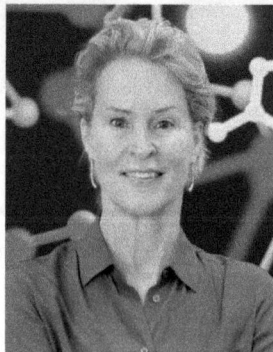

Frances Arnold
Credit — Wikimedia Commons

Vitamins as Coenzymes

Many water-soluble vitamins—especially the B vitamins—turn into coenzymes in your body. For example, vitamin B3 (niacin) becomes $NAD^+/NADH$, and vitamin B2 (riboflavin) becomes $FAD^+/FADH_2$. Both help your cells convert food into energy. Without enough of these vitamins, those chemical reactions slow down, and you can feel run-down.

PAMELA ANDERSON

Actress **Pamela Anderson** got into running because she wanted a new challenge and a healthy way to support causes she cared about. After finishing the 2013 New York City Marathon, she kept up the same training routine for a while. But the next year, she felt weirdly exhausted, and her race times started slipping. A blood test showed she was low in vitamin B12 and folate. Her doctor recommended a B-complex supplement, plus more leafy greens and protein sources in her meals. Within a couple of months, **Pamela** was back to feeling strong and trimmed several minutes off her marathon time.

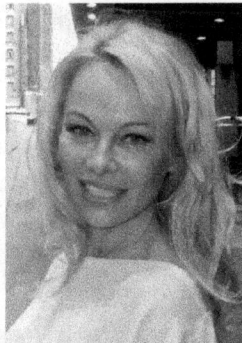

Pamela Anderson
Credit – Wikimedia Commons

Minerals Also Play a Role

Minerals like magnesium are called cofactors and are crucial for hundreds of processes, including making protein and energy. Think of vitamins and minerals as the spark that lets enzymes work at full speed. If you're short on these nutrients, your metabolism can stall, and that can lead to all sorts of problems—fatigue, trouble thinking, or even bigger health issues if it goes on too long.

Better-Absorbed Coenzyme Forms

Some vitamins come in different forms, and the "coenzyme" or "activated" versions can sometimes be absorbed better. For example, methylcobalamin (a form of B12) doesn't need extra steps to work in your body. Pyridoxal-5'-phosphate (P5P) is a similar version of vitamin B6. If you have genetic traits or health issues that affect how well you convert nutrients, you might get extra benefits from these more active forms.

I.2.3: OXIDATIVE STRESS AND ANTIOXIDANTS

Scientists studying how to live longer soon discovered that antioxidants play a big role in keeping cells healthy. But it's all about balance and figuring out what works best for you as an individual.

Free Radicals vs. Antioxidants

Free radicals are unstable molecules made during normal body processes or picked up from pollution, radiation, or cigarette smoke. They can harm your cells by stealing electrons from other molecules, damaging DNA and cell membranes in the process. Antioxidants step in by donating electrons to these free radicals, neutralizing them before they can cause serious harm.

Vitamin C and E

Vitamin C (ascorbic acid) and Vitamin E (tocopherols and tocotrienols) are two famous antioxidants. Vitamin C is water-soluble and works in places like your blood, while Vitamin E is fat-soluble and helps protect cell membranes and other fatty tissues. Both are heavily studied and are known for supporting the immune system, protecting skin, and helping cells stay healthy.

Newer Antioxidants (Astaxanthin, NAD+ Boosters)

Lately, people have been talking about other antioxidants, like astaxanthin (found in salmon and algae) and NAD+ boosters (like nicotinamide riboside). Astaxanthin might be even more powerful than some classic antioxidants. NAD+ boosters aim to raise your NAD+ levels, which helps with DNA repair and energy production—both of which drop as we age. Early research on these is promising, but we still need more human studies to say for sure how well they work long term.

Glutathione—Your Body's In-House Superhero

Glutathione is like your body's own mighty superhero. Made from three amino acids (glutamine, cysteine, and glycine), it shields cells from damage by neutralizing harmful molecules (free radicals) and even helps recycle other antioxidants like Vitamins C and E. It also helps the liver detox and keeps your body's internal balance in check—big reasons why it's often called the "master antioxidant."

Case Study: Antioxidants and Skin Health

A 2021 study in the *Journal of Cosmetic Dermatology* found that people who used a mix of antioxidants, including Vitamin C and astaxanthin, saw better skin elasticity, more hydration, and fewer wrinkles over 12 weeks. More research is needed, but it's an exciting look at how different antioxidants might work together to help keep skin looking youthful.

Don't Overdo It

Free radicals aren't always bad; your body uses some for things like signaling the immune system or adjusting to exercise. Taking too many antioxidants can throw off that balance, a situation sometimes called "reductive stress." So, the best plan is a balanced, nutrient-rich diet plus carefully chosen supplements. That way, you're giving your body the protection it needs without messing up its natural processes.

By focusing on a balanced diet (for both macros and micros), understanding how enzymes and coenzymes work, and paying attention to antioxidants, you're already on the path to better health and maybe even a longer life. Remember: there are no shortcuts—only smart choices and consistent effort.

Although there is much to learn about how our bodies function, it's critical to know as much as you can, just like the importance of performing preventative maintenance on your car. My friend **Khloe Kardashian** said:

"I just think that knowing about your body at any age, whether it's educating yourself on fertility, getting mammograms, going through puberty – whatever it may be, is really important. I just really encourage women empowerment and being comfortable talking about these issues."

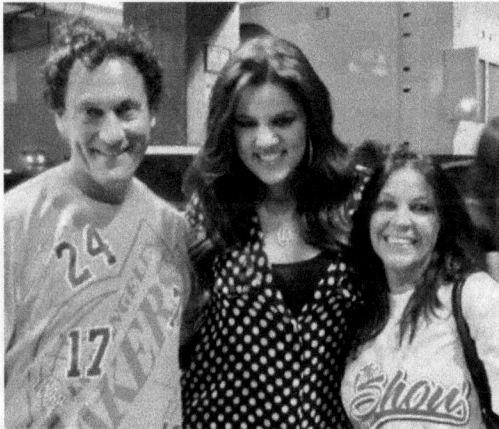

Tad Sisler with Khloe Kardashian and Robin Dougan
Source – Sisler Private Collection

SECTION THREE: SAFETY, REGULATION, & QUALITY
1.3.1: UNDERSTANDING LABELS AND CLAIMS

When you walk through the supplement aisle (or browse online), it's easy to get overwhelmed by all the fancy labels. You'll see words like "organic," "non-GMO," or "standardized extract." You might also notice different kinds of "facts" labels—like Nutrition Facts or Supplement Facts. Here's how to make sense of it all so you don't get tricked by marketing hype.

TERMS LIKE "ORGANIC", "NON-GMO," AND "STANDARDIZED EXTRACT" CAN INDICATE QUALITY

Organic: If a supplement or herb says "organic," it typically means the ingredients were grown without synthetic fertilizers, pesticides, or genetic engineering. It doesn't guarantee the product is perfect, but it usually signals higher-quality ingredients and better manufacturing practices.

Non-GMO: This tells you the ingredients weren't genetically modified. Some people like knowing their supplements come from more natural sources.

Standardized Extract: This is especially important for herbal supplements. It means the active compounds (like curcuminoids in turmeric) are present at consistent levels in every batch. If you see a supplement labeled as "standardized," you know it should have the same amount of the key beneficial substance each time you buy it.

"NUTRITIONAL FACTS" VS. "SUPPLEMENT FACTS"

Nutrition Facts Label: This is what you'll find on regular foods and drinks. It lists things like calories, fats, carbs, and specific vitamins or minerals. It's designed to help you see if you're getting too much sugar, sodium, or other nutrients in your daily meals.

Supplement Facts Label: This is the panel you'll see on bottles of vitamins, minerals, and herbs. It should list the amounts of each active ingredient, plus the percent Daily Value (%DV) if available. Supplement labels often include disclaimers like "These statements have not been evaluated by the FDA" because they're not as strictly regulated as medicines.

BE WARY OF MARKETING BUZZWORDS

When I was in sixth grade, I had a teacher who showed us how to spot propaganda. Even an eleven-year-old can see through sketchy marketing if they know what to look for. Words like "miracle," "wonder," or "cure-all" are red flags. In many places, it's illegal to make bold health claims without real proof. So if a label sounds too good to be true—like it fixes every disease under the sun—it probably is.

WILL FERRELL

Will Ferrell isn't just a funny actor—he's also run marathons and loves challenging himself. One day, he stumbled upon an online ad for a "fat-burning miracle" pill. It promised to melt away extra pounds, so he ordered it to boost his running performance. After a few weeks, he noticed zero improvements and started feeling sick and dizzy during his daily jogs. Worried, **Will** finally did some research and discovered the brand was shady. Tests revealed the pills had mystery ingredients not listed on the label. He immediately threw them away and got back to focusing on a healthy diet and real training. Whatever you take, make sure you're buying from **trusted sources**, reading labels carefully, and looking for **third-party certifications** that verify authenticity.

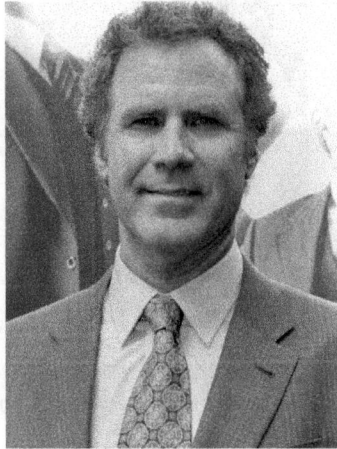

Will Ferrell
Credit – Wikimedia Commons

I also had a friend named **Peppy** who tragically died from taking Phen-Fen, a diet craze around the turn of the 21st century. It was supposed to help people lose weight, but it came with serious risks. Today, Ozempic is a big weight-loss drug, and it might work for some, but always be aware of side effects—some people lose muscle instead of just fat, which isn't healthy.

One time, I was tired and a friend gave me an energy drink. I love coffee, but that energy drink made me feel sick and jittery. Later, I saw that it contained guarana—a plant from the Amazon that acts like a strong stimulant. That stuff just didn't agree with me!

ALWAYS LOOK FOR CERTIFICATIONS (NSF, USP, and Others)

NSF International (NSF): This group tests supplements to make sure they meet health and safety standards. If you see the NSF mark, it usually means the company cares about quality and consistency.

United States Pharmacopeia (USP): USP sets strict standards for purity and potency. If a supplement has the USP seal, it's been tested for quality.

Other Third-Party Tests: Seals from groups like Informed Choice, ConsumerLab, or UL also show that the supplement's contents have been verified by an independent lab. It's never a 100% guarantee of a "miracle," but it does mean the product is a lot more likely to be safe and accurately labeled.

"The safety of the people shall be the highest law."
– Marcus Tullius Cicero

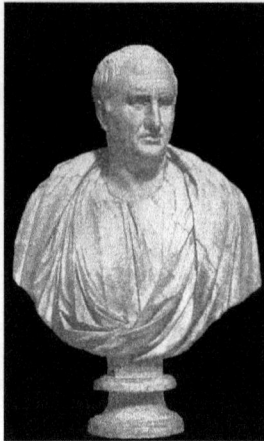

Marcus Tullius Cicero
Credit: PICRYL/creativecommons.org

I.3.2: THIRD-PARTY TESTING AND GMP STANDARDS

Not all supplements are created equal. Some follow strict rules and testing; others don't. If you're serious about your health, you'll want to understand how to pick safer products and dodge ones that might be contaminated or mislabeled.

REPUTABLE BRANDS FOLLOW GOOD MANUFACTURING PRACTICES (GMP)

Good Manufacturing Practices (GMP) are rules set by agencies like the FDA (in the U.S.) to ensure products are made in a clean, well-run facility. Companies that follow GMP have to document their processes and test each batch to ensure it meets the right standards. If you choose GMP-compliant brands, you're more likely to get a supplement without hidden nasties.

THIRD-PARTY TESTING ENSURES PURITY, POTENCY, AND ABSENCE OF CONTAMINANTS

Even if a company follows GMP, it's still smart to check if they use independent labs to test their products. These labs confirm the supplement actually has what the label says it does—and that it's free from heavy metals, bacteria, or sketchy chemicals. This extra layer of testing helps you separate serious brands from those that rely on flashy marketing.

HEAVY METALS, PESTICIDES, OR ADULTERANTS CAN APPEAR IN POORLY REGULATED PRODUCTS

I've been to conferences in Las Vegas where anyone with money could "white label" supplements by sticking their own brand on some factory-made product. If the factory isn't reputable, contaminants like mercury or hidden steroids can end up in the pills. That's scary. If you ever consider creating your own supplement line, work with a certified supplier who does thorough testing. Remember, your health (and your customers' health) depends on it. For information on how to do a simple blood test for heavy metal contamination, check the section on this subject in my book **Stay Healthy, Stay Youthful: The Science of Living to 150.**

CASE STUDY:

In 2015, an investigation found that several popular herbal supplements had zero trace of the herbs they claimed to contain. Understandably, people were upset and demanded stricter testing. In response, many trustworthy brands started investing more in third-party certifications to prove their products were legit.

CHECK FOR RECOGNIZED SEALS (NSF, ConsumerLab)

As mentioned, organizations like **NSF International, ConsumerLab, USP,** and **UL** do rigorous testing. If a supplement bottle proudly shows one of these seals, an independent group has confirmed it meets certain standards for purity and quality. While that doesn't mean it's magical, it does mean it's less likely to be a fraud or contain hidden dangers.

"Our rights are not absolute. Our rights can be curtailed in the interest of public safety." President John F. Kennedy

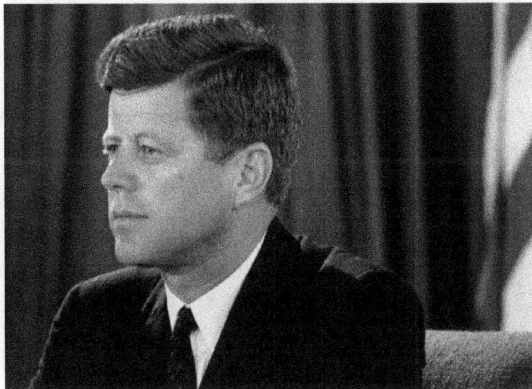

President John F. Kennedy
Credit: PICRYL/creativecommons.org

I.3.3: KEY REGULATORY BODIES

Supplements and vitamins are regulated differently around the world. Knowing a bit about these rules can help you avoid legal headaches or health risks, especially if you travel or order products from other countries.

FDA (U.S.) VS. EFSA (Europe) VS. WHO GUIDELINES

FDA (U.S.): The Food and Drug Administration checks that supplements follow the Dietary Supplement Health and Education Act (DSHEA).

Companies must follow good manufacturing practices, but they don't have to prove their supplements work the way prescription drugs do.

EFSA (Europe): The European Food Safety Authority sets rules for health claims and labeling throughout EU member states. The approval process is typically stricter, and claims must meet higher evidence standards.

WHO (Worldwide): The World Health Organization offers guidelines for traditional medicines and herbal products. They don't enforce laws directly, but they issue recommendations to help countries create safer systems.

PRESCRIPTION, OVER-THE-COUNTER, AND SUPPLEMENTS

How a product is classified (prescription drug vs. OTC vs. supplement) affects its availability, how it's marketed, and how tightly it's regulated. Prescription drugs go through rigorous clinical trials. Over-the-counter meds are deemed safe enough for self-use. Supplements sit in a sort of "gray area." They don't need the same type of proof that drugs do, which is why you should be extra cautious when picking a brand.

DIFFERENT COUNTRIES HAVE DIFFERENT RULES

Some substances—like DHEA or high-dose melatonin—are sold as normal supplements in certain places but require a prescription in others. Hormone-based supplements can raise extra concern about misuse or unknown risks. If you're traveling, remember that what's legal in one country might be banned in another.

CASE STUDY:

Mark was shocked when he discovered that while he could buy melatonin off the shelf in the United States, he needed a prescription for it in parts of Europe. He was used to taking it for jet lag, but overseas pharmacies wouldn't sell it without a doctor's note. That's when he realized local rules can totally change how easy it is to get a supplement—even one that seems pretty harmless.

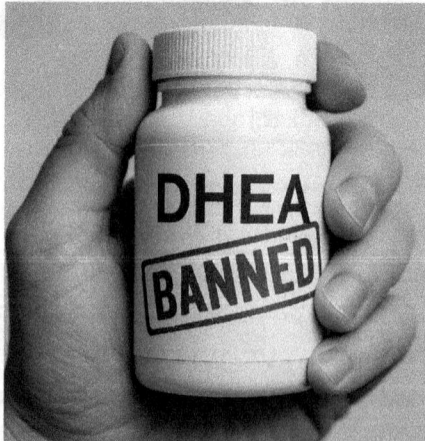

BE AWARE OF LOCAL LAWS TO AVOID TROUBLE

Knowing your own country's supplement rules—and the rules of any place you plan to visit—keeps you from accidentally breaking laws or using unsafe products. This is especially true for importing supplements or ordering them online from international sellers. Think of it like food safety: you don't want to risk your health or your legal standing just because a product wasn't allowed in the place you're traveling.

"Food safety involves everybody in the food chain." – Mike Johanns

1.3.4: CONSULTING HEALTHCARE PROFESSIONALS

Vitamins, supplements, and herbs can enhance your health, but they're not a one-size-fits-all solution. Consulting a healthcare professional before starting or changing your regimen ensures safety, effectiveness, and alignment with your unique needs. Here's why it's necessary and who can guide you.

WHY IT'S IMPORTANT

Avoiding Interactions: Supplements can interact with medications, altering their effects or causing side effects. For example, vitamin K may reduce the effectiveness of blood thinners like warfarin, while St. John's Wort can interfere with antidepressants. A 2025 study found 20% of supplement users experienced mild interactions.

Tailoring to Health Needs: Your health status—whether you're pregnant, managing diabetes, or over 60—affects supplement safety. High doses of vitamin A can harm the liver, and iron supplements may worsen hemochromatosis. Professionals personalize your plan.

Ensuring Proper Dosage: Too little of a supplement may be ineffective, while too much can cause toxicity, like vitamin D leading to kidney issues. Guidance ensures the right dose.

Choosing Quality Products: Not all supplements are equal; some may contain contaminants or lack claimed ingredients. Professionals recommend brands with third-party testing (e.g., USP, NSF) for purity and potency.

Special Populations: Pregnant women need folate, children require safe doses, and older adults may need B12 due to reduced absorption. A 2025 review emphasizes tailored advice for these groups.

TYPES OF HEALTHCARE PROFESSIONALS

Primary Care Physicians (PCPs): Familiar with your medical history, they assess supplement safety and coordinate care.

Registered Dietitians (RDs): Nutrition experts who align supplements with dietary needs for optimal health.

Naturopathic Doctors (NDs): Specialize in natural therapies, offering expertise in herbs and holistic approaches.

Pharmacists: Identify drug-supplement interactions and recommend safe, high-quality products.

Specialists: For specific conditions (e.g., cardiologists for heart health, endocrinologists for diabetes), they provide targeted supplement advice.

PRACTICAL STEPS

Discuss Your Health: Share your medical history, medications, and goals with a professional to create a safe plan.

Get Tested: Blood tests for nutrient levels (e.g., vitamin D, B12) guide supplement choices.

Choose Quality: Select products with third-party certifications (USP, NSF) to ensure purity and potency.

Monitor and Adjust: Regular check-ins with professionals help refine your regimen based on health changes.

Consulting a healthcare professional is a small step that maximizes the benefits of your supplement plan while minimizing risks, keeping you on track for a healthier, longer life.

With these basics in mind, let's move on to the real superstars—our vitamins themselves. Get ready for an A-to-K tour of nutrients that can help you feel your best!

CHAPTER TWO
THE CORE VITAMINS (A, B-COMPLEX, C, D, E, K)

J ust one single deficiency can derail your entire body. Discover how these 'alphabet vitamins' each play a significant role in keeping you energized, immune-strong, and youthful.

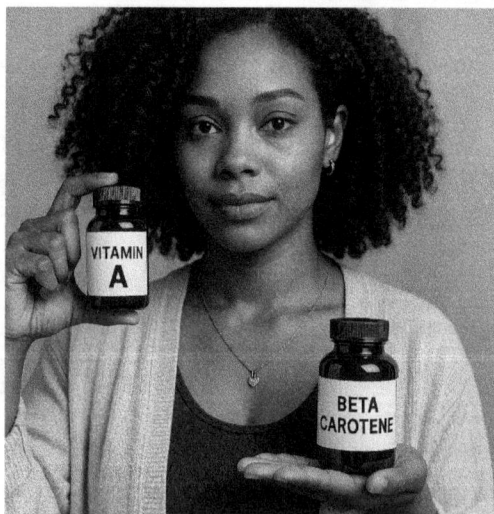

SECTION ONE: VITAMIN A AND THE B-COMPLEX
2.1.1: VITAMIN A (RETINOL, BETA-CAROTENE)

So much information is required to completely understand supplements. If you're confused, you're not alone. It can be akin to what my old friend, **President Gerald R. Ford** said:

"History and experience tell us that moral progress comes not in comfortable and complacent times, but out of trial and confusion."

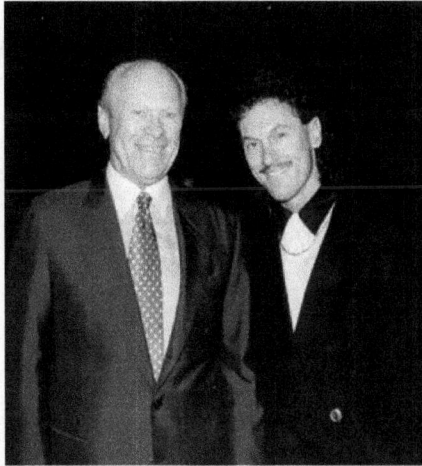

President Gerald R. Ford and Tad Sisler
Source – Sisler Private Collection

Remember, just by reading this book, you are learning volumes and making huge progress.

Each vitamin has magical properties that work to make our bodies healthier. Think of Vitamin A like a flashlight that helps you see in the dark. It's important for your eyes, especially at night, and it also keeps your skin and immune system healthy. Just like you need a good flashlight to explore a dark room, your body needs Vitamin A to help you see and stay strong.

VITAMIN A: TWO MAIN FORMS
Vitamin A is a fat-soluble nutrient that comes in two main types:
Preformed Vitamin A (Retinol)
• Found in animal-based foods (liver, fish oil, dairy).
• Your body uses it right away, so it can become toxic if you take too much.
Provitamin A Carotenoids (like Beta-Carotene)
• Found in colorful fruits and vegetables (carrots, sweet potatoes, spinach).
• Your body turns these carotenoids into Vitamin A only as needed, which lowers the risk of taking too much.

Even though these two forms are different, they both end up doing the same jobs in your body. That's why they're grouped together under the name "Vitamin A."

BEST SOURCES OF VITAMIN A

Animal (Retinol): Liver (beef or chicken), egg yolks, dairy products.

Plant (Carotenoids): Carrots, sweet potatoes, spinach, kale, pumpkin, red peppers.

WHY VITAMIN A MATTERS

Vision: Vitamin A helps make a pigment called rhodopsin in your eyes, which lets you see in low light. If you don't get enough, you may have trouble seeing at night (night blindness).

Immune Function: It keeps the lining of your eyes, nose, and skin strong, helping you fight off germs.

Gene Expression (Retinoic Acid): When your body turns Vitamin A into retinoic acid, it helps control certain genes that affect cell growth and development.

HOW MUCH TO TAKE (DOSAGE AND SAFETY)

Recommended Dietary Allowance (RDA):

• Adult Men: about 900 micrograms RAE (Retinol Activity Equivalents) daily.
• Adult Women: about 700 micrograms RAE daily.

Tolerable Upper Intake Level (UL): Around 3,000 micrograms RAE per day for adults (from preformed retinol). Consistently going above this can cause Vitamin A toxicity (hypervitaminosis A).

Absorption Tip: Since Vitamin A is fat-soluble, take it with a meal that has some healthy fats (like avocado, nuts, or olive oil).

Carotenoids: Beta-carotene (from plants) is less likely to cause toxicity because your body controls how much it converts.

FAT-SOLUBLE AND TOXICITY RISK

Because it's stored in your liver and fat tissue, extra Vitamin A can build up. Too much can lead to side effects like nausea, headaches, dizziness, and in serious cases, liver damage.

WORKS WELL WITH OTHER NUTRIENTS

Zinc: Helps transport Vitamin A in the body.

Vitamins D, E, and K2: Often balanced with Vitamin A to keep everything in harmony. But watch out—too much of one fat-soluble vitamin can throw the others off.

HELEN KELLER INTERNATIONAL

Helen Keller was born blind and deaf. Her story is documented in the heartfelt book and movie *The Miracle Worker. Helen Keller International (HKI)* is a global nonprofit co-founded by **Helen Keller** that focuses extensively on preventing blindness and reducing malnutrition. One of *HKI's* major programs involves vitamin A supplementation to prevent night blindness and other severe effects of deficiency in children. There are few documented stories of Vitamin A deficiency because it generally happens in third-world countries. However, **Helen Keller's** story is a testament to how most of us take our vision for granted, and we should cherish the ability to see and protect it with good nutrition. Sometimes, when your body is telling you something isn't right, it pays to listen, find out why, and make the healthy choice that gets you back in the game. Suppose you experience a loss of vision, especially before dawn or after dusk. In that case, a medical professional may suggest you take retinol and add foods packed with beta-carotene, like carrots, spinach, and sweet potatoes, to your meals.

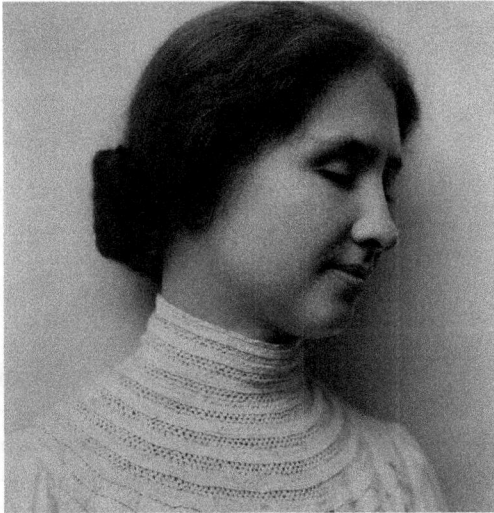

Helen Keller

Recreated from an Image at LOC's Public Domain Image Collections – Get Archive

"I got cocky and I stopped taking my vitamins. It was an inconvenience to have a suitcase full of vitamins with me on the road. About two years ago, it caught up with me."
— *Mary Ann Mobley, Miss America 1959*

Key Takeaways:
• Take Vitamin A with meals.
• Don't go overboard—avoid mega-doses of preformed Vitamin A.
• Some people (like pregnant women or older adults) need special advice from a healthcare provider.

By understanding how **vitamin A** works, when to supplement, and how much is safe, you can harness its wide-ranging benefits—particularly for **vision, immune health, and cellular functions**—while minimizing the risk of toxicity.

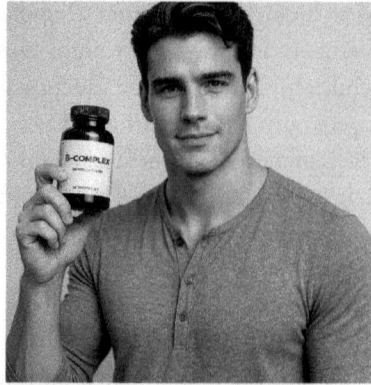

2.1.2: THE B-COMPLEX OVERVIEW

Think of the **B vitamins** as a team of construction workers who turn the food you eat into energy. Each vitamin (B1, B2, B3, B5, B6, B7, B9, and B12) has its own specific job, but together they keep your nerves, muscles, and brain running smoothly—like a busy city that always needs power.

All B vitamins are water-soluble, which means your body doesn't store a lot of them. If you take more than you need, you'll usually pee out the extra. Still, a few B vitamins can cause problems if you take very high amounts for a long time, so it's good to know the safe ranges.

Common B Vitamins and Their Food Sources

• **B1 (Thiamin):** Whole grains (brown rice, whole wheat), legumes, pork, sunflower seeds.

• **B2 (Riboflavin):** Dairy (milk, yogurt), eggs, lean meats, spinach, almonds.

• **B3 (Niacin):** Poultry, fish (tuna, salmon), peanuts, mushrooms, fortified cereals.

• **B5 (Pantothenic Acid):** Mushrooms, avocados, chicken, eggs, whole grains.

• **B6 (Pyridoxine):** Poultry, fish, potatoes, bananas, chickpeas.

• **B7 (Biotin):** Eggs, almonds, walnuts, sunflower seeds, salmon.

• **B9 (Folate/Folic Acid):** Leafy greens (spinach, kale), legumes (beans, lentils), oranges, fortified grains.

• **B12 (Cobalamin):** Animal products (meat, dairy, eggs), shellfish (clams), fortified plant-based milk or cereals (for vegans).

HOW THE B VITAMINS WORK

Coenzymes in Energy Metabolism: B vitamins help enzymes break down carbs, proteins, and fats into energy (ATP).

Nerve Function: Certain B vitamins (B1, B6, B12) are critical for healthy nerves.
DNA and RNA Synthesis: Folate (B9) and B12 help make and repair DNA and RNA.
Homocysteine Regulation: B6, B9, and B12 help control homocysteine, an amino acid. Too much homocysteine may increase the risk of heart and nerve problems.

WHAT THE RESEARCH SAYS

Deficiency Correction: Fixing low levels of B vitamins can boost energy, mood, and overall health.
Neurological Benefits: B6, B9, and B12 support the brain and nerve cells. Some studies suggest they may help with cognition and help keep homocysteine in check.
Feeling of Vitality: While they're not "energy drinks," B vitamins help your body stay energized if you're low on them to begin with.

KEEPING B VITAMINS BALANCED

Since B vitamins dissolve in water, it's hard to overdose on most of them. But watch out for these exceptions:
• **Niacin (B3):** More than 35 mg a day can cause skin flushing, liver problems, and stomach issues.
• **B6 (Pyridoxine):** Taking over 100 mg daily for a long time can cause nerve damage.
• **Folate (B9):** Too much can hide a B12 deficiency, which can delay treatment for serious nerve problems.

SYNERGY WITH OTHER SUBSTANCES

Take with Food: Helps reduce any stomach upset and may improve absorption.
Pair with Minerals: Some people take B vitamins with magnesium or zinc because they often work well together.
Homocysteine Help: B6, B9, and B12 together help keep homocysteine levels healthy, which can protect your heart and brain.

SIMON COWELL

Simon Cowell, the TV judge with the blunt opinions, was once so drained that he said he couldn't even concentrate on important meetings. He felt fuzzy-headed and was getting tired way too fast, especially with late-night filming schedules. After talking with his doctors, Simon decided to try vitamin B12 injections. He later shared that he felt a huge difference, like his tiredness switched off and he could think clearly again. He went back to being his sharp, quick-talking self on camera.

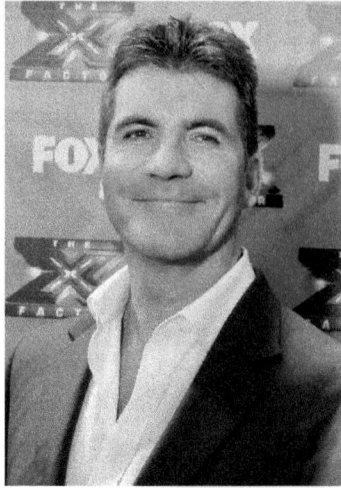

Simon Cowell
Credit – Wikimedia Commons

2.1.3: INDIVIDUAL B-VITAMINS

Below is a more detailed look at each B vitamin: its key roles, daily dosage guidelines, and possible issues if you take too much.

THIAMINE (B1)

• Helps turn carbs into energy.
• Important for your brain and nerve function.
Deficiency Disease: Beriberi (affects the heart and nervous system).
Suggested Daily Dosage (RDA):
• Women: ~1.1 mg/day
• Men: ~1.2 mg/day
Toxicity: There's no set upper limit; it's rare to have too much B1.
Works Well With: Magnesium (which supports energy production).

RIBOFLAVIN (B2)

• Helps your body produce energy (ATP).
• Supports antioxidant actions (helps regenerate glutathione, a key antioxidant).
Deficiency Sign: Ariboflavinosis (dry, cracked lips, sore throat, inflamed tongue).
Suggested Daily Dosage (RDA):
• Women: ~1.1 mg/day
• Men: ~1.3 mg/day
Toxicity: No upper limit established. Extra B2 turns pee bright yellow.
Works Well With: Other B vitamins, especially B6 and B9.

NIACIN (B3)

• Forms NAD and NADP, which help release energy from food.

• At high doses (under medical supervision), it can improve cholesterol by lowering LDL and raising HDL.

High Doses and Flushing:
• Can cause redness, itching, and warmth on the skin.
• Extended-release forms may reduce flushing but can stress the liver if overused.

Suggested Daily Dosage (RDA): (NE = Niacin Equivalents)
• Women: ~14 mg NE/day
• Men: ~16 mg NE/day

Upper Limit (UL): 35 mg/day. Going above this can lead to severe flushing or liver trouble.

Works Well With: Taking it with food can lessen flushing. Sometimes vitamin C or E helps reduce the flush.

PANTOTHENIC ACID (B5)

• Helps make Coenzyme A (CoA), which is needed to break down carbs, fats, and proteins for energy.
• Needed to make hormones and neurotransmitters (like acetylcholine).

Deficiency: Rare, but can cause fatigue, irritability, or muscle cramps.

Suggested Daily Dosage (AI): ~5 mg/day for adults.

Toxicity: No established upper limit; generally very safe.

Works Well With: Vitamin C for adrenal support; other B vitamins for overall metabolism.

PYRIDOXINE (B6)

• Helps your body handle protein and produce neurotransmitters like serotonin and dopamine.
• Teams up with B9 and B12 to control homocysteine (linked to heart health).

Deficiency Signs: Irritability, confusion, depression, weak immune function, anemia, or neuropathy.

Suggested Daily Dosage (RDA):
• ~1.3 mg/day for most adults (19–50).
• Higher for older adults, pregnant or breastfeeding women.

Upper Limit (UL): 100 mg/day. Going above this for a long time can harm your nerves.

Works Well With: B9 and B12 for homocysteine; magnesium for metabolism and nerve health.

BIOTIN (B7)

• Helps break down fats, proteins, and carbs.
• Supports healthy hair, skin, and nails.

Deficiency: Rare, but can cause thinning hair or brittle nails. Some antibiotics or genetic issues can lead to lower biotin levels.

Suggested Daily Dosage (AI): ~30 mcg/day for adults.

Toxicity: No upper limit set; generally safe.

Works Well With: Other B vitamins for energy; enough protein also helps strengthen hair and nails.

FOLATE / FOLIC ACID (B9)

• Crucial for making and repairing DNA, especially important during pregnancy.

• Prevents neural tube defects like spina bifida.

Deficiency:

• Can cause megaloblastic anemia (large, immature red blood cells).

• In pregnancy, low folate greatly increases the risk of birth defects.

Suggested Daily Dosage (RDA):

• Most adults: 400 mcg DFE/day

• Pregnant women: 600 mcg/day

• Breastfeeding: 500 mcg/day

Upper Limit (UL): 1,000 mcg/day from supplements or fortified foods. Too much can hide a B12 deficiency.

Works Well With: B6 and B12 for managing homocysteine. Vitamin C helps convert folate into its active form.

VITAMIN B12 (COBALAMIN)

• Helps form red blood cells (along with folate).

• Maintains the myelin sheath around nerves, crucial for healthy nerve signals.

Forms of B12:

Methylcobalamin: A coenzyme form that's more directly active in the body.

Cyanocobalamin: A common synthetic form that your body converts to an active form.

Absorption Tip: Requires "intrinsic factor" from your stomach. Some people (especially older adults) may need higher doses or even shots if they can't absorb it well.

Suggested Daily Dosage (RDA): ~2.4 mcg/day for adults. Higher for pregnant or breastfeeding women.

Toxicity: No upper limit. Generally very safe.

Works Well With: B9 and B6 for homocysteine control. Often recommended for older adults, vegans, or vegetarians.

CASE STUDY

Rebecca had high homocysteine levels, which can increase the risk of heart and nerve problems. Tests showed she was slightly low in B6, B9, and B12. She started taking supplements to bring those levels up.

Result: Her homocysteine levels dropped to a healthier range, her energy improved, and she may have reduced some of her health risks. This proves how important B6, B9, and B12 are for controlling homocysteine.

Key Reminder:

• Take your B vitamins with meals.

• Combine them thoughtfully with other nutrients (like magnesium or zinc) if you need extra metabolic or nerve support.

• Don't hesitate to ask a health professional for help if you're going to try high doses.

By staying aware of how Vitamin A and the B vitamins work—and by knowing the right amounts to take—you can support better health, feel more energized, and avoid problems that come from taking too little or too much.

SECTION TWO: VITAMINS C AND D

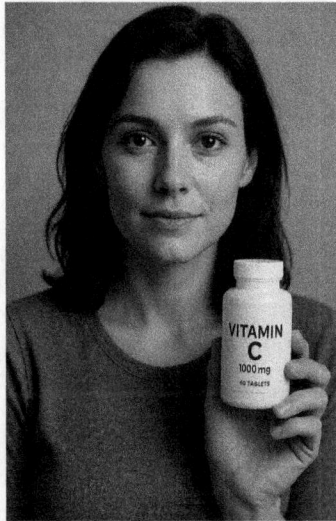

2.2.1: VITAMIN C (ASCORBIC ACID)

Vitamin C is like a dedicated "fix-it" crew that helps keep your body strong. It not only supports your immune system but also repairs and heals small breaks or wounds you might get every day. Think of it like having a handyman inside you, constantly working to keep everything in top shape!

BEST SOURCES OF VITAMIN C: Citrus fruits (oranges, grapefruit), bell peppers, strawberries, broccoli, kiwifruit, tomatoes.

CHEMICAL/PHYSICAL PROPERTIES

Water-Soluble Antioxidant: Vitamin C dissolves easily in water inside your body. Extra amounts are flushed out in your urine, which means it's harder (but not impossible) to take too much.

Easily Oxidized: Vitamin C can lose its strength when it's exposed to air, heat, or light. For example, if you leave orange juice sitting out for a long time or cook vegetables at very high temperatures, you might lose some Vitamin C.

MECHANISM OF ACTION

Collagen Production: Vitamin C is crucial for making collagen (the stuff that keeps your skin, bones, and joints strong). It helps certain amino acids do their job in building sturdy tissues.

Immune Support: Vitamin C can give your immune cells a boost, helping them deal with damage or stress. Although it might not completely stop colds, it could shorten how long they last.

Other Roles: It helps refresh other antioxidants (like Vitamin E) and can also help your body absorb iron more effectively, especially if you don't eat meat.

SUGGESTED DAILY DOSAGE

General Guidelines:
- Adult men: around 90 mg/day
- Adult women: around 75 mg/day
- Pregnant or breastfeeding women: 85–120 mg/day

Higher Doses: Some people take 1,000 mg or more per day to help reduce cold symptoms or boost immunity. However, the usual advice is not to exceed 2,000 mg a day (2 g) to avoid stomach troubles.

TIMING AND COMBINATION

When to Take It: You can take Vitamin C with or without food, but having it with a meal might cut down on any chance of an upset stomach.

Iron Absorption: Combine Vitamin C with iron-rich foods (like spinach) or iron supplements to help your body use that iron better.

Pair with Other Antioxidants: Vitamins C and E often work well together to fight oxidative stress.

SAFETY

Generally Safe: Most people do fine with normal amounts.

Mega-Doses: Taking way too much can cause diarrhea, nausea, and cramps. If you're prone to kidney stones, high doses may raise your risk (though studies differ on this).

Overdose: It's rare because extra Vitamin C usually just leaves your body through urine. Still, taking huge amounts every day isn't recommended long term.

CLINICAL CASE STUDY:

Hospitals sometimes use high-dose Vitamin C (through an IV) for certain patients to help with inflammation or stress in the body. Some early research looks promising, but we need more large-scale studies to know for sure how well it works. What's clear is that Vitamin C is a key player in healing and supporting your immune cells.

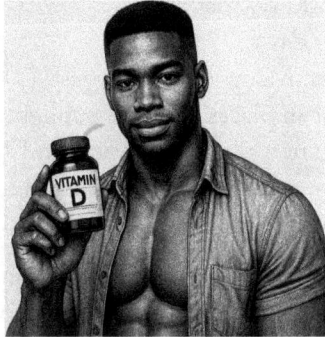

2.2.2: VITAMIN D2 (Ergocalciferol) vs. D3 (Cholecalciferol)

Vitamin D is like bottled sunshine. Your skin naturally makes it when you're out in the sun. It helps your bones grow strong, and many experts say Vitamin D3 (especially with Vitamin K2) is great for overall longevity. A May 2025 study from Mass General Brigham (MGB) and the Medical College of Georgia reveals that taking Vitamin D supplements may protect against biological aging by slowing the shortening of telomeres (*Fox News*).

BEST SOURCES OF VITAMIN D:

D2 (Ergocalciferol): Mushrooms exposed to UV light, fortified plant milks, certain supplements.

D3 (Cholecalciferol): Fatty fish (salmon, mackerel), egg yolks, fortified dairy, and sunlight.

MECHANISM OF ACTION

Calcium & Phosphorus Regulation: Vitamin D makes sure your body absorbs enough calcium and phosphorus to keep bones strong.

Bone Health: Adequate Vitamin D levels can keep bones from becoming soft or brittle, preventing diseases like rickets (in kids) and osteoporosis (in adults).

Other Roles: Scientists think Vitamin D helps regulate the immune system, support mood, and may even influence metabolism.

NATURAL SOURCES OF VITAMIN D

Vitamin D3 (Cholecalciferol) from Sunlight: Your skin makes D3 when exposed to UVB rays. Factors like location, skin color, and sunscreen can affect how much D3 you produce. You can also get it from fish, egg yolks, and fortified milks.

Vitamin D2 (Ergocalciferol) from Mushrooms: Mushrooms exposed to UV light are a natural source of D2. Some brands boost D2 levels by purposely giving mushrooms more UV exposure.

SUGGESTED DAILY DOSAGE
Recommended Daily Intake (RDI):
- Adults up to 70 years: 600 IU/day
- Adults over 70: 800 IU/day

Higher Recommendations: Many experts suggest 1,000–2,000 IU for adults, especially during winter or in places with less sunlight.

Therapeutic Doses: If you're really low in Vitamin D, doctors might prescribe 2,000–5,000 IU daily (or sometimes 50,000 IU weekly for a short time) to catch you up.

SOLUBILITY: Vitamin D is fat-soluble. That means it absorbs better if you take it with a meal containing healthy fats. A lot of people take Vitamin D with vitamins A, E, and K, and especially with Vitamin K2 to help the calcium go into your bones (instead of floating around where it shouldn't).

SAFETY AND TOXICITY
Upper Limits: Most adults shouldn't exceed 4,000 IU of Vitamin D per day without a doctor's guidance.

Overdose Potential: Too much Vitamin D can push your calcium levels too high (hypercalcemia), leading to symptoms like nausea, vomiting, weakness, or confusion. This is rare, but it can happen if you take extremely high doses for a long time.

Monitoring: If you're taking high doses, it's wise to get your blood tested for Vitamin D and calcium levels.

SYNERGY WITH OTHER SUBSTANCES
With Meals Containing Fat: Helps your body soak up the vitamin.

With Vitamin K2: Boosts the chance that calcium gets into your bones and not in your arteries.

With Magnesium: Your body uses magnesium to help activate Vitamin D, so if you're low on magnesium, Vitamin D might not do its job as well.

TORI SPELLING
Tori Spelling, famous from TV shows and real-life reality series, experienced a rough patch when she felt constantly worn out after having her children. At first, she thought it was just normal "mom exhaustion." Later, a doctor visit revealed that her vitamin D levels were too low. **Tori** shared that after she added extra vitamin D into her daily routine—like taking walks in the sunshine and using supplements—she noticed a big improvement in her mood and energy. It's a reminder that new moms (and really anyone) should keep track of their health, even for something as simple as a vitamin check.

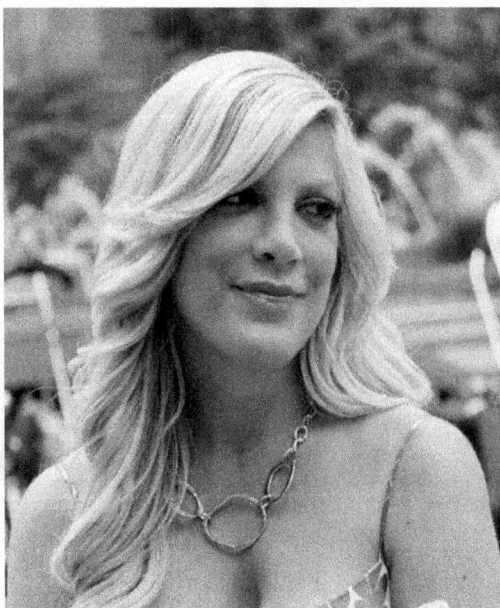

Tori Spelling
Credit – Wikimedia Commons

My friend **Manny** was also severely deficient in Vitamin D (less than 10 ng/mL). With a doctor's help, he took 5,000 IU of D3 daily plus Vitamin K2 and magnesium. After six months, his blood levels were back in a healthy range of 30–50 ng/mL, and he noticed improvements in energy, mood, and even bone density. Everyone's different, but **Tori's** and **Manny's** stories highlight how working closely with a healthcare professional can help fix deficiencies.

2.2.3: EMERGING RESEARCH ON VITAMIN D

Scientists now see Vitamin D as more than just a bone-builder. It may play a part in immune health, mood regulation, and even reduce the impact of some respiratory infections.

POTENTIAL IMMUNE BENEFITS BEYOND BONE HEALTH

Immune Cell Function: Many cells that protect you from illness have Vitamin D receptors, which means Vitamin D can help them work better.

Autoimmune Conditions: Low Vitamin D levels might be linked to higher chances of autoimmune diseases (like multiple sclerosis).

Respiratory Infections: People with low Vitamin D could be more at risk for issues like colds or the flu.

POSSIBLE ROLE IN MOOD REGULATION

Seasonal Affective Disorder (SAD): When sunlight is low in winter, Vitamin D production can drop, which might affect mood and serotonin (a "feel-good" brain chemical).

Research: While some studies say Vitamin D supplementation can lift mild depressive symptoms, others show mixed results. It's important to look at overall lifestyle, including light therapy, healthy fats (like omega-3s), and good eating habits.

STUDIES ON HIGHER VS. LOWER THRESHOLDS FOR OPTIMAL D LEVELS (30–50 ng/mL Debate)

Different health organizations suggest different "best" levels of Vitamin D in your blood:

Institute of Medicine (IOM): 20 ng/mL for most bone-health needs.

Endocrine Society: Over 30 ng/mL, and possibly up to 50 ng/mL for more general health benefits.

Because people are unique—due to genetics, age, or how their bodies absorb vitamins—these ranges might vary. Doctors often test your 25-hydroxyvitamin D levels to see if you need more or less supplementation.

INTERACTION WITH MAGNESIUM

Why Magnesium Matters: Vitamin D has to go through two main steps in your liver and kidneys to become "active," and those steps require magnesium.

Synergy: If you're low on magnesium, it can seem like your Vitamin D is low too because it can't be activated properly. Eating leafy greens, nuts, seeds, and whole grains can help boost magnesium, and supplements are an option if you're still not getting enough.

CLINICAL CASE STUDIES:

In the context of COVID-19, some researchers noted a possible link between low Vitamin D and more severe illness. That doesn't mean taking Vitamin D automatically prevents serious complications—it's just a reminder that balanced Vitamin D levels might support a healthier immune response. More studies are underway to see exactly how Vitamin D works during infections.

Bottom Line:

Vitamin C is a champion for healing and immune support.

Vitamin D (especially D3) is like liquid sunshine for your bones and might help with mood and immunity as well.

Both are vital for anyone looking to stay healthier and possibly ward off certain illnesses.

Always talk to a trusted healthcare professional about the right dosage and timing for you, especially if you're taking higher amounts or have special health concerns.

SECTION THREE: VITAMINS E AND K, AMINO ACIDS

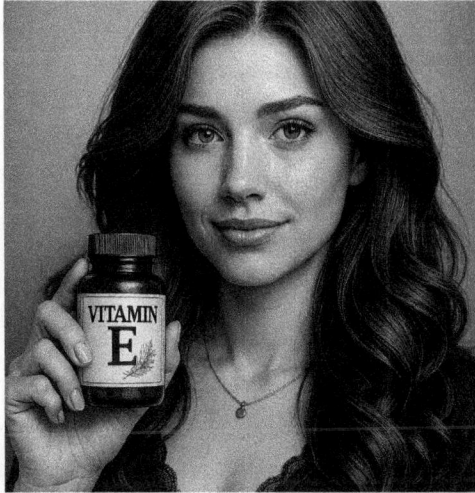

2.3.1: VITAMIN E (TOCOPHEROLS & TOCOTRIENOLS)

Vitamin E is like a superhero shield for your cells. It's an antioxidant, which means it protects your cells from damage caused by things like pollution or stress. If you imagine each cell as a little city, Vitamin E is the force field that guards it against invaders. Vitamin E has amazing capabilities for overall health, potential skin benefits, and long-term longevity.

BEST SOURCES OF VITAMIN E: Nuts (almonds, hazelnuts), seeds (sunflower seeds), vegetable oils (sunflower, safflower), spinach, avocado.

Vitamin E Family: This nutrient is not a single compound but a family of eight structurally related molecules: **Tocopherols:** Alpha-, beta-, gamma-, and delta-tocopherol. **Tocotrienols:** Alpha-, beta-, gamma-, and delta-tocotrienol
Primary Forms: Alpha-tocopherol is the most biologically active form in humans and the one typically measured in blood tests. However, research increasingly suggests gamma-tocopherol and tocotrienols also provide unique health benefits.

ANTIOXIDANT THAT PROTECTS CELL MEMBRANES

Vitamin E is like a personal bodyguard for your cells. It's **fat-soluble**, which means it hangs out in the fatty parts of your cell membranes (the outer walls of your cells) and fights off harmful substances called **free radicals**. By protecting these membranes, Vitamin E helps keep cells healthy and strong.

SUGGESTED DAILY DOSAGE

RDA (Recommended Dietary Allowance) for Adults (19+): 15 mg of alpha-tocopherol daily *(That's about 22.4 IU of natural Vitamin E or 33.3 IU of synthetic Vitamin E.)*

Common Supplement Range: 200–400 IU per day, though some special products go higher.

Upper Intake Level (UL): 1,000 mg of alpha-tocopherol daily (about 1,500 IU in natural form). Going over this regularly might lead to health problems.

SOLUBILITY

Since Vitamin E is **fat-soluble**, you absorb it best when you eat it with a little fat—like avocado, nuts, or olive oil.

INTERACTIONS AND CAUTIONS

Blood Thinning: Vitamin E can make your blood less likely to clot. This might help some people keep their hearts healthy, but it can be dangerous if you're also on blood thinners like warfarin or if you're taking other blood-thinning supplements (such as high-dose fish oil or garlic).

High Doses & Vitamin K: Lots of Vitamin E can interfere with how Vitamin K works, which could increase your chance of bleeding. Talk to a doctor if you take any medication that thins your blood.

OVERDOSE POTENTIAL

Over 400 IU/day: May increase risk of bleeding by interfering with Vitamin K.

Toxicity (Rare): Your body usually regulates Vitamin E levels. But if you go above 1,000 mg per day (UL) for a long time, you could experience problems like bleeding issues, tiredness, or blurred vision.

Signs of Overdoing It: Nausea, diarrhea, fatigue, or blurred vision. If you notice these, lower your dose or stop using it and check with a healthcare pro.

SYNERGY WITH OTHER SUBSTANCES

Vitamin C: Helps recharge Vitamin E so it can keep acting as an antioxidant.

Healthy Fats: Improve absorption (since Vitamin E is fat-soluble).

Polyphenols & Carotenoids (from fruits, veggies, whole grains): Combine with Vitamin E to boost your total antioxidant defenses.

VITAMIN E FOR SKIN HEALTH AND SCAR HEALING:

Some studies (and plenty of personal experiences) suggest that Vitamin E—used on the skin or taken as a supplement—may help scars fade, speed up wound healing, and improve skin texture.

Topical Application: Vitamin E is often mixed with other soothing ingredients like aloe vera to help with scars and irritation.

Oral Supplements: Keeping your Vitamin E levels up might help skin heal better overall, possibly by protecting cell membranes from damage.

(We still need more big, well-designed studies for firm proof, but many doctors and surgeons already suggest Vitamin E for scar care.)

———

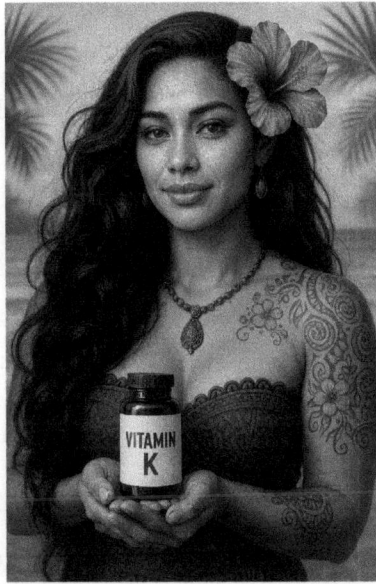

2.3.2: VITAMIN K1 VS. K2

Vitamin K is like the traffic controller for your blood. It helps your blood know when to form clots—so if you get a cut, it helps stop the bleeding. It also works with other nutrients to keep your bones healthy. Picture a traffic light that keeps cars from crashing; Vitamin K does the same thing for your blood cells and bones.

Vitamin K1 is found in leafy green vegetables, like broccoli. I love broccoli, but my friend, former **President George H.W. Bush**, got in big trouble with the broccoli farmers (and with his wife **Barbara!**) when he said:

"I do not like broccoli. And I haven't liked it since I was a little kid and my mother made me eat it. And I'm President of the United States and I'm not going to eat any more broccoli."

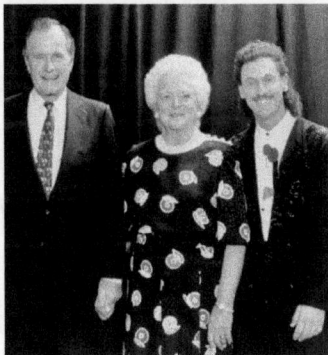

President George H.W. Bush and Barbara Bush with Tad Sisler
Source – Sisler Private Collection

I think the former President's statement is hilarious, but the truth is that broccoli (and particularly broccoli sprouts) contains unbelievable properties that are believed to slow or prevent certain cancers. The K Vitamins have other great benefits as well:

BEST SOURCES OF VITAMIN K:

Vitamin K1 (Phylloquinone): Found in leafy green veggies like kale, spinach, and broccoli.

Vitamin K2 (Menaquinones): Comes from fermented foods (like natto and some cheeses), egg yolks, and organ meats (like liver). Subtypes include MK-4, MK-7, MK-9, etc.

MK-7 (from natto) is often researched for heart and bone health.

MECHANISM OF ACTION

Blood Clotting: Vitamin K kicks off the creation of clotting factors (like prothrombin). It activates proteins that latch onto calcium, helping blood clot properly.

Bone Building: Vitamin K2 activates osteocalcin, a protein that hooks calcium onto your bones. Adequate K2 supports bone density and lowers fracture risk.

EVIDENCE-BASED USES

Heart Health: Vitamin K2 (especially MK-7) may help reduce plaque in arteries and keep them more flexible. Some studies link it with a lower chance of heart disease.

Bone Strength: Vitamin K2 seems to boost bone mineral density and prevent fractures. It teams up with Vitamin D to make sure more calcium goes into bones instead of arteries.

DOSAGE RECOMMENDATIONS

General Guidelines (Adequate Intake, AI):
• Adult women: ~90 mcg/day
• Adult men: ~120 mcg/day

K2 (MK-7) Supplements: Many studies use 100–200 mcg/day for bone and heart health. Some go higher (up to 360 mcg/day) with no major problems, but 100–200 mcg/day is a common starting point.

No Official Upper Limit (UL): Vitamin K doesn't have a widely recognized toxicity level. Still, more isn't always better, especially if you're on blood thinners.

SOLUBILITY

Like Vitamin E, Vitamin K is **fat-soluble**, so take it with a meal that includes healthy fats (think avocado, nuts, or olive oil).

SYNERGY WITH OTHER SUBSTANCES

Vitamin D3: D helps your body absorb calcium, K sends that calcium to your bones.

Calcium & Magnesium: Vitamin K "locks" calcium into bone, but calcium and magnesium also need to be at healthy levels.

OVERDOSE POTENTIAL: Vitamin K toxicity is super rare. Your liver doesn't store much of it, and the body efficiently recycles what you do take in.

MEDICATION INTERACTIONS

Blood Thinners (e.g., Warfarin): Vitamin K intake can decrease the effectiveness of anticoagulants. Dosages and diet must be carefully managed to maintain stable Vitamin K levels. Always consult a healthcare provider before supplementing if you take blood-thinning medication.

SAFETY AND TOXICITY

Blood Thinners (e.g., Warfarin): Vitamin K can reduce how well these drugs work. If you take such meds, you have to keep your Vitamin K intake consistent and talk with a healthcare provider before taking any extra.

CASE STUDY: Improved Bone Density in Older Adults

In one study, older adults who took about 180 mcg of K2 (MK-7) every day for a year noticed better bone density and fewer joint complaints—especially those who also got enough calcium and Vitamin D.

"To me, supplements are a necessity, not a luxury. I think of them as medicine: Instead of asking a doctor to prescribe me a drug when I'm ill, I'd rather take something that can help me avoid getting sick in the first place." –
Laird Hamilton

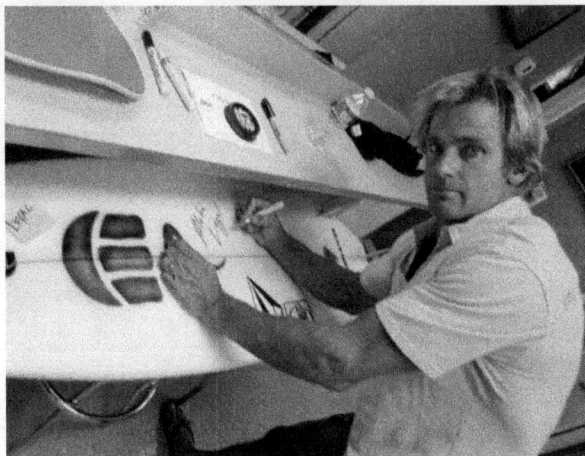

Laird Hamilton
Credit – Wikimedia Commons

2.3.3: SYNERGY IN THE ALPHABET VITAMINS

These four (A, D, E, and K) are all **fat-soluble** and can be stored in your body. That's good news if you miss a day, but it also means you shouldn't take massive amounts for too long.

BALANCING FAT-SOLUBLE VITAMINS TO AVOID DEFICIENCES OR TOXICITIES

Vitamin A: Too little can cause night blindness, immune issues, and skin problems; too much (over ~10,000 IU a day for a long time) can harm your liver and cause headaches.

Vitamin D: Not enough can weaken bones and mess with your immune system. Too much (way above ~10,000 IU a day) can lead to high calcium levels in your blood, causing nausea or kidney damage.

Vitamin E: Deficiency is rare, but extreme overuse (1,000 mg/day+) can thin the blood too much.

Vitamin K: Deficiency can make you bruise easily or bleed more; large amounts rarely cause problems, but can interfere with blood thinners.

PAIRING VITAMIN D3 WITH K2 FOR BETTER CALCIUM UTILIZATION

Vitamin D3 increases how much calcium you absorb from food.

Vitamin K2 directs calcium into your bones rather than letting it build up in your arteries.

Typical Daily Combo:
• Vitamin D3: 1,000–2,000 IU (25–50 mcg)
• Vitamin K2 (MK-7): 90–200 mcg

VITAMIN E AND OTHER ANTIOXIDANTS

Vitamin E often teams up with Vitamin C, selenium, or polyphenols (found in fruits and veggies). Together, they can offer stronger protection against cell damage.

HOW TO COMBINE THESE VITAMINS IN DAILY ROUTINES

Take with Food: A bit of fat (like olive oil, nuts, or avocado) helps you absorb these vitamins.

Don't Double-Dip: If you're already taking a multivitamin plus single supplements, make sure you're not going over the safe limits.

Check Medication Interactions: Especially blood thinners with Vitamin K or high-dose Vitamin E.

Adjust as Needed: Get blood tests sometimes (like a 25-hydroxy Vitamin D test) to ensure your levels are healthy—neither too low nor too high.

2.3.4: THE ROLE OF AMINO ACIDS

Amino acids aren't vitamins, but they're often mentioned along with vitamins and supplements because they're so crucial to how our bodies work. The pioneer of the discovery of DNA, **Francis Crick** (along with his friend **James Watson**) said: *"The sequence of amino acids in a protein is determined by the sequence of bases in some region of a particular nucleic acid molecule,"* basically summarizing the central dogma of molecular biology: Genetic information flows from DNA to RNA to protein, with the amino acid sequence being the key component of a protein. With all we're learning today about DNA and RNA, it's amazing to think that it all centers around the role of amino acids!

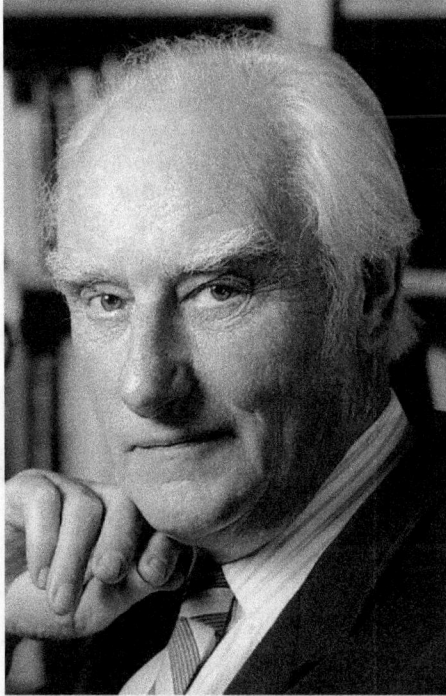

Francis Crick
Credit - Wikimedia Commons

AMINO ACIDS: BUILDING BLOCKS OF PROTEINS

Think of amino acids as tiny building blocks that snap together to form proteins. These proteins help repair muscles, run chemical reactions, transport nutrients, and do pretty much every important job in your body.

Most amino acids dissolve easily in water and travel through your bloodstream. If you eat a balanced diet—enough protein from meats, fish, dairy, eggs, beans, etc.—you generally get all the amino acids you need. Still, certain groups (like athletes or older adults) may benefit from supplements.

ESSENTIAL AMINO ACIDS (EAAs)

"Essential" means your body can't make them on its own, so you **must** get them from food (like meat or beans). They help keep your muscles strong, your brain working right, and your immune system ready for battle.

Examples: Leucine, Isoleucine, Valine, Lysine, Methionine, Phenylalanine, Threonine, Tryptophan, and sometimes Histidine.

Daily Protein Needs:
About **0.8 grams of protein per kilogram of body weight** per day for most healthy adults (though athletes or older adults may aim for 1.2–1.6 g/kg).

Supplement Doses (EAAs/BCAAs): Often 5–10 g per serving. Too much of any single amino acid can lead to imbalances or stomach issues.

OVERDOSE POTENTIAL: While no strict "UL" (Tolerable Upper Intake Level) exists for each essential amino acid, **excessive single-amino-acid supplementation** can cause imbalances or gastrointestinal discomfort.

Leucine in very high doses has been associated with hyperammonemia (excess ammonia in the blood), but this is rare under normal use.

SYNERGY WITH OTHER SUBSTANCES

Carbohydrates: Consuming EAAs or BCAAs with some carbs can improve muscle uptake and reduce muscle breakdown.

Vitamin B6: Involved in amino acid metabolism (e.g., transamination reactions).

NON-ESSENTIAL AMINO ACIDS

These are the amino acids your body **can** produce on its own. But they're still important for recovery, immune health, and more.

Examples: Glutamine, Arginine, Proline, Alanine, Glycine.

Conditionally Essential: In times of stress or illness, your body might need more of these than it can make by itself.

Supplement Examples:

Glutamine: About 5 g/day supports gut and immune health. Athletes may take more.

Arginine: 3–6 g/day for circulation.

Glycine: ~3 g before bed can help with sleep.

Watch for GI upset if you take large amounts.

SYNERGY WITH OTHER SUBSTANCES

Glutamine + Probiotics: This may support gut lining and beneficial bacteria.

Arginine + Citrulline: Often taken together for enhanced nitric oxide support.

SPECIALIZED AMINO ACIDS

Some amino acids have unique "superpowers":

Taurine: Good for heart health, often in energy drinks.

Citrulline: Boosts nitric oxide for better blood flow and exercise performance.
Ornithine: Helps remove ammonia from the body (part of the "urea cycle").
Beta-Alanine: Raises carnosine levels in muscles, helping you power through intense workouts.

SUGGESTED DAILY DOSAGE
Taurine: 500–2,000 mg/day (some take more under medical supervision).
Citrulline: 3–6 g/day (often as "L-citrulline malate").
Beta-Alanine: 2–4 g/day; can cause a tingling feeling in the skin (paresthesia), which isn't dangerous but can be odd.

SYNERGY WITH OTHER SUBSTANCES
Taurine + Magnesium: Sometimes used together to support relaxation and cardiovascular health.
Citrulline + Arginine: Potentiates nitric oxide production more effectively than either alone in some studies.
Beta-Alanine + Creatine: Frequently combined in athletic performance supplements for complementary effects on strength and endurance.

PRACTICAL TIPS FOR AMINO ACID SUPPLEMENTATION
Food First: Try to meet your protein goals with whole foods.
Check for Synergy: Some amino acids work better with carbs or B vitamins (for example, B6 helps with amino acid metabolism).
Moderation Matters: Too much of one amino acid can throw off the balance of others in your body.
Individual Needs: Athletes, older adults, or people recovering from illness might need more specialized supplements.
Possible Side Effects: Large doses can trigger stomach problems or other issues. Listen to your body and talk with a healthcare professional if something feels off.

Now that we've looked at vitamins and amino acids, let's explore the essential minerals that help build our bones, power our muscles, and support many enzyme-driven processes in the body.

In this world of information overload, it's easy to get lost in the wealth of information coming at you. I take comfort in the words of my great friend, legendary *Academy-Award Nominated* Actor **Elliott Gould:**

> *"I find it so easy to get distracted – I try not to do more than one thing at any one time."*

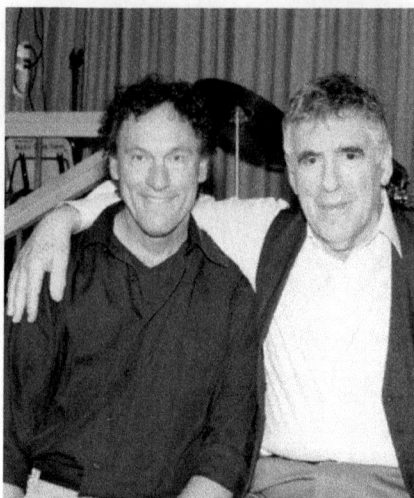

Tad Sisler and Elliott Gould

2.3.5: VITAMIN DEFICIENCIES AND SYMPTOMS

Vitamins like A, B-complex, C, D, E, and K are like the superheroes of your body, keeping everything from your eyes to your bones in top shape. But what happens when these heroes go missing? I've touched on defiencies throughout each chapter and I will continue to do so, but it's good to have a reference to go to, because you want to be ready when your body starts sending out SOS signals in the form of deficiency symptoms. Let's dive into the most common vitamin deficiencies, what signs to watch for, and how to keep your body humming along, all based on the latest 2025 science.

COMMON VITAMIN DEFICIENCIES AND THEIR SIGNS
Vitamin D: The Sunshine Vitamin

Vitamin D is your body's sunshine-powered fuel, crucial for strong bones and a tough immune system. If you're not getting enough sun, fatty fish, or fortified foods, you might be one of the 40% of folks in the U.S. with low levels. Symptoms can include achy bones, weak muscles, or catching every cold going around. In kids, severe deficiency can lead to rickets, where bones soften and bend, while adults might face osteomalacia, a milder version. To stay topped up, catch some rays (safely!), munch on salmon, or talk to your doctor about a D3 supplement, especially if you're in a cloudy area or have darker skin.

Vitamin B12: The Energy Booster

B12 is like the spark plug for your energy and nerves, found mostly in meat, dairy, and fortified cereals. Vegans, older adults, or those with digestive issues might miss out, affecting about 6% of younger folks and more seniors. Signs of low B12 include feeling wiped out, weak, constipated, or even tingling in your hands and feet. Serious cases can mess with memory or mood. If you're vegan or over 60, get your levels checked and consider a supplement to keep your spark alive.

Vitamin C: The Immune Defender

Vitamin C is your immune system's best friend, keeping your skin and gums healthy. While scurvy (yep, like old-timey sailors) is rare today, a diet low in fruits and veggies can still cause trouble. Look out for bleeding gums, easy bruising, or feeling run-down. Load up on oranges, strawberries, or bell peppers to keep your defenses strong and your smile bright.

Vitamin A: For Eyes and Skin

Vitamin A is your go-to for sharp vision and smooth skin, found in carrots, sweet potatoes, and spinach. Deficiency is more common in developing countries but can happen if your diet's lacking. Symptoms include trouble seeing in low light (night blindness), dry, flaky skin, or getting sick more often. Keep your eyes and skin glowing by adding colorful veggies to your plate.

Folate (Vitamin B9): The Cell Builder

Folate is a big deal for making DNA and new cells, especially if you're pregnant. Low levels can lead to anemia, making you tired, or increase birth defect risks in pregnancy. Since food fortification, it's less common, but leafy greens, beans, and fortified cereals keep you covered.

LESS COMMON DEFICIENCIES

Vitamin E: This one's rare, as nuts, seeds, and oils usually do the trick. But if you're low, you might notice nerve or muscle issues, like weakness or vision problems. Keep snacking on almonds to stay safe.

Vitamin K: Essential for blood clotting, deficiency can cause bleeding issues, like easy bruising or nosebleeds. Leafy greens like kale or broccoli usually have you covered, so it's rare in healthy folks.

SPOTTING AND FIXING DEFICIENCIES

Feeling tired or achy? It could be a vitamin deficiency, but symptoms can be sneaky and overlap with other issues. A blood test from your doctor is the gold standard to check your levels—don't guess! A varied diet packed with fruits, veggies, whole grains, and proteins is your best defense. If you're vegan, live in a cloudy place, or have health conditions like Crohn's, supplements might be your sidekick. But don't go overboard—too much of some vitamins (like A or D) can cause trouble. Always chat with your doctor before starting supplements, especially if you're on meds or have health issues.

QUICK REFERENCE GUIDE

Here's a handy table to keep it all straight:

Vitamin	Deficiency Symptoms	Common Sources
A	Night blindness, dry skin, infections	Carrots, sweet potatoes, spinach
B12	Fatigue, weakness, neurological issues	Meat, dairy, fortified cereals
C	Bleeding gums, bruising, fatigue	Citrus fruits, berries, peppers
D	Bone pain, muscle weakness	Sunlight, fatty fish, fortified milk
E	Nerve, muscle damage (rare)	Nuts, seeds, vegetable oils
K	Bleeding disorders	Leafy greens, broccoli

START SMALL, WIN BIG

You don't need to overhaul your life overnight. Swap a soda for water, toss some spinach in your smoothie, or take a quick walk in the sun. These small steps, backed by 2025 research, can keep your body youthful and ready for the longevity journey ahead. Stay curious, check in with your doctor, and let's keep those vitamin levels topped up to feel younger every day!

CHAPTER THREE
THE ESSENTIAL MINERALS

"Sometimes when we crave certain foods it's our body telling us that we're dehydrated or lacking certain minerals." – Joshua Rosenthal

If you've ever wondered why some people seem to have thick, strong hair or rarely feel wiped out, minerals might be their hidden helpers. My own mother developed osteoporosis later in life, and although she did take calcium, she might have had even sturdier bones if she'd started taking it earlier.

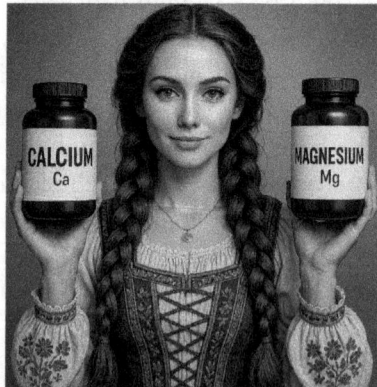

SECTION ONE: MACRO MINERALS
3.1.1: CALCIUM, MAGNESIUM, AND PHOSPHORUS
CALCIUM

Imagine your bones like the walls of a house. Calcium is the cement holding those walls together. When you eat foods with calcium (like milk, cheese, or leafy greens), you're giving your bones the "cement" they need to stay strong. Without enough calcium, those walls can weaken, making it easier for them to crack or break.

MAGNESIUM

Think of magnesium as the friendly helper that keeps your body's "power lines" running. It helps your muscles relax after they flex, and it helps your heart keep a steady beat. Magnesium also helps your body make energy, so you can stay active and alert throughout the day.

PHOSPHORUS

Picture phosphorus as the bright lightbulb in each of your cells. It's a big part of a molecule called ATP, which your body uses for fuel—kind of like a car needs gas. Together with calcium, phosphorus also helps build strong bones and teeth, making them great partners for a healthy skeleton and a great smile.

BEST SOURCES OF CALCIUM, MAGNESIUM, AND PHOSPHORUS

Calcium: Dairy products (milk, yogurt, cheese), fortified plant-based milks (soy, almond), dark leafy greens (collard greens, kale), canned fish with bones (sardines, salmon)

Magnesium: Dark leafy greens (spinach, Swiss chard), nuts (almonds, cashews), seeds (pumpkin seeds), whole grains (brown rice)

Phosphorus: Dairy products, meat (chicken, beef), fish, legumes (lentils, chickpeas), nuts, whole grains

CLASSIFICATION: ESSENTIAL MAJOR MINERALS

Calcium: Helps keep bones and teeth strong, supports muscle contraction, and plays a part in sending nerve signals.

Magnesium: A cofactor in hundreds of chemical reactions, critical for muscle relaxation, nerve function, and making energy.

Phosphorus: Builds bones (together with calcium) and is a key player in ATP, your body's main energy molecule.

HOW THEY WORK: BONE DENSITY, MUSCLE FUNCTION, AND ENERGY

Bone Density: Calcium and phosphorus form crystals in bones to keep them sturdy. Magnesium helps manage bone mineral balance and supports overall bone strength.

Muscle Function: Calcium kicks off muscle contraction; magnesium helps your muscles relax afterward, stopping painful cramps.

ATP Energy (Phosphorus): Phosphorus helps build ATP, the fuel your cells rely on for energy. It also helps with cell signals and metabolism.

SUGGESTED DAILY DOSAGE

Calcium: Around 1,000 mg/day for most adults (19–50); 1,200 mg/day for women 51+ and men 71+

Magnesium: About 310–320 mg/day for women; 400–420 mg/day for men

Phosphorus: About 700 mg/day for adults

Upper Limits (Approximate)

Calcium: About 2,000–2,500 mg/day (going above this may raise the risk of kidney stones)

Magnesium (from supplements): About 350 mg/day (extra magnesium from food is usually not a problem)

Phosphorus: Around 3,000–4,000 mg/day (too much can throw off your calcium balance)

SOLUBILITY

These major minerals dissolve or break down into ions in your body's fluids. Unlike the fat-soluble vitamins (A, D, E, and K), these minerals mix easily with water.

SYNERGY WITH OTHER NUTRIENTS

Calcium + Vitamin D: Vitamin D helps your body absorb calcium better.

Magnesium + Vitamin D: You need enough magnesium for Vitamin D to work properly.

Calcium + Phosphorus: Both help strengthen bones; the right balance is crucial.

OVERDOSE POTENTIAL

Excess Calcium = Possible Kidney Stones: Taking more than about 2,000–2,500 mg a day for a long time can cause kidney stone issues or block the absorption of other minerals like iron and zinc.

Magnesium Overload = Stomach Trouble: If you take over 350 mg/day of magnesium from supplements (on top of foods), it can cause diarrhea or stomach cramps. Extremely high amounts could even mess with your heartbeat or blood pressure.

Too Much Phosphorus: Eating lots of processed foods or drinking a lot of soda can raise phosphorus levels and weaken bones over time, especially if your kidneys have trouble filtering it out.

CLINICAL TRIAL

In one small study, people who had mild trouble sleeping said they slept better after taking 300–400 mg of magnesium glycinate each night for about eight weeks. Researchers think this happened because magnesium helps muscles relax, supports healthy nerves, and might help the body control melatonin (a hormone that regulates sleep).

As we're revealing the amazing properties of minerals, exciting new developments and discoveries may come soon with space exploration and mineral mining on asteroids and other planets. This reminds me of a statement made by my dear friend, multi-platinum recording artist **Kenny Rogers**:

"I'm so totally future oriented that, for me, I don't know what the future's about, but I can promise you it's gonna be exciting!"

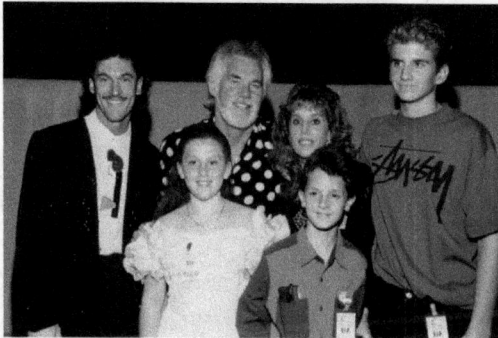

Tad Sisler and Family with Kenny Rogers
Source – Sisler Private Collection

3.1.2: POTASSIUM AND SODIUM
POTASSIUM

Think of potassium like the battery inside each of your cells. It sends out tiny electrical signals that help your muscles move and your heart pump. Foods like bananas, potatoes, or avocados "charge" these batteries. If you don't get enough potassium, you can feel weak or tired because your "batteries" aren't getting enough juice.

SODIUM

Picture sodium as a traffic cop, directing cars along a busy street. It controls how much fluid flows in and out of your cells so they don't swell up or dry out. Sodium also helps electrical signals travel through your nerves. When you eat salty foods, you're sending more "traffic signals" into your body, but having too much sodium can make your heart and blood vessels work overtime.

BEST SOURCES OF POTASSIUM AND SODIUM

Potassium: Bananas, potatoes (with skin), tomatoes, beans, avocados, oranges

Sodium: Table salt and plenty of processed foods (most people actually get too much sodium already)

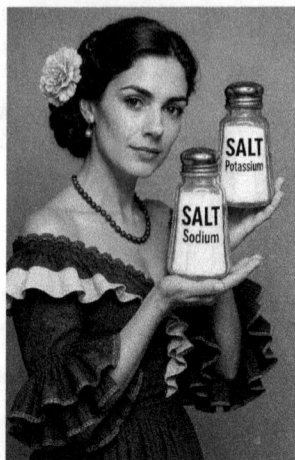

KEEPING BLOOD PRESSURE IN CHECK

Sodium and potassium team up to balance fluids in your body. Too much sodium often raises blood pressure, while enough potassium can help counteract sodium's effects.

Sodium: Many experts suggest fewer than 2,300 mg/day. Some say 1,500 mg/day is best if you have high blood pressure risks.

Potassium: Most adults need around 2,600–3,400 mg/day. Getting it from whole foods (bananas, avocados, beans, potatoes) is ideal.

EXCESS AND BALANCE

Too Much Sodium: Can lead to high blood pressure and strain on your heart.

High Potassium Intake: Usually safe unless you have kidney problems; then it can become dangerous, causing a condition called hyperkalemia that affects your heart rhythm.

PAULA RADCLIFFE (British Marathon Legend)

Imagine you're running on a very hot day and you sweat so much that your clothes stick to your skin. That's what happened to **Paula Radcliffe**, one of the fastest marathon runners in the world. She didn't realize at first that the sweat dripping off her was carrying away a lot of important minerals—like sodium and potassium—that her body needed. Because she trained so hard, especially in warm weather, she sometimes felt weak and got bad cramps. After talking with her doctors, **Paula** added sports drinks and more salty snacks to her routine. This helped her feel stronger during races and recover faster afterward.

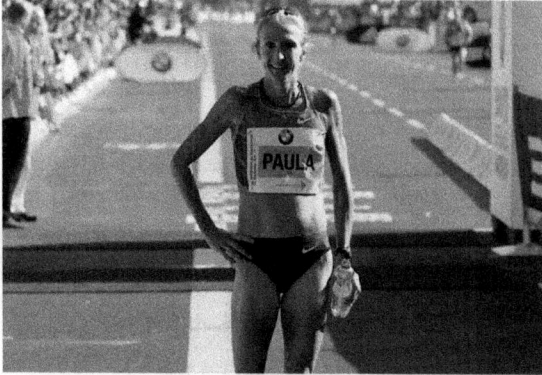

Paula Radcliffe
Credit – Wikimedia Commons

"Companies are experimenting with replacing sodium chloride with potassium chloride, because most of the health problems come from sodium. It works for some products, but if you diminish the amount of sodium, people want sugar and fat instead." – Michael Moss

3.1.3: BIOAVAILABILITY AND INTERACTIONS

Sometimes, taking a supplement doesn't mean your body uses all of it. Several things matter: the mineral's form, competition with other nutrients, and even timing. Imagine your body is a city bus, and minerals like calcium and magnesium are passengers. Some hop on easily (like magnesium citrate), while others (like magnesium oxide) can have a tough time. If too many calcium passengers jump on at once, magnesium might get left behind since there are only so many seats.

MINERALS CAN COMPETE FOR ABSORPTION

Taking large amounts of calcium can interfere with the absorption of magnesium (and vice versa) because they use some of the same "bus seats" in your gut.

Tip: If you need high doses of two minerals, you might take them at different times of day or ask a healthcare professional for the best schedule.

CERTAIN FORMS ARE MORE EASILY USED BY THE BODY

"Citrate," "glycinate," or "malate" forms usually absorb better than "oxide." For example, **magnesium citrate** is known to be more bioavailable (easy to absorb) than magnesium oxide.

Study Example: One study compared magnesium oxide to magnesium citrate, and the citrate version was absorbed much better. People who took it showed higher magnesium levels in their blood and urine afterward.

TIMING MATTERS

Some minerals should be taken with meals to avoid stomach upset; others might absorb better on an empty stomach. For instance:

Iron + Vitamin C: Taking iron with something high in vitamin C (like orange juice) can improve absorption.

Calcium + High Fiber: A lot of fiber at the same time can reduce calcium absorption, so some folks space them out.

BEWARE OF TOO MUCH

Too much of one mineral can throw others out of balance. For example, excessive magnesium might lead to diarrhea or reduce other minerals. Taking mega doses of calcium can increase your risk of kidney stones.

SECTION TWO: TRACE MINERALS
3.2.1: IRON, ZINC, COPPER

"A cardio workout increases blood flow and acts as a filter system. It brings nutrients like oxygen, protein, and iron into the muscles that you've been training and helps them recover faster." – Harley Pasternak

IRON

Picture your body like a big city, with oxygen as the mail that needs to reach every "house" (your cells). Iron is the mail truck carrying that oxygen to your muscles and organs. If you're low on iron, it's like having fewer mail trucks— your cells don't get enough oxygen, so you feel tired or weak.

ZINC

Think of your body as a castle under attack by germs. Zinc acts like the loyal guard, helping your immune system fight off invaders. It also repairs worn-down parts of the castle (like wounds). Not enough zinc, and it's easier for germs to sneak in.

COPPER

Imagine your body as a huge power station, with wires that carry tiny electric signals. Copper is part of those wires, helping your body create energy, keep blood vessels strong, and make healthy bones. Without enough copper, those "wires" can get frayed, and things stop working smoothly.

Iron is an element that helps your body to generate strength. Great athletes use whatever they need, internally and externally, to find enormous strength to overcome all odds. My dear friend **Frank Hamblen**, 7-time Championship-Winning *NBA* Coach, said:

"You just refuse to lose. True success is found in the relentless pursuit of excellence and the unwavering belief in your own potential."

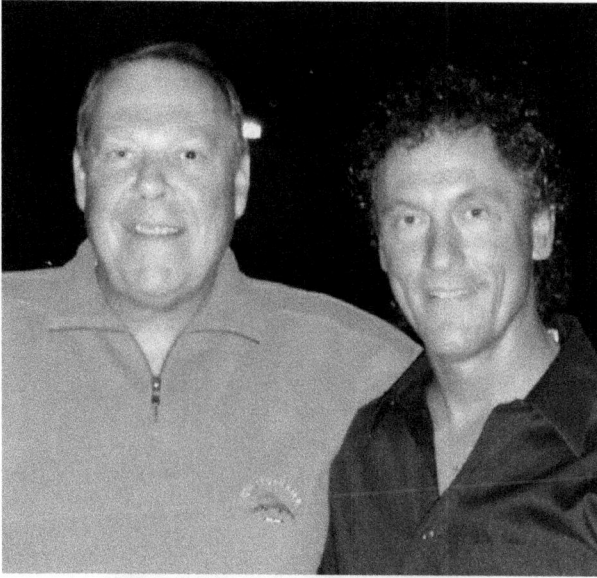

Frank Hamblen and Tad Sisler
Source: Tad Sisler's Personal Collection

CLASSIFICATION

All three—iron, zinc, and copper—are "trace minerals," meaning your body needs them in small amounts, but that small amount is still super important for:

Iron: Building red blood cells to carry oxygen.

Zinc: Supporting your immune system, growth, and healing.

Copper: Helping certain enzymes with energy production and strong connective tissue.

BEST SOURCES

Iron:
- Heme iron (found in animal foods): Red meat, poultry, fish
- Non-heme iron (from plants): Spinach, lentils, beans, fortified cereals

Tip: Vitamin C (like in bell peppers or oranges) helps your body use iron better.

Zinc: Oysters, red meat, poultry, beans, nuts, seeds (pumpkin, sesame)

Copper: Organ meats (liver), shellfish, nuts (cashews, walnuts), seeds (sesame), whole grains

HOW THEY HELP

Iron: Part of hemoglobin, which carries oxygen to cells. Low iron can cause fatigue or even anemia.

Zinc: Boosts immune function, helps with DNA and protein building, and aids in growth and repair.

Copper: A cofactor for many enzymes that help with energy, collagen (for skin and connective tissue), and iron absorption.

SUGGESTED DAILY DOSAGE AND TOXICITY

Iron
- Men: ~8 mg/day
- Women (19–50 years): ~18 mg/day (due to monthly blood loss), dropping to ~8 mg/day after menopause
- Upper Limit: ~45 mg/day for adults (too much can harm the liver and other organs)

Zinc
- Men: ~11 mg/day
- Women: ~8 mg/day
- Upper Limit: ~40 mg/day (excess zinc can lower copper levels and weaken immunity)

Copper
- Adults: ~0.9 mg/day
- Upper Limit: ~10 mg/day (too much can damage the liver or cause stomach problems)

SOLUBILITY & ABSORPTION

Unlike fat-soluble vitamins (A, D, E, K), these minerals aren't stored in big fatty areas. They're generally water-soluble, meaning the body will get rid of extra amounts mostly through urine or bile (though iron is a bit more complicated because the body recycles it).

SYNERGY & REAL-LIFE EXAMPLES

Iron + Vitamin C: Helps iron stay in a form your body can absorb.

Zinc & Copper: Taking a lot of zinc for a long time can block copper absorption, so some supplements include both.

STAYING IN BALANCE

Too much iron can cause damage to organs because of oxidative stress.

Too much zinc can block copper and weaken your immune system.

Too much copper can damage your liver.

PADMA LAKSHMI (Author, TV Host)

Padma Lakshmi always seemed to feel worn-out, like she was running on empty. Even if she got plenty of sleep, she had little energy and found herself out of breath doing everyday things. After visiting her doctor, she found out she had iron-deficiency anemia. This meant her blood didn't have enough iron to carry oxygen around her body. **Padma** started eating more iron-rich foods—like spinach and beans—and took an iron supplement with vitamin C (which helps her body use iron better). Before long, she noticed a big change in how she felt—she wasn't nearly as tired, and she could go about her busy life with new energy.

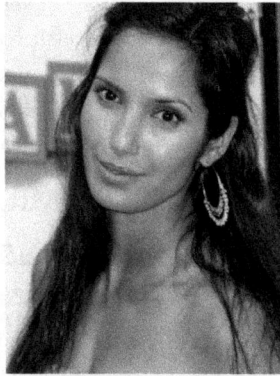

Padma Lakshmi

You should consult healthcare professionals for personalized guidance if you're considering high-dose or long-term supplementation. Everybody has their own unique dietary intake, health status, and biochemical needs.

And…achieving optimal health should not be a goal you make just for yourself. Everyone around you, including family, friends, and business associates, benefits when you can give all you've got due to a healthy lifestyle. It's also not just about playing your part; it's about connecting with others and learning from the experience. Like a football player, you need a team and support system to keep yourself accountable. My dear friend, legendary *Hall of Fame* **NFL** lineman **Junior Seau** said:

"I didn't play the game for the money or the fame. I played because I loved the game. It was my sanctuary, my escape, and my way of connecting with something greater than myself. Football taught me discipline, resilience, and the importance of teamwork. It shaped me into the person I am today, and for that, I will forever be grateful."

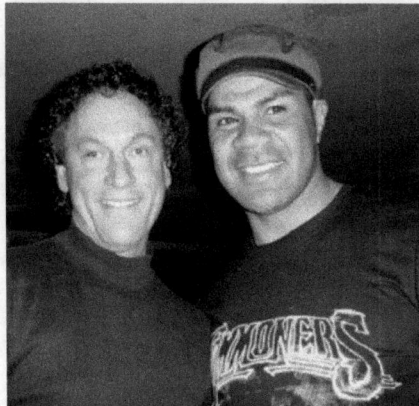

Tad Sisler with NFL Hall of Famer Junior Seau
Source – Sisler Private Collection

Junior was a fantastic person, and I'm so grateful for my close friendship with him while he was still with us. You could easily substitute the word "Football" in his quote with "a healthy lifestyle," "my life's work," or a few other things. Remember, you never have to do anything alone if you choose.

3.2.2: SELENIUM, IODINE, CHROMIUM

"God sleeps in the minerals, awakens in plants, walks in animals, and thinks in man." – Arthur Young

SELENIUM
Think of your body as a castle that needs protecting from "free radicals" (the sneaky attackers that damage your cells). Selenium teams up with enzymes—like brave knights—to block these attackers. It also helps your thyroid (the body's energy center) run smoothly.

IODINE
Your thyroid is like the director of a big theater production, managing your growth, energy, and even how your brain works. Iodine is the script the director reads. Not enough iodine, and the show goes off-script—your metabolism and energy can drop, causing problems like weight gain or fatigue.

CHROMIUM
Imagine your blood as a train track delivering sugar (fuel) to cells. Insulin is the train conductor who makes sure the sugar arrives where it should. Chromium is like the map guiding the conductor. Enough chromium helps your cells get the fuel they need for energy.

BEST SOURCES
Selenium: Brazil nuts (just one or two can meet your daily need), seafood (tuna, salmon), whole grains, organ meats
Iodine: Iodized salt, seaweed (kelp, nori), fish (cod, tuna), dairy (milk, cheese)
Chromium: Broccoli, whole grains, lean meats, eggs, nuts

KEY ROLES
Selenium: Works with enzymes (like glutathione peroxidase) to fight cell damage and support the thyroid.
Iodine: Needed to make thyroid hormones (T3 and T4), which control metabolism and growth.
Chromium: Helps insulin move sugar from your blood into your cells, supporting balanced energy and healthy blood sugar levels.

DAILY DOSAGE & TOXICITY
Selenium
• RDA: 55 mcg/day

- Upper Limit: About 400 mcg/day (too much can cause hair loss, brittle nails, or nerve issues)

Iodine
- RDA: 150 mcg/day for adults
- Upper Limit: About 1,100 mcg/day (excess could trigger thyroid issues)

Chromium
- Adequate Intake (AI): ~35 mcg/day for men, ~25 mcg/day for women
- No well-established Upper Limit for trivalent chromium (the safe form), but stay cautious with high-dose supplements.

OVERDOSE POTENTIAL

Selenium: Toxicity is called selenosis—hair loss, nail problems, or even nerve damage.

Iodine: Too much can flip your thyroid from underactive to overactive or vice versa.

Chromium: Rarely toxic unless taken in industrial forms (hexavalent chromium) not found in common foods.

Remember: More isn't always better! Stick with recommended levels or talk with a healthcare provider.

"The cure for anything is salt water: sweat, tears, or the sea."
— Karen Blixen

3.2.3: MANGANESE, MOLYBDENUM, BORON

"In nature, there is no separation between design, engineering, and fabrication; the bone does it all." — Neri Oxman

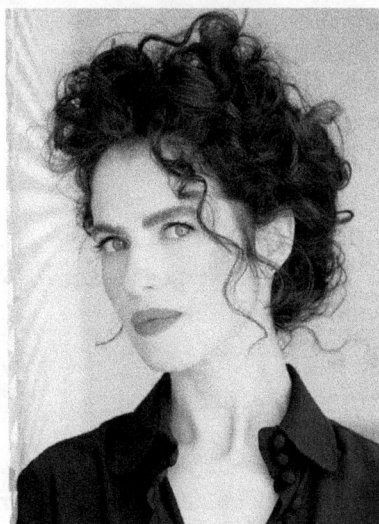

Neri Oxman
Credit — Noah Kalina — Wikimedia Commons

MANGANESE

Think of your bones as a construction site. Manganese is like the foreman, making sure your "builders" (enzymes) have what they need to keep bones strong and help your body produce energy.

MOLYBDENUM

Imagine your body as a giant puzzle. Molybdenum is a tiny but crucial piece that helps certain enzymes "click" into place. These enzymes break down and remove harmful stuff in your system, so even though you need only a little bit of molybdenum, it's still vital.

BORON

Think of your bones and hormones like a dance team. Boron keeps them moving in perfect rhythm, helping bones stay solid and hormones stay balanced. It also helps minerals like calcium and magnesium get to where they're needed.

BEST SOURCES

Manganese: Whole grains (oats, brown rice), nuts (hazelnuts, pecans), leafy greens, pineapple, tea

Molybdenum: Legumes (beans, lentils), grains (whole wheat, oats), nuts, leafy veggies

Boron: Fruits (apples, pears, grapes), nuts (almonds, walnuts), avocados, beans, dried fruits

KEY ROLES & DOSAGE

Manganese
• AI: ~2.3 mg/day for men, ~1.8 mg/day for women
• UL: ~11 mg/day (too much can be toxic, affecting the nervous system)

Molybdenum
• RDA: 45 mcg/day
• UL: 2,000 mcg/day (2 mg) (very high doses can affect copper levels or cause joint pain)

Boron
• No official RDA; many experts suggest 1–3 mg/day is okay.
• Some say up to 20 mg/day may be safe, but research is ongoing. Too much can cause digestive trouble or other issues.

SECTION THREE: PRACTICAL USE OF MINERALS
3.3.1: OPTIMAL PAIRINGS

"There are tons of vitamins and minerals you'll get in plant-based foods that are not soluble if you don't eat fat." – Damaris Phillips

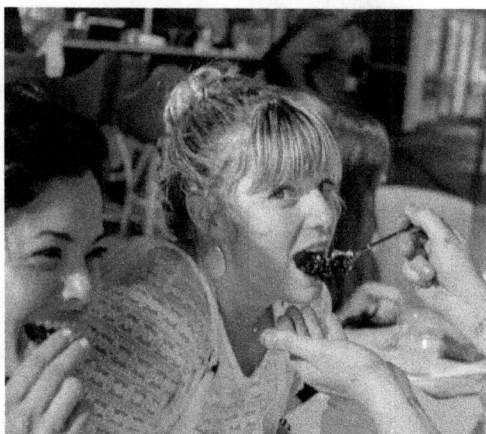

Damaris Phillips
Credit – Wikimedia Commons (cropped)

Just like some actors perform better together, certain minerals and vitamins work best when they appear at the same time. Here are a few examples:

Calcium + Vitamin D + Vitamin K2: A trio for bone health. Calcium builds bones, Vitamin D helps absorb calcium, and Vitamin K2 helps direct calcium into the bones (not the arteries!).

Iron + Vitamin C: Vitamin C turns iron into a form your body absorbs more easily.

Magnesium + Vitamin B6: Can help reduce stress and improve muscle relaxation.

JESSICA ALBA (Actress and Entrepreneur)

When **Jessica Alba** was pregnant, she found that she felt extra tired if she didn't get enough iron in her meals. But she also knew she needed plenty of calcium to help her baby's bones grow strong. At first, she tried taking both supplements at the same time, but her doctor suggested splitting them up:

Morning: Iron pills with something high in vitamin C (like orange juice) to help her body use the iron.

Evening: Calcium pills with dinner, so the calcium wouldn't block her iron.

Once **Jessica** made this simple schedule, she felt more energetic, and she knew her baby was getting what it needed. And, as time went on, she kept her children a priority in her life.

"I wish there were two of me and 48-hour days so I could get everything done. But for me, I have to not try and think that everything has to be 100% perfect all the time and leave room for error. As long as my kids feel loved and a priority, everything really is secondary." – Jessica Alba

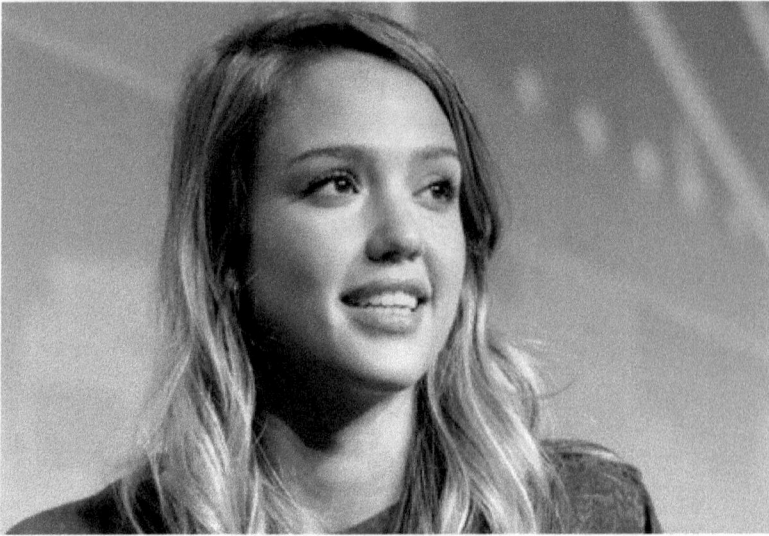
Jessica Alba
Credit – Wikimedia Commons

AVOID HIGH-FIBER MEALS WITH IRON SUPPLEMTATION TO IMPROVE UPTAKE

Why fiber matters: While fiber is very important for digestion and overall health, very high-fiber foods (like bran cereal or certain whole grains) can bind to iron and reduce the amount absorbed.

TIPS FOR SUCCESS: If you're relying on an iron supplement, aim to take it at a time separate from your highest-fiber meal of the day—maybe 1–2 hours before or after. You can still enjoy a balanced diet with fiber; just be mindful of **timing** to ensure that your iron is absorbed effectively.

KEY TAKEAWAY: By pairing the right vitamins and minerals together—and being mindful of **timing** and **dietary fat** for the fat-soluble nutrients—you can boost your body's ability to absorb and use these essential compounds. This balanced approach helps you get the most out of supplements and supports your long-term health goals.

3.3.2: SAFETY AND CONTRAINDICATIONS

My dear old friend, philanthropist **T. Denny Sanford**, has done more to advance noble causes in health and medicine than almost anyone on the planet. The foundation of his, and all, research is to push the limits of knowledge while focusing on safety. All great medical studies begin with what doesn't work, and this is where contraindications come into play.

"People who are crazy enough to think they can change the world are the ones who do." – T. Denny Sanford

72

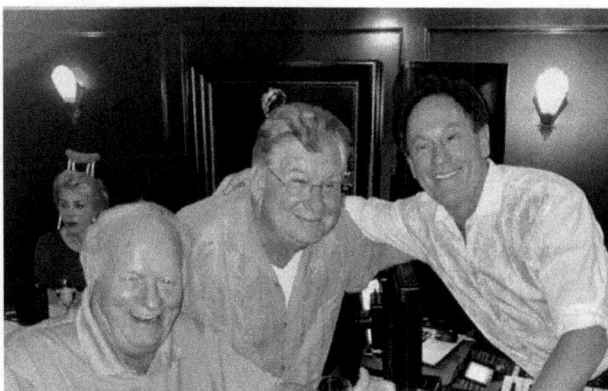

T. Denny Sanford with Ron Zagami and Tad Sisler
Source – Sisler Private Collection

Safety is key, and contraindications—times you shouldn't take something—matter.

EXAMPLES

Hemochromatosis: A genetic disorder causing too much iron absorption. People with this issue should avoid iron supplements unless a doctor says otherwise.

Kidney or Heart Conditions: Too much calcium can stress the kidneys or cause heart rhythm problems. Ask your doctor if you have a history of stones or heart trouble.

DRUG INTERACTIONS

Zinc can reduce the absorption of certain antibiotics.

Calcium can interfere with thyroid medication.

Tip: Separate mineral supplements from medications by at least a couple of hours.

START SLOW

If you're unsure, start with lower doses or just meet recommended amounts. If you need higher amounts, talk to a doctor. More isn't always better.

"At the end of the day, the goals are simple: safety and security."
– Jodi Rell

3.3.3: FOOD VS. SUPPLEMENT SOURCES

What's the best way to get minerals? Through food or supplements—or both?

Whole Foods: Fruits, vegetables, grains, and meats offer minerals plus other helpful nutrients like fiber and vitamins.

Supplements: Can fill in the gaps when your diet isn't enough. They're also helpful for people with special needs (like pregnant women, athletes, or older adults).

EXAMPLE MEAL PLAN RICH IN ESSENTIAL MINERALS:

Breakfast: Oatmeal with chia seeds (magnesium, manganese), topped with almonds (calcium, magnesium) and berries (vitamin C)

Lunch: Spinach salad (iron, calcium) with bell peppers (vitamin C), feta cheese (calcium), pumpkin seeds (zinc, magnesium), whole-grain bread (selenium if soil is rich)

Snack: Yogurt or plant-based yogurt (calcium, potassium) + a Brazil nut (selenium)

Dinner: Grilled salmon (iodine, selenium) or tofu (if vegetarian), broccoli (calcium, chromium), sweet potato (potassium), brown rice (manganese)

Dessert (Optional): A little dark chocolate (magnesium, iron)

ORGANIC VS. CONVENTIONAL

Mineral content varies based on soil quality, not just an "organic" label. Some organic farms have richer soils, but conventional farms can also produce nutrient-dense foods. Eating a rainbow of fruits and veggies is a great way to cover your bases. For instance:

White: Tofu, potatoes, garlic, onions, oats, cauliflower

Purple: Eggplant, blackberries, currants, blueberries, red cabbage, beeets

Green: Peppers, beans, spinach, kale, limes, avocado, cabbage, beans, pears, celery, zucchini, pesto, apples

Yellow: Squash, corn, lemons, eggs, legumes, banana, mushrooms, pineapple, grapefruit, macadamia nuts, sesame seeds, cashews, quinoa, chickpeas, peanuts, almonds, walnuts, pecans, brown rice, beans, ginger, peppers

Orange: Carrots, oranges, pumpkins, peaches, sweet potatoes, yams, cantaloupe, apricots, mango, peaches

Red: Tomatoes, peppers, raspberries, strawberries, apples, cranberries, beans

3.3.4: MINERAL DEFICIENCIES AND TOXICITIES

Minerals are essential for numerous bodily functions, from building strong bones to supporting heart rhythm. Deficiencies or excesses can disrupt health, so recognizing their symptoms is crucial for maintaining vitality. Below, we outline deficiencies and toxicities for key minerals, their symptoms, and dietary sources, based on 2025 research. Here's your "one-stop" reference shop for deficiencies and toxicities:

COMMON MINERAL DEFICIENCIES

Calcium: Vital for bones, muscles, and nerves. Deficiency can lead to osteoporosis, muscle cramps, or dental issues, common in those with low dairy or vitamin D intake. Sources include dairy, leafy greens, and fortified foods.

Magnesium: Supports over 300 enzymatic reactions, including energy production. Low levels may cause muscle twitches, fatigue, or irregular heartbeat, often linked to poor diet or digestive issues. Found in nuts, seeds, and whole grains.

Iron: Essential for oxygen transport. Deficiency causes anemia, with fatigue, weakness, and pale skin, prevalent in women and vegetarians. Red meat, beans, and fortified cereals are key sources.

Zinc: Crucial for immunity and wound healing. Deficiency leads to immune issues, hair loss, or slow healing, seen in poor diets or malabsorption. Oysters, beef, and pumpkin seeds are rich sources.

Iodine: Needed for thyroid hormones. Deficiency causes goiter or hypothyroidism, with weight gain and fatigue, common in low-iodine areas. Seafood and iodized salt provide ample amounts.

Selenium: An antioxidant supporting thyroid function. Deficiency may cause muscle weakness or infection risk, though rare. Brazil nuts and fish are top sources.

LESS COMMON DEFICIENCIES

Phosphorus: Supports bone health; deficiency is rare but can cause bone pain or weakness. Found in meat and dairy.

Potassium: Regulates fluid balance and heart rhythm; low levels from excessive loss (e.g., vomiting) cause muscle weakness or cramps. Bananas and potatoes are sources.

Sodium: Maintains fluid balance; deficiency is rare but can cause confusion or seizures from overhydration. Found in salt and processed foods.

Copper, Chromium, Manganese, Molybdenum, Boron: Deficiencies are uncommon but can affect blood, metabolism, or bone health if low.

MINERAL TOXICITIES

Excessive intake, often from supplements, can be harmful:

Calcium: High levels cause kidney stones or constipation

Iron: Overload (hemochromatosis) damages organs like the liver

Zinc: Excess causes nausea or copper deficiency

Selenium: High doses lead to hair loss or neurological issues

Iodine: Overuse disrupts thyroid function

Magnesium: High doses from supplements cause diarrhea or cramping

QUICK REFERENCE TABLE

Mineral	Deficiency Symptoms	Toxicity Symptoms	Common Sources
Calcium	Osteoporosis, muscle cramps	Kidney stones, constipation	Dairy, leafy greens
Magnesium	Twitches, fatigue, arrhythmia	Diarrhea, cramping	Nuts, seeds, grains

Iron	Anemia, fatigue, pale skin	Organ damage	Red meat, beans
Zinc	Immune issues, hair loss	Nausea, copper deficiency	Oysters, beef, seeds
Iodine	Goiter, hypothyroidism	Thyroid dysfunction	Seafood, iodized salt
Selenium	Muscle weakness, infections	Hair loss, neurological	Brazil nuts, fish

3.3.5: MINERAL INTERACTIONS AND ABSORPTION OPTIMIZATION

Minerals interact with each other and other nutrients, affecting how well your body absorbs them. Understanding these interactions ensures you get the most from your diet or supplements.

KEY INTERACTIONS

Calcium and Iron: High calcium intake can reduce iron absorption, impacting anemia prevention. Take iron-rich foods or supplements separately from calcium.

Zinc and Copper: Excess zinc can lower copper levels, affecting nerve health. Balance zinc supplements with copper-rich foods like liver.

Magnesium and Calcium: These compete for absorption, so high doses of one may limit the other. Maintain a balanced intake.

Vitamin D and Calcium: Vitamin D enhances calcium absorption, essential for bone health. Ensure adequate vitamin D from sun or supplements.

Phytates and Oxalates: Found in grains and spinach, these bind minerals like iron and zinc, reducing absorption. Soaking or fermenting foods improves bioavailability.

OPTIMIZING ABSORPTION

Eat a Varied Diet: Include a mix of mineral-rich foods to avoid imbalances.

Time Supplements: Take competing minerals (e.g., calcium and iron) at different times of day.

Check with a Doctor: Blood tests confirm mineral levels, especially if you have health conditions or take medications.

Prepare Foods Wisely: Soak grains or cook spinach to reduce phytates and oxalates, boosting mineral uptake.

By addressing these interactions and following these strategies, you can ensure your body gets the minerals needed for health and longevity.

DON'T RELY ON SUPPLEMENTS ALONE

I have a nephew who believed he could eat anything as long as he took enough supplements. He ended up gaining too much weight and eventually needed surgery. You can't out-supplement a bad diet without consequences. Pills can help, but real, whole foods are still the backbone of good health. Combining a nutritious, mineral-rich diet with targeted supplementation—when truly necessary—is generally the safest strategy.

I'm a big believer in supplements, but relying on pills alone misses the holistic benefits of whole foods and can risk nutrient imbalances. Aim for a balanced diet as the foundation of good health. Developing good habits will get you there. My friend, former **United States Secretary of State, General Colin Powell** said:

"If you are going to achieve excellence in big things, you develop the habit in little matters. Excellence is not an exception, it's a prevailing attitude."

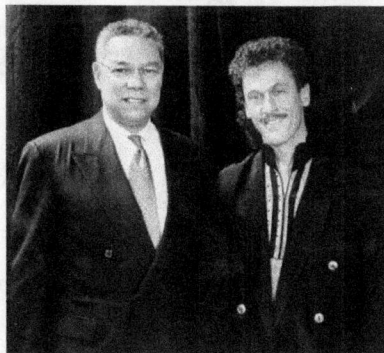

Secretary of State, General Colin Powell and Tad Sisler
Source – Sisler Private Collection

A well-balanced diet is a daily habit that leads to overall excellence in health. When you add supplements in a careful, thoughtful way—especially if you have a deficiency or higher needs—you'll be covering all your mineral bases without risking harmful side effects.

Ready to keep exploring nature's pharmacy? In the next chapter, we'll dive into the world of herbs and how they can give you an extra boost for better health and a longer life.

CHAPTER FOUR
HARNESSING THE POWER OF HERBS

From ancient poultices to modern extracts, herbs have helped people heal for thousands of years. Curious about the secrets they hold? Let's explore how different herbal and botanical extracts may strengthen our health, support our immune systems, boost our energy, and even calm our minds.

EXAMPLES OF HERBAL AND BOTANICAL EXTRACTS

Herbs and plant extracts can offer a wide variety of benefits:

Adaptogens help our bodies cope with stress.

Immune-support herbs strengthen our natural defenses.

Anti-inflammatory plants help ease swelling and discomfort.

Blood sugar support herbs keep our energy levels steady by helping balance glucose.

Cognitive enhancers can improve focus and clear thinking.

Digestive aids support a healthy gut and better digestion.

Metabolism boosters may give a gentle energy lift while supporting weight management.

Circulation and heart health herbs keep blood flowing smoothly and help maintain healthy blood pressure.

Soluble fiber (found in things like psyllium husk) forms a gel in your stomach, helping regulate blood sugar and cholesterol.

Insoluble fiber (like wheat bran) adds bulk to keep digestion moving.

Polyphenols are protective plant compounds that help cells stay healthy.

Lecithin is a fatty substance that helps oily and watery ingredients blend together in our cells.

SECTION ONE: ADAPTOGENS AND TONIC HERBS

"All those spices and herbs in your spice rack can do more than provide calorie-free, natural flavorings to enhance and make food delicious. They're also an incredible source of antioxidants and help rev up your metabolism and improve your health at the same time." – Suzanne Somers

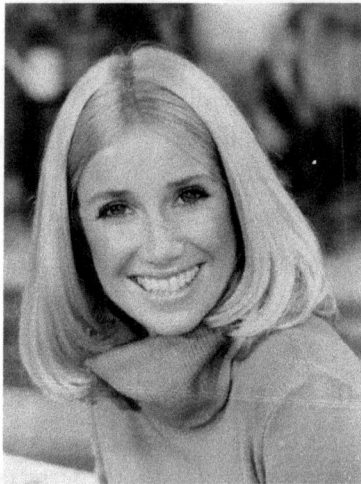

Suzanne Somers
Credit – Picryl / creativecommons.org

4.1.1: ASHWAGANDHA AND RHODIOLA ROSEA

ASHWAGANDHA

Imagine carrying a heavy backpack full of stress. Ashwagandha helps lighten that load so you don't feel exhausted all the time. It's an ancient herb known for helping calm the mind, encourage better sleep, and improve mood. Think of it as a supportive friend who keeps you steady when life gets tough.

RHODIOLA ROSEA

Picture your energy and focus like a campfire. Rhodiola Rosea is the steady stream of firewood that keeps that fire burning bright. This herb grows in cold, rocky regions but is surprisingly good at helping you feel alert, adapt to stress, and avoid that "crash" when you're super busy.

WHY THEY'RE CALLED ADAPTOGENS

Both Ashwagandha and Rhodiola are "adaptogens," meaning they help the body handle stress and stay balanced without being too energizing or too calming. They work with our body's main stress system (the hypothalamic-pituitary-adrenal axis), and research shows they may help keep the stress hormone cortisol under control.

Ashwagandha: May lower cortisol levels, support sleep quality, and even help with energy.

Rhodiola Rosea: May boost the cell's ability to create and use energy. This can lead to better mental and physical stamina.

EVIDENCE-BASED USES

Stress Reduction:

Ashwagandha: Studies show it can help healthy adults feel less stressed or anxious.

Rhodiola Rosea: Often cited for improving mood and reducing mental fatigue during challenging work or study.

Endurance & Physical Performance:

Ashwagandha: Some research suggests it may boost muscle strength and workout recovery.

Rhodiola Rosea: Small studies say it can help you exercise longer and recover faster.

VALERY POLYAKOV
THE RECORD-SETTING SPACE TRAVELER

Valery Polyakov is a Russian cosmonaut who spent 437 days aboard the MIR space station—the longest single space-flight in history.

Imagine living on a giant science-lab in space for more than a year, where every day feels like gym class with no gravity. **Dr. Polyakov** wanted to stay strong and clear-headed, so he packed an herbal combo called **ADAPT** that contained Rhodiola Rosea. He took it every day. Just like the runner in your story, **Polyakov** said the herb kept his energy up, helped him bounce back from tough space-workouts, and made long, stressful days feel easier. When he finally landed, he told the scientists who monitored him that Rhodiola had helped him handle the marathon mission without burning out.

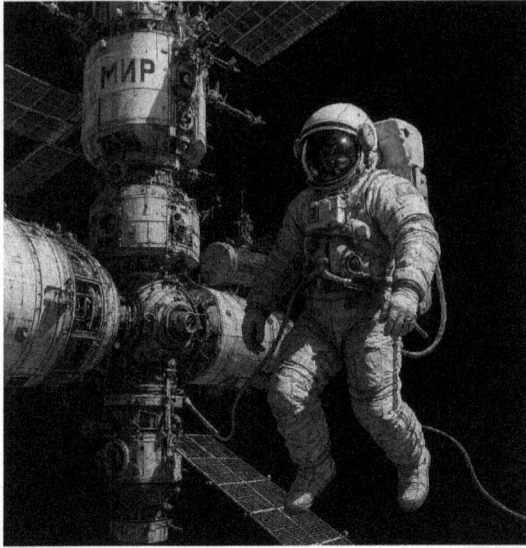

GENERALLY WELL-TOLERATED
Generally safe at recommended doses.

Ashwagandha: Might lower blood pressure or blood sugar, so people on meds for these conditions should watch their levels.
Rhodiola Rosea: May interact with drugs for mood or blood pressure.

If you're pregnant, nursing, or on prescription meds, talk to a healthcare provider first.

By combining **Ashwagandha** and **Rhodiola Rosea** with a balanced lifestyle— adequate sleep, good nutrition, and stress-management techniques—many individuals can better handle daily challenges and maintain more stable energy levels. My friend, iconic actor **Lorenzo Lamas** is the son of legendary actor **Fernando Lamas**. **Lorenzo** experienced an enormous amount of stress naturally throughout his career as a television actor on popular shows like *Renegade* and *Falcon Crest*. **Lorenzo** shared a reflection regarding how he handled it:

> *"The most important thing I learned from Dad about show business was never take myself seriously and never stop having fun with my craft."*

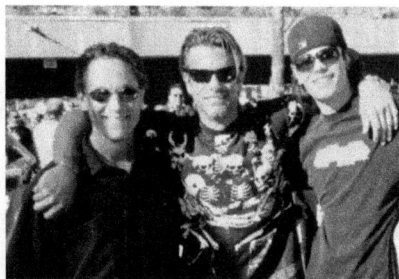

Tad Sisler with Lorenzo Lamas and A.J. Lamas
Source: Tad Sisler's Personal Collection

Not learning how to overcome stress can take years off your life. We have many tools to deal with this, and herbal remedies can be a part of your toolbox.

4.1.2: GINSENG (PANAX) AND ELEUTHERO

GINSENG (Panax)

Imagine a high-quality phone charger that quickly recharges your energy and focus. That's Panax ginseng. It may give you a small mental boost and help you feel less tired, especially during homework, sports, or a busy day.

ELEUTHERO

Think of Eleuthero as a friendly coach for your whole body. It won't give you superpowers, but it can help you bounce back from hard workouts or stressful days. People often say it helps them stay balanced and keep going when life gets hectic.

SOO JOO PARK

Runway model **Soo Joo Park** flies from New York to Paris and Seoul on a tight schedule. Before fashion month one winter, she started taking a spoonful of Korean red-ginseng extract every morning, a habit she picked up at Seoul's duty-free shops. Over the next month of back-to-back shows, she noticed fewer colds, steadier energy during late fittings, and calmer nerves when call-times were 6 a.m. She now swears by the adaptogenic root, along with meditation and Pilates, to keep stress low and focus high.

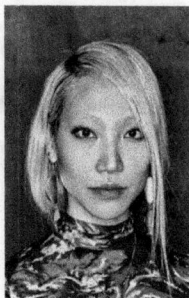

Soo Joo Park
Credit — Wikimedia Commons

TRADITIONAL ROOTS

Panax Ginseng (Asian or Korean Ginseng) has been a key part of Traditional Chinese Medicine for centuries, known for restoring energy (qi) and supporting overall vitality.

Eleuthero (sometimes called Siberian Ginseng) isn't a "true ginseng," but it shares similar adaptogenic benefits. Traditionally used in Russia and parts of Asia to reduce fatigue and boost endurance.

BENEFITS

Cognitive Function: Panax ginseng might sharpen mental clarity. Eleuthero could help reduce mental fatigue, though fewer studies back it up than Panax ginseng.

Energy and Stamina: Both can combat tiredness and improve vitality without the jitters of caffeine.

Immune Support: Some studies say they might help the immune system respond better to stress, though neither is a cure-all.

POTENTIAL INTERACTIONS

Both Panax ginseng and Eleuthero can affect blood pressure and blood sugar. If you have hypertension or diabetes, check with your doctor. Always look for standardization and quality certification to avoid mislabeled or weak products.

My friend **Mark Redman**, one of the great *Major League Baseball* pitchers, found himself pitching in the World Series. His performances generally highlighted **Mark's** outstanding cognitive function and energy, but they were naturally filled with stress. **Mark** said:

"It came to the point where you try to do too much out there. You give up a couple of runs and in the back of your head, because of the way things have gone all year, I just tried to battle. It can be wearing on a person, but I've been there before."

Mark Redman stayed in the battle of the moment and prevailed. If you find yourself in similar situations, you may find some help in herbal remedies.

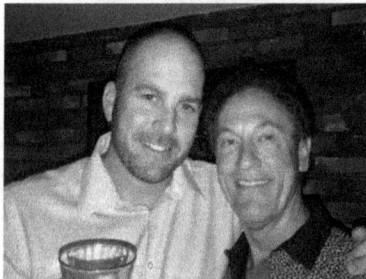

Mark Redman and Tad Sisler
Source – Sisler Private Collection

4.1.3: HOLY BASIL (TULSI) AND MACA

HOLY BASIL (Tulsi)

Picture a gentle shield that keeps stress and worries from overwhelming you. Holy basil, or Tulsi, is known to help people feel calmer, and it can also support your immune system. In places like India, people often drink Tulsi tea daily for a calmer mindset and stronger health.

MACA

Imagine your energy level as a small campfire. Maca is like extra-high-quality firewood from the Andes that makes the flame burn brighter and steadier. It's often used for boosting stamina and focus, giving a gentle nudge to keep you going through the day.

AYURVEDIC STAPLE (Tulsi) AND PERUVIAN POWER (Maca)

Holy Basil (Tulsi): A key herb in Ayurveda, known for calming stress and supporting clear breathing.

Maca: Grown in Peru's Andes, used for energy, endurance, and possible hormone balance. Many users say it helps them stay strong and focused.

MOOD & VITALITY

Holy Basil: Often brewed as tea to promote a balanced mood and reduce anxiety.

Maca: Many people report feeling more energetic and upbeat with consistent use.

ELLIE GOULDING

Pop singer **Ellie Goulding** loves tough workouts—boxing rounds, sprint drills, and Barry's Bootcamp classes. To keep from crashing halfway through, she whirls up a morning smoothie loaded with greens, vegan protein, and—her favorite booster—maca powder. She told *Well + Good* that maca makes the shake "really filling" and gives her steady energy so she can hit every high note and every burpee without feeling wiped out.

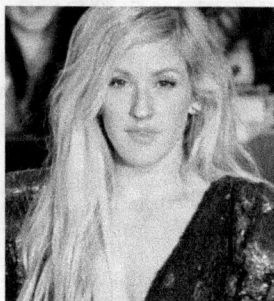

Ellie Goulding
Credit – Wikimedia Commons

QUALITY MATTERS

Maca: Watch out for products mixed with cheap fillers. Look for transparent labeling (Lepidium meyenii) and testing by reputable brands.

Holy Basil (Tulsi): Widely available as teas, capsules, or extracts. Go for well-known companies that test for purity.

Both Tulsi and Maca have deep cultural roots—in India and Peru—and are treasured for their ability to promote health, calm, and vitality.

My good friend, legendary actress **Dyan Cannon**, had enormous success and accolades, but her journey was sometimes stifled by fear and emotional distress. **Dyan,** like most of us, always wondered if the other shoe was going to drop:

"Have you noticed when you start getting happy, you say, uh-uh, I'd better watch out. I feel too good. Something's going to happen."

Finding ways to manage stress—whether through herbs, mindfulness, or positive thinking—can help break that cycle of worrying about the "other shoe" dropping.

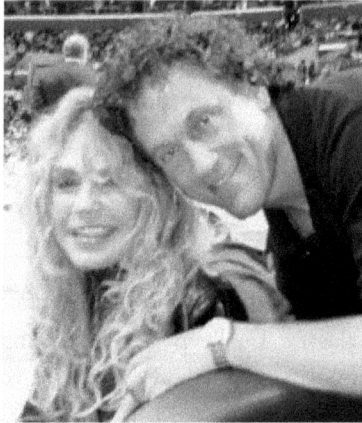

Dyan Cannon and Tad Sisler
Source: Tad Sisler's Personal Collection

4.1.4: HERB-DRUG INTERACTIONS

Adaptogens and tonic herbs like ashwagandha, rhodiola, ginseng, eleuthero, holy basil, and maca can enhance your health, but they may interact with medications, altering their effectiveness or causing side effects. Always consult your healthcare provider before combining these herbs with prescriptions, especially if you have chronic conditions. Below, we outline potential interactions for each herb, based on 2025 research.

Ashwagandha: May lower blood sugar and blood pressure, potentially amplifying diabetes or hypertension medications, risking hypoglycemia or hypotension. It could also affect thyroid medications, sedatives, or immunosuppressants, increasing side effects (*NCCIH*). A 2025 study notes mild interactions with at least 29 drugs, including SSRIs (*Health.com*).

Rhodiola: Can reduce blood sugar or blood pressure, enhancing related medications, which may lead to excessively low levels. It may interact with antidepressants, increasing serotonergic effects, or drugs metabolized by liver enzymes (CYP3A4, CYP2C9) (*NCCIH*). A 2025 case study reported restlessness with rhodiola and paroxetine (*PubMed*).

Ginseng: Might interact with calcium channel blockers, statins, antidepressants, or blood thinners like warfarin, though warfarin effects are inconsistent (*NCCIH*). A 2025 review suggests monitoring for cognitive or cardiovascular drug interactions (*Planta Medica*).

Eleuthero (Siberian Ginseng): May affect heart medications like digoxin, increasing levels, or interact with diabetes drugs, blood thinners, immunosuppressants, or drugs metabolized by CYP2D6/CYP3A4 (*WebMD*). A 2025 study notes potential liver enzyme inhibition (*Planta Medica*).

Holy Basil (Tulsi): Could slow blood clotting, increasing bleeding risk with anticoagulants (e.g., warfarin) or antiplatelets (e.g., aspirin). It may enhance sedatives like pentobarbital or affect thyroid medications (*RxList*). A 2025 study suggests moderate interaction risks (*Merck Manual*).

Maca: Limited data on interactions, but some products may contain hidden sildenafil, interacting with nitrates (e.g., nitroglycerin) and causing dangerous blood pressure drops (FDA). A 2025 study indicates potential CYP3A4 interactions (*PubMed*).

Consult your doctor to tailor herb use to your medications and health needs, ensuring safe integration for longevity benefits.

4.1.5: HERBAL SUPPLEMENTS STANDARDIZATION

Standardization ensures herbal supplements deliver consistent amounts of active ingredients, critical for reliable health benefits. For example, ashwagandha may be standardized to 5% withanolides, rhodiola to 3% rosavins, or ginseng to 4% ginsenosides. Variations in growing conditions, harvest time, or processing can affect potency, so standardized extracts provide a predictable dose, enhancing safety and effectiveness. A 2025 review emphasizes standardization for consistent therapeutic outcomes (*Planta Medica*).

Look for labels stating "standardized extract" with specific percentages of active compounds. Choose brands with third-party testing (e.g., USP, NSF) to verify purity and avoid contaminants like heavy metals or hidden drugs. Reputable products offer transparency, ensuring you get the intended benefits without risks. Check for certifications and avoid products with vague claims or missing ingredient details (*NCCIH*).

SECTION TWO: MEDICINAL MUSHROOMS
4.2.I: REISHI, CHAGA, AND CORDYCEPS

REISHI

Reishi is often called the "mushroom of immortality." Think of it as a wise, gentle teacher that helps you relax, manage stress, and sometimes sleep better. It's not going to make you live forever, but many believe it helps the body find its calm center.

CHAGA

Chaga is like a sturdy shield for your immune system. It grows on birch trees in cold climates and is packed with powerful compounds that may help your body's defenses work better. Some people say it's like armor that helps them stay healthier.

CORDYCEPS

Cordyceps is like a personal trainer that cheers you on when you're running or playing sports. It's known for boosting energy and endurance, helping you go the extra mile without feeling exhausted.

WHY THEY'RE CALLED FUNCTIONAL FUNGI

Reishi, Chaga, and Cordyceps contain special compounds (like polysaccharides) that can help our bodies adjust to stress. Studies suggest they may also offer antioxidant benefits, scavenge free radicals, and possibly support the immune system in staying alert and ready.

PRELIMINARY RESEARCH

Immune Boost: Some animal and lab studies show these mushrooms may increase certain immune cells.

Respiratory Health: Cordyceps is popular among athletes for its potential to improve how the body uses oxygen.

Gastrointestinal Upset: In large doses, these mushrooms could cause stomach problems. If you take immunosuppressants, talk to a doctor before trying them. A 2012 study in *The American Journal of Chinese Medicine* found that polysaccharides in Reishi improved immune responses in animal models. While more human research is needed, it's a good sign that these mushrooms might help us stay healthier.

"Today, reishi stands out as one of the most valuable of all polypore mushrooms in nature for the benefit of our health. Many naturopaths and doctors prefer organically-grown reishi from pristine environments because they are more pure." – Paul Stamets

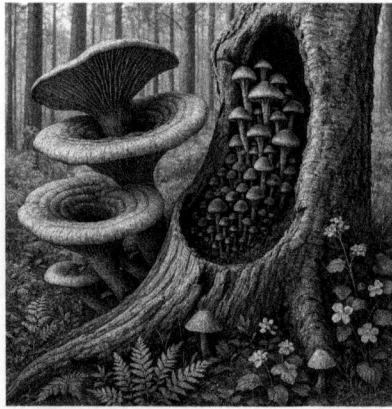

4.2.2: LION'S MANE AND TURKEY TAIL

LION'S MANE

Lion's Mane is often called "food for the brain." Picture your brain like a busy city with roads that need repairs. Lion's Mane may help fix and build those "roads" by promoting the production of Nerve Growth Factor (NGF). Early studies say it could support memory and focus, especially for people with mild cognitive issues.

TURKEY TAIL

Think of your immune system as a team of superheroes. Turkey Tail is like an advanced training camp, helping boost those superheroes' fighting skills. Rich in beta-glucans (special sugars that can affect immune cells), Turkey Tail may support people during challenging times like cancer treatments, making their immune system more resilient.

LION'S MANE FOR COGNITIVE HEALTH

Unique Compounds: Hericenones and erinacines in Lion's Mane may spark more NGF production.

NGF Helps Neurons: NGF is vital for the growth and survival of some types of brain cells.

Early Studies: Preliminary research hints at memory and focus benefits.

TURKEY TAIL FOR IMMUNE SUPPORT

Beta-Glucans: Turkey Tail contains high levels of these immune-boosting sugars.

Polysaccharide-K (PSK) & PSP: In places like Japan, extracts from Turkey Tail are sometimes used alongside medical treatments to help strengthen the body's defenses.

One small study in Japan found older adults with mild cognitive impairment showed better scores on memory tests after taking Lion's Mane extract. Once they stopped taking it, their scores went back toward normal levels—suggesting Lion's Mane needs consistent use.

QUALITY AND PURITY

Mushrooms can soak up heavy metals if they grow in polluted soil. Look for brands that test for contaminants. Standardized extracts list how much of each active compound you're getting.

"Turkey tail mushrooms have been used to treat various maladies for hundreds of years in Aisa, Europe, and by indigenous peoples in North America. Records of turkey tail brewed as medicinal tea date from the early 15th century, during the Ming Dynasty in China." – Paul Stamets

4.2.3: PSILOCYBIN MUSHROOMS - BENEFITS AND RISKS

Sometimes called "magic mushrooms," psilocybin mushrooms contain a psychoactive compound (psilocybin) that can change how you see, think, or feel. People have used them in spiritual ceremonies for centuries, and researchers today are studying how psilocybin might help with depression, anxiety, and addiction. However, laws about psilocybin differ depending on where you live, and it carries risks like "bad trips" if taken incorrectly.

Micro-dosing: Taking very small amounts to boost creativity or mood without a strong psychedelic effect. **Always check legal status and be aware of potential side effects.**

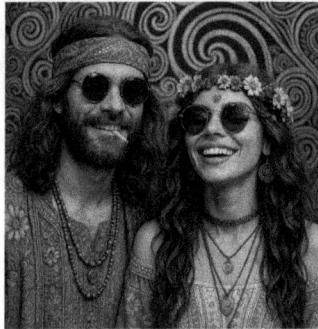

"Mushrooms are miniature pharmaceutical factories, and of the thousands of mushroom species in nature, our ancestors and modern scientists have identified several dozen that have a unique combination of talents that improve our health." – Paul Stamets

4.2.4: PRACTICAL TIPS FOR USING MUSHROOMS - CAPSULE VS. POWDER VS. WHOLE MUSHROOMS:

Whole Mushrooms: You get all the nutrients, but cooking can be time-consuming. Some medicinal varieties taste bitter.

Powders: Easy to add to drinks or food, but the flavor might not appeal to everyone, and the potency can vary.

Capsules: Very convenient with no taste, but can be pricier.

PAIRING WITH VITAMIN C

Sometimes taking mushroom extracts with Vitamin C (like orange juice) might help your body use the healthy compounds better.

TRADITIONAL TCM DECOCTIONS

In Traditional Chinese Medicine, people simmer mushrooms like Reishi for about an hour to draw out their good stuff. It's a slow, soothing process that has been used for generations.

CHECK LABELS FOR FRUIT BODIES VS. MYCELIUM ON GRAIN

Fruiting Body: Contains more beneficial compounds.

Mycelium: Sometimes grown on grain, which can dilute the potency.

FLAVOR COUNTS

Certain mushrooms—like Shiitake, Lion's Mane, Maitake—are great in cooking. Reishi is usually too bitter for everyday meals, so it's often made into tea or capsules.

SAFETY NOTE

If you aren't 100% sure about a mushroom growing in the wild, don't eat it! Many are poisonous.

Regarding, psilocybin, think twice before you jump into using "magic mushrooms." I'm all for finding new ways to expand your consciousness, but I also believe that you shouldn't have to alter your consciousness through drinking or drugs in order to cope with life. Many of my friends learned that the hard way, including my dear friend, legendary *multi-platinum* artist **Glen Campbell.** **Glen** was such a good man, and he eventually conquered his addictions. **Glen** said:

"I spent some time in hell. God saved me."

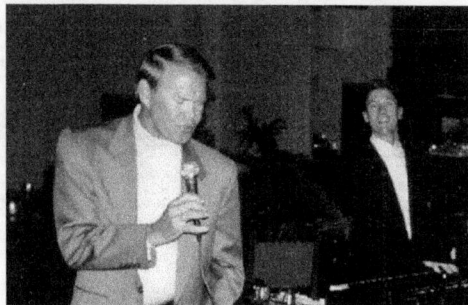

Glen Campbell performing with Tad Sisler
Source – Sisler Private Collection

SECTION THREE: TRADITIONAL POULTICES, TEAS, AND TOPICAL REMEDIES

TRADITIONAL POULTICES

A poultice is like a soft paste made from mashed herbs or other natural materials. You spread it on a cloth and place it over sore muscles, wounds, or irritated skin. The warmth and moisture can help with blood flow, draw out fluids, and soothe pain. It's an old-fashioned remedy that's still used today because it often works.

TOPICAL REMEDIES

These are treatments you put on the outside of your body—such as creams, gels, and lotions—to help with skin irritations or muscle aches. Different cultures have their own recipes, often using oils, waxes, and herbs.

4.3.1: MUSTARD, CASTOR OIL, AND CLAY POULTICES

MUSTARD POULTICES

Mustard poultices create gentle heat on the skin, helping with sore muscles or chest congestion. It's like putting a small heating pad on your body. Just be careful not to burn your skin by leaving it on too long.

CASTOR OIL POULTICES

Castor oil poultices are like a sponge drawing out unwanted stuff from your body. You soak a cloth in castor oil and place it on the area you want to soothe (like your joints or abdomen). Many people find it reduces swelling and discomfort.

CLAY POULTICES

Clay acts like a magnet for impurities and toxins. You apply it to the skin, let it dry, and then wash it off. It's a natural way to clean and soothe your skin—like giving it a gentle facial.

A FAMILY TRADITION

Sarah, dealing with a nagging cough, remembered her grandma's mustard poultice. She warmed a simple mustard mixture on the stove, placed it on her chest, and felt almost immediate relief from congestion—just like Grandma used to do.

BE CAUTIOUS WITH SKIN IRRITATION OR BURNS

Always be careful: mustard can irritate the skin, and castor oil or clay might bother some people. Start with a thin layer, watch for redness or itching, and wash it off if it starts to sting.

"My mom and grandma, growing up, one thing they emphasized was that you need to make sure that anything you put on your skin is also digestible by the body. For example, if something isn't safe for me to eat or consume, it's probably not good for your face. So I do a lot of natural remedies." – Halima Aden

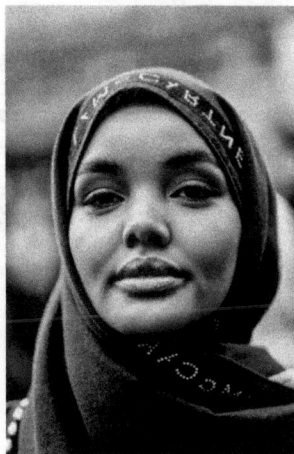

Halima Aden
Credit – Wikimedia Commons

4.3.2: HERBAL COMPRESSES (ARNICA, PLANTAIN, CALENDULA)

An herbal compress is like a "tea bag for your skin." You soak a cloth in herbs or a tea made from herbs, then apply it to a sore or irritated area.

ARNICA COMPRESS

Arnica, a yellow flower, can help with bruises or swelling (but never put it on broken skin or swallow it). It's like a gentle ice pack made of flowers, reducing bruises and helping them fade faster.

PLANTAIN COMPRESS

Not the banana-like plantain, but the common backyard weed. Plantain leaves can soothe bug bites, minor cuts, or rashes. Crush or brew the leaves, apply them to the skin, and let the plant's anti-itch powers do the rest.

CALENDULA COMPRESS

Calendula (a bright orange-yellow flower) can soothe cuts, scrapes, or irritated skin. Steeping the petals in warm water and placing them on the sore area is like wrapping your skin in a soft, healing hug.

A Historical Snapshot:

Long ago, a midwife named **Kathleen** brewed calendula petals for new mothers. She used arnica on bruises (making sure skin wasn't broken) and plantain to calm bug bites. This simple, natural approach was a lifeline for families who didn't have access to modern medicine.

SAFETY FIRST

Arnica: For external use only.

Plantain: Make sure you have the right plant. Some plants look alike but can irritate the skin.

Calendula: Very gentle, but always check for allergies.

"We have finally started to notice that there is real curative value in local herbs and remedies. In fact, we are also becoming aware that there are little or no side effects to most natural remedies, and that they are often more effective than Western medicine." — Anne Wilson Schaef

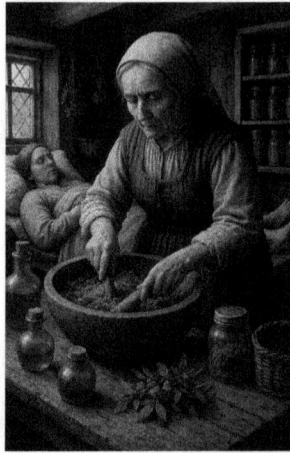

4.3.3: BEST TOPICAL HERBS FOR EXTERNAL USE

Remember, don't put anything on your body that might give you an allergic or toxic reaction. Always check with a healthcare professional before using anything new.

WOUND AND SKIN CARE

Few botanicals rival **Aloe vera** when it comes to first-aid fame: the plant's clear gel is packed with polysaccharides that form a cool, protective film over minor burns, razor nicks, and sun-scorched shoulders. Bright-orange **Calendula** (already mentioned in this chapter) blossoms follow close behind; infused into oil or cream, their carotenoid-rich resins speed epithelial repair and tame redness—perfect for chapped lips, diaper rash, or a freshly inked tattoo. **Yarrow** earns its spot for "field-dressing" scrapes; the feathery leaves contain achillein, astringent tannins, and natural antiseptics that help slow bleeding and kick-start tissue knitting.

PAIN, BRUISES AND SWELLING

When you bang a shin or roll an ankle, reach for **Arnica montana** (as we also just mentioned)—its sesquiterpene lactones (especially helenalin) calm inflammation, disperse pooled blood, and cut bruise recovery time in half for many users. For deeper aches, the allantoin in **Comfrey** (often labeled "knitbone") supports bone and tendon mending; modern salves use the leaf rather than the pyrrolizidine-alkaloid-heavy root, and only on unbroken skin. Pair either herb with a warm **Chamomile** compress—the same calming flowers you sip also contain azulene, a blue compound that comforts muscle tension and irritated joints.

ANTIMICROBIAL AND ACNE CONTROL

Tea Tree (Melaleuca alternifolia) oil is nearly synonymous with natural antisepsis; a 5 % gel rivals over-the-counter benzoyl peroxide for mild acne yet leaves skin less flaky. For fungal foes—athlete's foot, ringworm, under-breast rash—blend tea tree with **Witch Hazel** distillate. This bark-derived astringent tightens pores, dries excess moisture, and leaves behind pro-anthocyanidins that calm post-shave bumps. A dab of **Lavender** essential oil (one of the few that can be used neat in tiny amounts) not only lends a clean scent but also adds extra gram-positive–bacteria punch and speeds the sting out of insect bites.

CIRCULATION-BOOSTING AND MUSCLE-RUB BOTANICALS

Weekend warriors swear by **Rosemary** infused in olive or coconut oil—the camphor and cineole warm stiff shoulders, while rosmarinic acid delivers antioxidant defense to overworked tissues. Massage therapists often finish with a dot of **Ginger** or **Cayenne (Capsaicin)** ointment; these spices crank up micro-circulation, drawing fresh blood—and nutrients—into fatigued quads or cold hands. Used sparingly, they create a pleasant, lingering heat without the synthetic scent of commercial liniments.

TOPICAL-USE QUICK GUIDE

Prep	Primary Uses	How to Apply
Gel (*Aloe vera*)	Minor burns, razor nicks, sunburn	Split a fresh leaf, scoop out the clear gel, smooth over skin 1–3 × daily.
Oil infusion (*Calendula, Rosemary, Ginger*)	Dry or irritated skin; massage rub	Warm-steep dried herb in carrier oil 2–3 h (or sun-infuse 2 weeks); strain and apply as needed.
Compress (*Chamomile, Yarrow*)	Swelling, bruises, sore eyes	Brew a strong tea, soak a clean cloth, wring out, apply 10 min; repeat twice daily.

Prep	Primary Uses	How to Apply
Salve *(Arnica, Comfrey—leaf only)*	Sprains, stiff joints, bruising	Melt I part beeswax into 4 parts infused oil, cool, rub in 2 × daily; keep off broken skin.
Hydrosol / distillate *(Witch Hazel)*	Acne, razor burn, hot-weather chafing	Mist directly on clean skin or swipe with a cotton pad morning & night.
Essential-oil spot dab *(Tea Tree, Lavender)*	Single pimples, insect bites, fungal spots	Dilute I drop EO in 4–5 drops carrier (lavender may be used neat); dab twice daily.

SAFETY REMINDERS:
- Always patch-test a new herb on the inner forearm for 24 hours.
- Avoid arnica or comfrey on broken skin.
- Dilute essential oils properly—nature is potent!

4.3.4: BEST HERBAL TEAS

Nothing soothes us more than a nice, warm cup of herbal tea. Check steeping times on any particular tea to make sure you get the full benefits of the herbs. Also make sure before you ingest anything that you are not allergic.

CALMING AND SLEEP-SUPPORT

When the day winds down, nothing beats a cup that whispers "bedtime." **Chamomile** reigns supreme here—its apple-scented blossoms contain apigenin, a gentle compound that coaxes the nervous system into rest mode. **Lemon balm** follows close behind; steep the fresh-cut leaves for five minutes and you'll smell why herbalists call it "the balm that makes the heart merry." **Lavender's** floral notes add a spa-like layer and pair beautifully with chamomile in a I : I blend. For those who wrestle with stubborn insomnia, **valerian root** and **hops** create an earthy, mildly sedative duo that can shorten the time it takes to drift off. Brew **valerian** no longer than seven minutes to dodge its musky aftertaste, then sip slowly while the steam rises—it's a warm lullaby in a mug.

DIGESTIVE AND GUT-SOOTHING

Peppermint is the rock-star of post-meal comfort: **menthol** relaxes intestinal muscles, easing bloat and crampy "food baby" moments. Combine it with **ginger** and you get a two-pronged remedy that settles nausea *and* steady-state indigestion. **Fennel seed** adds a sweet, licorice kiss that many Mediterranean families swear by for gas relief—simply crush a teaspoon of seeds before steeping to unlock its aromatic oils. **Dandelion root**, roasted until it smells like chicory coffee, stimulates bile flow and is the liver's best friend after a heavy dinner. Finish with **lemongrass** for a bright citrus finish; its light antimicrobial punch keeps the whole digestive orchestra in tune.

IMMUNE AND RESPIRATORY

When sniffle season strikes, **hibiscus** brews up a tart, ruby-red shield rich in anthocyanins that help tame blood-pressure spikes while supporting vascular health. **Elderberry** and **elderflower**—dark berries paired with fragrant blooms—are famed for shortening the duration of colds; steep with a touch of **raw honey and lemon** for a comforting cough elixir. **Echinacea** joins the lineup as an immune primer, best taken at the *first* tickle in the throat, while **thyme's** piney leaves (loaded with **thymol**) act like a botanical vapor rub for the lungs. A **peppermint-licorice** "throat comfort" blend rounds off the chapter, coating raspy vocal cords as **peppermint** opens the nasal passages so you can breathe— and sleep—better.

ANTI-INFLAMMATORY, ENERGY AND METABOLISM

Need a lift without caffeine jitters? **Ginseng (Panax)** offers a clean, clarifying buzz—brew only three minutes to avoid bitterness. **Rooibos,** the red jewel of South Africa, is naturally caffeine-free yet rich in aspalathin and quercetin, compounds linked to smoother blood-sugar curves. A **cinnamon-spice** mélange (**cinnamon, clove, ginger**) enhances insulin sensitivity while satisfying dessert cravings with its bakery-warm aroma. **Turmeric-ginger** "golden" tea turns bright yellow in milk, thanks to curcumin—add a pinch of **black pepper** so your body absorbs up to 2,000 % more of this inflammation-tamer. Finally, **moringa leaf**—sometimes called the "miracle tree"—steeps into an emerald tonic packed with iron and calcium for all-day vitality.

HORMONE AND WOMEN'S HEALTH

Red clover blossoms supply gentle plant estrogens that ease hot flashes and mood swings in the menopause transition, while **spearmint** showcases intriguing science for women with hormonal acne or excess androgen symptoms: two cups a day lowered free testosterone in small studies. **Raspberry leaf** has been the midwife's ally for generations—rich in uterine-toning tannins, it's traditionally sipped in late pregnancy and for menstrual cramp relief. **Sage leaf** stands out for cognitive clarity and temperature regulation; its subtle savory flavor pairs nicely with **lemon balm** for a pleasant, slightly minty afternoon refresher.

ADAPTOGENS AND STRESS-RESILIENCE

Tulsi (holy basil) stars as an Ayurvedic adaptogen; you'll taste hints of clove and pepper as it steadies cortisol swings and encourages calm focus. **Ashwagandha root**—nutty, almost malt-like—works on the same stress axis but leans more toward evening relaxation; serve it with warm **oat milk** and a drizzle of **honey** for a nourishing nightcap. **Chaga mushroom**, slow-simmered rather than briskly steeped, yields a woodsy, vanilla-tinged decoction brimming with **beta-glucans**—ideal for fortifying immunity during high-stress weeks. **Cardamom-rose chai**, meanwhile, wraps the nerves in aromatic comfort while aiding digestion, making it a luxurious study-break brew.

BREWING TIPS
Leafy herbs (**lemon balm, nettle, raspberry**): 3–5 min at ≈ 200 °F.
Seeds & roots (**fennel, ginger, turmeric**): 8–10 min simmer or gentle boil.
Barks & mushrooms (**cinnamon, chaga**): 15 min low simmer or slow-cooker batch.

Sweeten lightly with **raw honey** or **maple**, and experiment with **citrus slices** or a splash of **plant milk** to create signature house blends your friends and relatives will remember.

In the next section, we'll check out nutraceuticals—specialized compounds that can help us take an even more advanced approach to health. Combined with herbal knowledge, these cutting-edge formulas may offer a new level of wellness and vitality.

4.3.5: BEST PRACTICES AND WARNINGS
Research or Consult a Pro
Know the exact plant species you're using. Learn about side effects. Get tips from certified herbalists, reputable books, or scientific sources.
Potential Allergies
Even natural herbs can cause reactions. Do a small patch test on your arm before using a new herb on a bigger area. If you see redness or swelling, stop right away.
Cautionary Tale
Sarah once grabbed what she thought was plantain while hiking. She ended up picking wild nettle by mistake and had a painful, itchy reaction. Moral of the story? Double-check the plant's identity!
Cleanliness Matters
Wash your hands before preparing poultices or compresses. Sterilize your tools. Use fresh or correctly dried herbs. Store your mixtures safely and for a short time only.
Respect Local Traditions and Modern Science
Each region has its own herbal customs—learn from local experts. But also look for scientific validation to back up what you've learned. Practice ethical gathering methods so you don't harm the environment.

My friend, iconic rapper **Snoop Dogg**, is known for having a fondness for a particular herb that I only touch on briefly later in this book. His music has gone from showcasing the realities of life on the street to a new place, reflecting that he is primarily a peaceful, loving individual. Lately, **Snoop** has focused on being a good example for boys and young men. He said:

> *"It's so easy for a kid to join a gang, to do drugs... we should make it that easy to be involved in football and academics."*

Remember, more importantly than what herbs you prefer, the world will be a better place if you spread love and kindness.

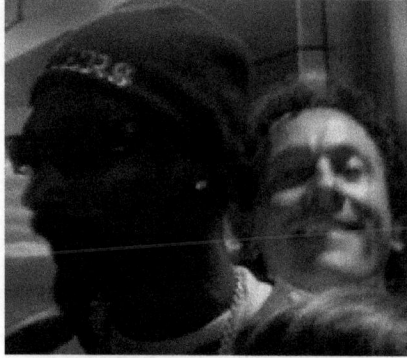

Snoop Dogg and Tad Sisler
Source – Sisler Private Collection

CHAPTER FIVE
SPECIALTY NUTRACEUTICALS & FUNCTIONAL COMPOUNDS

Modern research labs are churning out powerful extracts – like CoQ10, alpha-lipoic acid, and more – that can optimize energy, cognition, and aging. I've elaborated greatly on this in my book **"Stay Healthy, Stay Youthful: The Science of Living to 150"**. I'm excited about the idea that we may be able to actually reverse aging in the near future, and this chapter is full of great compounds that will help us to move more quickly in that direction.

> *"Only 20 percent of our longevity is genetically determined. The rest is what we do, how we live our lives and increasingly the molecules that we take. It's not the loss of our DNA that causes aging, it's the problems in reading the information, the epigenetic noise."*
> *– Dr. David Andrew Sinclair*

SECTION ONE: CoQ10, ALPHA-LIPOIC ACID, PQQ, BETA-GLUCANS, CANNABINOIDS, AND PHOSPHATIDYLSERINE

5.1.1: CoQ10 (UBIQUINONE VS. UBIQUINOL)
A Spark Plug for Your Cell's Energy

Imagine that every cell in your body is a tiny power plant. For these power plants to run, they need a spark plug—and that's basically what CoQ10 does. It helps your cells produce energy so you can stay active and feel steady throughout the day. Without enough CoQ10, those little power plants don't work as well, and your energy might dip.

How It Works

CoQ10 is crucial for helping your cells make ATP (the main energy molecule). You'll often see it talked about alongside "mitochondria," which are the tiny engines in each cell. Think of CoQ10 as the key that starts the engine. It also has antioxidant properties, meaning it shields your cells from harmful molecules and everyday wear and tear.

Who Should Consider It

People on statin drugs (statins lower CoQ10 levels in the body)
Anyone worried about heart health or feeling low energy
Older adults, since CoQ10 levels naturally drop as we age

SUGGESTED DAILY DOSAGE

Most people take **50–200 mg per day** of CoQ10 (often labeled as "ubiquinone"). Some doctors recommend higher doses—like **400–600 mg a day**—for special issues such as congestive heart failure. If you choose ubiquinol (the reduced form), your body usually absorbs it more easily, so you might not need as high a dose. But ubiquinol can cost more.

DIETARY SOURCES: Certain foods contain CoQ10, but usually in small amounts:
Organ meats (like beef heart or chicken liver)
Fatty fish (sardines, salmon, mackerel)
Nuts and seeds (peanuts, pistachios, sesame seeds)
Some veggies (spinach, broccoli, cauliflower)

The thing is, cooking can reduce CoQ10, and it can be hard to eat enough of these foods to get a truly beneficial dose. That's why many people prefer supplements.

SOLUBILITY:

CoQ10 dissolves in fat, so it's smart to take your pill with a meal that contains healthy fats—maybe some avocado, nuts, or olive oil. If you buy CoQ10 in oil-based capsules (softgels), absorption can be even better.

DR. TRAVIS STORK

Dr. Travis Stork is an ER physician & Emmy-winning host of *The Doctors*.
After seeing many heart-failure patients, he began monitoring his own cholesterol and energy. When his LDL crept up and he felt sluggish on busy ER shifts, a cardiologist friend recommended CoQ10. **Dr. Stork** now appears in Qunol ads taking 100 mg daily (3× better-absorbed form). He says adding

CoQI0 "re-charged" his stamina on long hospital days and during workouts, and he now recommends it to statin users for the same reason.

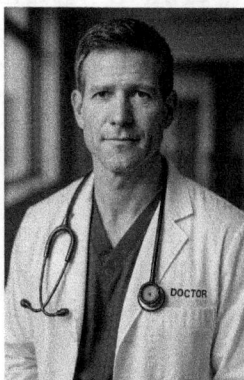

SYNERGY WITH OTHER SUBSTANCES
Omega-3 fatty acids (fish oil): May help further support cardiovascular health and improve CoQI0 absorption.

Vitamin E is also fat-soluble and an antioxidant, so that it can complement CoQI0's protective effects on cells.

SAFETY AND SIDE EFFECTS
CoQI0 is considered quite safe. Side effects are usually mild—like slight stomach upset—if you take more than 200–300 mg daily. If you're on blood thinners or other heart medications, check with your healthcare provider before starting CoQI0. Always store oil-based capsules in a cool, dry place.

"For me, training is my meditation, my yoga, hiking, biking all rolled into one. Wake up early in the morning, generally around 4 o'clock, and I'll do my cardio on an empty stomach. Stretch, have a big breakfast, and then I'll go train." – Dwayne "The Rock" Johnson

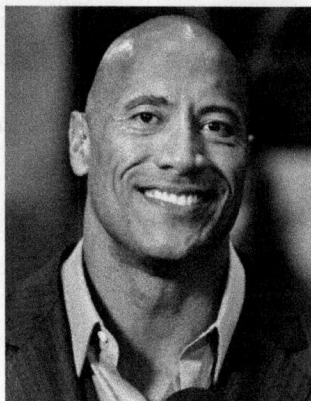

Dwayne Johnson
Credit – Wikimedia Commons

5.1.2: ALPHA-LIPOIC ACID (ALA)
UNIVERSAL ANTIOXIDANT AND METABOLIC HELPER
Think about your body as a busy city full of "sparks" (free radicals) that can damage cells if they run wild. Alpha-lipoic acid (ALA) acts like a master firefighter: not only does it put out those sparks, but it also helps other antioxidants (like vitamins C and E) recharge so they can keep fighting.

BOTH WATER- AND FAT-SOLUBLE
Most antioxidants work either in water or in fat, but ALA can work in both environments. That's why people call it a "universal antioxidant." It helps protect cells in many different parts of your body, including your brain, because it can cross the blood-brain barrier. It also regenerates other antioxidants like Vitamins C and E.

POTENTIAL FOR BLOOD SUGAR MANAGEMENT IN NEUROPATHY
Blood Sugar Support: ALA seems to help cells use sugar (glucose) better, which can be good news for people with type 2 diabetes or those who worry about high blood sugar.

Nerve Health: Some research suggests ALA can reduce the tingling or burning feeling (neuropathy) that often comes with diabetes.

STEWART BRAND
Whole Earth Catalog Founder **Stewart Brand** experienced frequent tingling and burning in his extremities. Stewart took a popular formula named *Juvenon*, created by **Bruce Ames** (main ingredients: **ALA + acetyl-L-carnitine**) for several months, noting better stamina and less "foot buzzing" that he attributed to ALA's antioxidant effect on peripheral nerves.

DOSAGE GUIDELINES AND MAXIMUM DOSAGE
Most people stick to around **300–600 mg a day**. Some medical studies go up to **1,200 mg** for certain short-term goals, like severe nerve discomfort, but that should be done under professional supervision.

DIETARY SOURCES
Small amounts of ALA appear in organ meats (liver, heart) and veggies like spinach and broccoli. However, it's tough to get enough from food alone to reach therapeutic levels.

WITH OR WITHOUT FOOD?
Some doctors suggest taking ALA on an empty stomach to avoid competing with other nutrients. Others say if it irritates your stomach, you can take it with a small meal. Either way, you'll likely still absorb it well because ALA can work in both water and fat.

POSSIBLE SIDE EFFECTS AT HIGHER DOSES

ALA is generally safe. At higher doses, a few people might get heartburn, a rash, or mild nausea. If you have diabetes or hypoglycemia, you'll want to watch your blood sugar levels closely, because ALA might lower them further.

Whatever you can do to avoid diabetes or to lessen the effects will help you hugely, and alpha-lipoic acid could be part of that regimen. My friend, legendary actress **Mary Tyler Moore,** struggled with diabetes, causing terrible physical problems that plagued her in later life. She said:

"My peripheral vision has been severely limited because of my diabetes, which means I can see just fine looking straight ahead. But if I am at a function with lots of people, I am constantly bumping into people — even kicking them!"

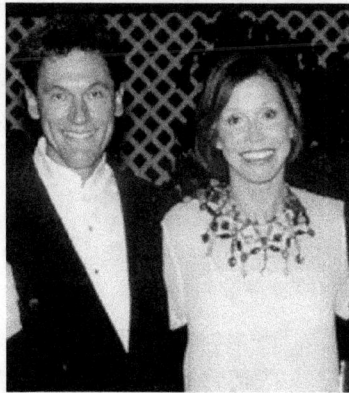

Tad Sisler with Mary Tyler Moore
Credit – Sisler Private Collection

5.1.3: PQQ (Pyrroloquinoline Quinone)
BUILDING NEW "POWER PLANTS" IN YOUR CELLS

Picture your cells as little cities that have special "buildings" (mitochondria) where energy is made. PQQ is like a construction crew that helps maintain and even build new mitochondria, potentially giving your body more energy capacity over time.

Energy Support: With healthier, stronger mitochondria, your cells can often produce more energy, which might help you feel more alert or active.

Brain Health: Early research hints that PQQ could help with focus or reduce "brain fog," possibly because of its antioxidant effect and support for nerve cells.

DOSAGES ARE STILL BEING RESEARCHED

Most supplements recommend **10–20 mg a day**, sometimes up to 40 mg in specific studies. There isn't a hard-and-fast "max dose" agreed upon yet, so if you go higher, do it with medical guidance.

OFTEN COMBINED WITH CoQ10 IN "MITOCHONDRIAL SUPPORT" FORMULAS

PQQ is often bundled with CoQ10 in a "mitochondrial support" formula. The idea is that CoQ10 helps each mitochondrion work well, while PQQ helps create more mitochondria. The synergy could mean better overall energy production.

SOLUBILITY: PQQ is generally **water-soluble**, meaning it dissolves in water-based environments. Many supplements come as capsules or tablets that can be taken with or without food.

OVERDOSE POTENTIAL: PQQ is typically well-tolerated. Some people report mild stomach upset or headaches if they exceed recommended amounts. If you take prescription meds, talk to a healthcare pro first.

DIETARY SOURCES: PQQ is naturally found in small amounts in foods like **kiwi, green peppers, and fermented soybeans**, although dietary levels are typically relatively low. Individuals looking to support overall energy levels, cognitive function, or healthy aging strategies may consider PQQ as part of a broader supplement regimen.

Whatever we can do to enhance brain health will have a profound effect on our lives, and PQQ may be a tool in that arsenal. **Deepak Chopra** said:

"Our minds influence the key activity of the brain, which then influences everything; perception, cognition, thoughts and feelings, personal relationships; they're all a projection of you."

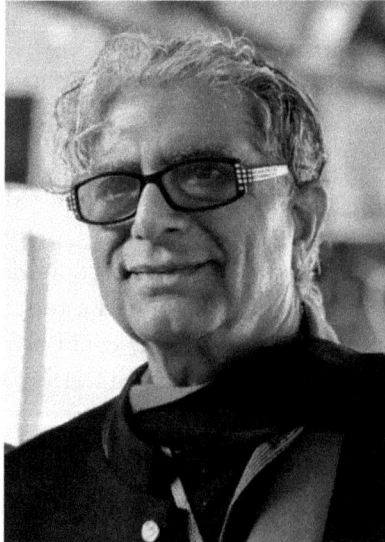

Deepak Chopra
Credit – Gage Skidmore/Wikimedia Commons

5.1.4: BETA-GLUCANS

Imagine your immune system as castle guards protecting you from germs. Beta-glucans (found in oats, barley, mushrooms) are like special training sessions that help those guards recognize invaders more quickly. They can also form a gel in your digestive tract that helps lower cholesterol.

TWO MAJOR TYPES

Mushroom-based: Found in shiitake, maitake, or reishi mushrooms. Often linked to better immune response.

Oat/barley-based: Linked to cholesterol-lowering benefits and better heart health.

RECOMMENDED DOSAGES

For Cholesterol: About 3 grams of oat beta-glucan daily (that's roughly 1½ cups of cooked oatmeal).

For Immune Support: 250–500 mg of mushroom beta-glucan extract; some people go as high as 1,000 mg.

DIETARY SOURCES

Mushrooms: Shiitake, Maitake, and Reishi mushrooms are particularly rich in beta-1,3/1,6-glucans, often linked to immune benefits.

Oats and Barley: Contain beta-1,3/1,4-glucans, best known for cholesterol-lowering effects.

Baker's Yeast: Beta-glucan extracted from yeast is also used in many immune-support supplements.

Eating oatmeal, barley, or mushrooms is a great start. But for bigger effects—like wanting to significantly lower LDL cholesterol or seriously boost immunity—some folks take concentrated beta-glucan supplements.

DEMI LOVATO

Award-winning singer **Demi Lovato** keeps Now Alchemy's "Limitless Mushrooms" tincture on her supplement shelf. The formula supplies a multi-mushroom blend (chaga, turkey tail, lion's mane, shiitake, etc.) that the company highlights as "high in beta-glucans." In a video on the brand's site, **Demi** explains that she's been taking the tincture for several months because it *"helps me stay healthy,"* crediting it with fewer sick-days and better overall vitality. **Demi** wants to be a healthy role model for her fans:

"I feel like I'm held more accountable to stay healthy now because now I'm a role model to young girls to not have eating issues and to not say, 'Hey, it's OK to starve yourself' or 'It's OK to throw up after your meals' - that's not OK." – Demi Lovato

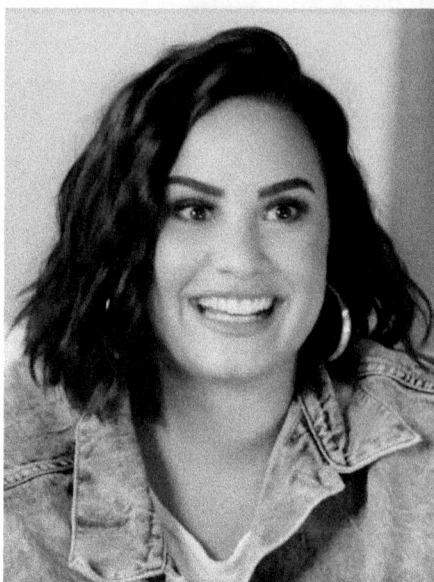

Demi Lovato
Credit – Wikimedia Commons

SOLUBILITY AND BEST PRACTICES
Water-Soluble Fiber: Beta-glucans from oats and barley are water-soluble, forming a gel-like substance in the intestine.
Mushroom Beta-Glucans: Also soluble, though their absorption pattern focuses more on immune cell activation via gut-associated lymphoid tissue.
COMBINING WITH OTHER SUPPLEMENTS
It's common to see beta-glucans combined with other nutritional compounds in "immune support" or "wellness" formulas. Potential synergists include:
Vitamin C and Zinc: Common immune-boosting duo that may complement beta-glucans' immune-modulating effects.
Probiotics: Since beta-glucans can support gut health, pairing them with probiotics may enhance digestive and immune benefits.

SAFETY AND OVERDOSE POTENTIAL
Beta-glucans are generally safe. If you suddenly eat a lot more fiber, you might feel bloated or gassy at first. Gradually increase your intake, and you'll likely adapt just fine.

"The most common objection that I hear to walking as exercise is that it's too easy, that only sweaty, strenuous activity offers real benefits. But there is abundant evidence that regular, brisk walking is associated with better health, including lower blood pressure, better moods and improved cholesterol rates."

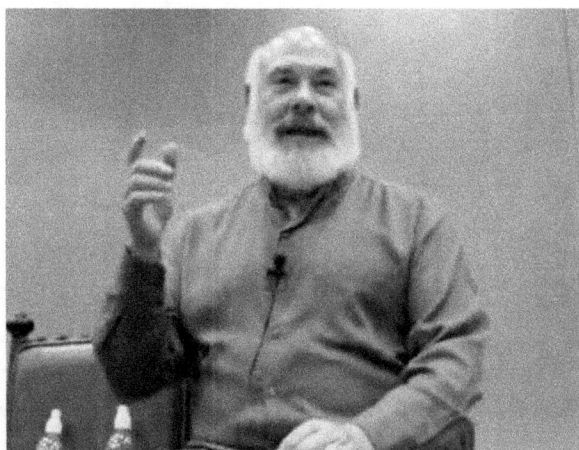

Andrew Weil
Credit – Creative Commons Attribution 3.0 License -
https://commons.wikimedia.org/wiki/File:Andrew_Weil_01.jpg

5.1.5: CANNABINOIDS (CBD)

Cannabinoids, like CBD from hemp, act as messengers that help maintain balance in your body (mood, sleep, pain, and more). Unlike THC (which can cause a "high"), CBD usually helps people relax or manage discomfort without intoxication.

COMMON BENEFITS

Stress & Anxiety Relief: May help you feel calmer and sleep better.
Pain & Inflammation: Some folks say it eases aching joints or muscle soreness.
Sleep Support: A portion of users report deeper rest or fewer night-time awakenings.

DOSAGES ARE STILL BEING RESEARCHED; TYPICAL RANGE

There's no one-size-fits-all:
Mild Stress: 10–30 mg/day
Higher Needs (pain/anxiety): 30–50 mg/day or more
Research doses: Sometimes up to 300–600 mg/day, but that's usually under clinical study conditions.

SOLUBILITY

CBD is **fat-soluble**, so taking it with a meal containing healthy fats can help your body absorb it better. You'll often see it as an oil-based tincture or in capsules. Some formulas add melatonin for sleep or turmeric for inflammation support.

SAFETY

CBD usually isn't linked with any major side effects at moderate doses. A high dose might make you drowsy, alter your appetite, or cause stomach upset. If you're on blood thinners or other meds, check with your doctor because CBD can interact with certain prescriptions.

DIFFERENCE BETWEEN CBD AND THC

CBD and THC are two primary cannabinoids derived from the cannabis plant with different effects:

CBD (Cannabidiol) is non-intoxicating and may support mood balance, stress management, pain modulation, and overall relaxation.

Legal status varies, but hemp-derived CBD (with less than 0.3% THC) is widely available.

THC (Tetrahydrocannabinol): Psychoactive—produces the "high" associated with marijuana. Potential **benefits** include pain relief, appetite stimulation, nausea reduction (e.g., in chemotherapy patients), and sleep support.

Health risks may include impaired judgment, anxiety or paranoia (especially at higher doses), and potential dependency or abuse with prolonged, heavy use. Legal status and regulations vary by region.

THC OVERDOSE POTENTIAL

While there is no documented case of a fatal THC overdose in humans, taking too much can lead to severe adverse effects commonly referred to as "green out." These include intense anxiety, paranoia, rapid heart rate, and, in some cases, hallucinations or disorientation. Such experiences, while extremely uncomfortable, are typically not life-threatening and tend to resolve as the THC metabolizes and wears off. However, chronic heavy use or excessively high doses can carry additional risks, especially in individuals with underlying mental health conditions. Consequently, moderation and responsible consumption are advised.

ADDITIONAL MAJOR POINTS : **Quality and Purity**: Look for **third-party lab testing** to ensure CBD products are free from contaminants (e.g., pesticides, heavy metals) and contain the advertised amount of CBD.

I do not personally recommend marijuana or THC for regular use, mainly because I've had this experience, and I believe that, in addition to the health risks, it slows you down from realizing your full potential as a human. I did not like what it did for my own general health, either. But I understand the allure, and I know many people who have used it medicinally successfully.

"Marijuana has many useful uses. I have fibromyalgia pain in this arm, and the only thing that offers any relief is marijuana." – Morgan Freeman

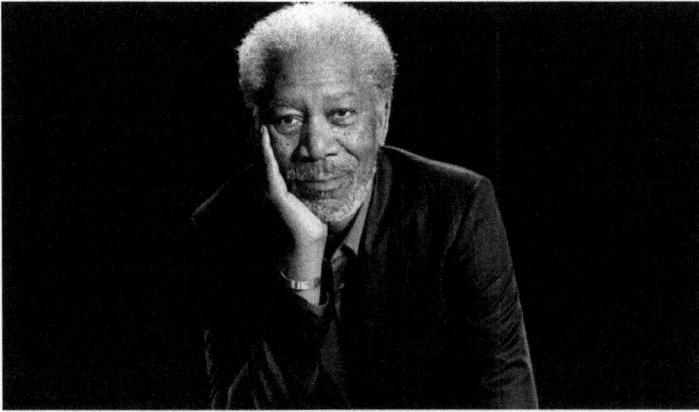

Morgan Freeman
Credit – Hdwallpapers.net/ https://creativecommons.org/licenses/by-sa/3.0/

5.1.6: PHOSPHATIDYLSERINE

Picture your brain like a classroom where the students (brain cells) need to share information. Phosphatidylserine (PS) helps keep that communication strong so things don't get chaotic. Studies suggest it may support memory, mental clarity, and even your ability to cope with stress.

SUPPORTS BRAIN FUNCTION

Brain Membrane Health: Your brain cells rely on healthy membranes to send signals correctly. PS helps keep these membranes flexible and functional.

Stress & Cortisol: Some research shows PS may help regulate cortisol, the "stress hormone." That can mean feeling calmer under pressure.

COMBINED WITH OTHER SUPPLEMENTS IN FORMULAS

Phosphatidylserine is frequently included in **nootropic ("brain-boosting") blends**, often combined with:

Omega-3 fatty acids (especially DHA): May enhance brain membrane fluidity and overall cognitive support.

Ginkgo biloba: Used in some formulas to improve blood flow to the brain and memory.

B-complex vitamins: Certain B vitamins (like B6, B9, and B12) support neurotransmitter synthesis, potentially amplifying PS's benefits.

JOE ROGAN

Comedian, UFC Commentator, and podcaster **Joe Rogan** has to remember hundreds of stats on live TV and during his podcasts, but he started noticing tip-of-the-tongue moments. He helped create **Onnit's "Alpha Brain,"** a nootropic that supplies about **100 mg of phosphatidylserine per serving**. Joe says he takes it before stand-up sets and fight nights; within a month he felt **"one step ahead,"** with words coming to him more smoothly.

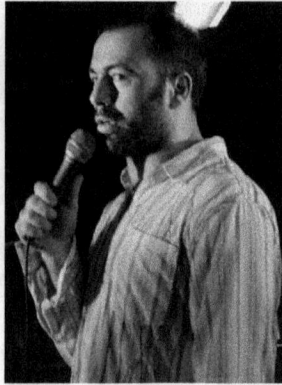

Joe Rogan
Credit – Wikimedia Commons

DOSAGES ARE STILL BEING RESEARCHED; TYPICAL RANGE

Many people take **100–300 mg** daily, sometimes split across two or three doses. For significant memory or focus issues, some go up to **400–600 mg** (short term, under a doctor's advice).

DIETARY SOURCES

Phosphatidylserine is found naturally in certain foods, though often in relatively **small amounts: Organ meats**, such as liver • **Fish**, particularly oily varieties like mackerel and herring • **White beans** and **soybeans** (plant-based sources) Given that typical diets may not provide substantial PS, many people interested in its cognitive benefits opt for supplements to reach higher doses.

SOLUBILITY AND BEST PRACTICES

Fat-Soluble: As a phospholipid, PS is more easily absorbed when ingested with a meal containing **healthy fats** (e.g., avocado, nuts, fish oil).
Timing: Some individuals prefer taking PS in the morning or early afternoon to support daytime cognition, while others may find it helpful later in the day to assist with stress regulation.

SAFETY AND OVERDOSE POTENTIAL

PS is usually safe, though more than 400 mg a day might cause mild digestive upset or difficulty sleeping. It's also good to remember changes in cognition often take several weeks to become noticeable.

There's no ceiling to how far you can go if you utilize your precious brain power. My dear friend **Jack Kemp** was a championship-winning *NFL* quarterback who became a **Congressman, Secretary of Housing and Urban Development,** and **Vice-Presidential** candidate. He was an outstanding human being, full of compassion and great ideas, a perfect example of a man who used his brain to the fullest. His advice and wisdom helped me realize I had no limitations in my journey to an extraordinary life. **Jack** said:

"There are no limits to our future if we don't put limits on our people."

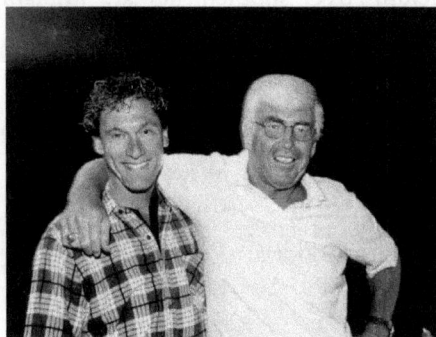

Tad Sisler with Secretary Jack Kemp
Source – Sisler Private Collection

5.1.7: EMERGING LONGEVITY COMPOUNDS

Certain compounds are gaining attention for their potential to extend healthy lifespan by supporting cellular health. Spermidine, urolithin A, and alpha-ketoglutarate (AKG) are among the most promising, backed by 2025 research. These nutrients may enhance longevity by promoting autophagy, improving mitochondrial function, and reducing inflammation. Consult a healthcare provider before use, as human studies are still emerging.

Spermidine: A polyamine found in wheat germ, soybeans, and aged cheese, spermidine promotes autophagy, a cellular process that clears damaged components. Animal studies show it extends lifespan and improves heart health, while a 2018 human study of 829 participants linked higher dietary intake to reduced all-cause mortality (HR 0.74, 95% CI: 0.66–0.83) (*American Journal of Clinical Nutrition*). A 2025 cohort study of 1,770 subjects aged 39–67 further supports reduced mortality (*Endocrine Abstracts*). Supplements like spermidineLIFE are available, but more human trials are needed.

Urolithin A: Produced by gut bacteria from ellagic acid in pomegranates, berries, and nuts, urolithin A enhances mitochondrial function through mitophagy. A 2024 systematic review of five human studies (250 participants) found that doses of 10–1000 mg/day for 28 days to 4 months improved muscle strength and reduced inflammation, with ongoing research into longevity benefits (*ScienceDirect*). Products like Mitopure offer urolithin A, but efficacy varies by individual gut microbiome.

Alpha-Ketoglutarate (AKG): A key metabolite in the tricarboxylic acid (TCA) cycle, AKG supports energy metabolism and reduces inflammation. A 2020 mouse study showed calcium-AKG extended lifespan and reduced frailty by lowering inflammatory cytokines (PubMed). A 2023 review highlights its role in epigenetic regulation and stem cell health, with human studies still limited (*ScienceDirect*). Calcium-AKG supplements are available, but professional guidance is advised.

QUICK REFERENCE TABLE

Compound	Key Benefits	Sources	Research Status
Spermidine	Promotes autophagy, heart health	Wheat germ, soybeans, cheese	Human studies ongoing
Urolithin A	Enhances mitochondria, muscle	Pomegranates, berries, nuts	Early human trials
AKG	Boosts energy, reduces inflammation	Supplements (calcium-AKG)	Limited human data

SECTION TWO: RESVERATROL, QUERCETIN, TRANS-PTEROSTILBENE, AND OTHER POLYPHENOLS

5.2.1: RESVERATROL

"Resveratrol does not act primarily as an antioxidant. It is far more interesting and powerful than that. Resveratrol turns on our body's genetic defenses against diseases and aging itself."
– Dr. David Andrew Sinclair

TINY BODYGUARDS FROM GRAPES AND BERRIES

Resveratrol is often called a "longevity molecule." It's found in red wine, grapes, and certain berries. Some scientists say it might activate "sirtuin" genes linked to healthy aging.

POTENTIAL PERKS

Heart and Metabolic Support: May help lower inflammation or support healthier blood vessels. One known safety consideration is that resveratrol can **influence platelet function** and may have a mild **blood-thinning** effect. Individuals taking anticoagulant or antiplatelet medications (e.g., warfarin or aspirin) should consult a healthcare provider before adding high-dose resveratrol. At typical supplement doses, side effects are usually minimal but can include mild gastrointestinal upset.

Animal Studies: In certain animal experiments, high doses extended lifespan. Human studies are less clear but still promising.

THE FRENCH PARADOX

Despite a diet rich in saturated fats—think buttery croissants and rich cheeses—the French historically demonstrated lower heart disease rates than other Western nations. This phenomenon, termed the 'French Paradox,' has been partially attributed to the fact that the French consume red wine regularly, containing resveratrol. While it's likely that other factors like overall lifestyle and portion sizes also play a role, this observation sparked global interest in resveratrol's potential heart-protective properties.

SUGGESTED DAILY DOSAGE AND MAXIMUM DOSAGE

100–250 mg daily for general well-being. Some protocols use higher doses (500–1,000 mg), but going high might require medical supervision because resveratrol can thin the blood a bit.

SOLUBILITY

Absorption: Better if taken with a little fat and sometimes with piperine (black pepper extract) to boost uptake.
If on blood thinners: Talk to your doctor first.

SYNERGY WITH OTHER SUBSTANCES

Quercetin and Pterostilbene: Often combined in "longevity" or "anti-aging" formulas for a more comprehensive polyphenol profile.
Omega-3 Fatty Acids: Pairing resveratrol with healthy fats might help with absorption and provide complementary cardiovascular benefits.
Quality and Purity: Always look for reputable brands that offer **third-party testing** to ensure the supplement is free from contaminants and accurately labeled. While resveratrol may offer certain health perks, it's not a substitute for foundational habits like a balanced diet, moderate exercise, and adequate sleep.

"Resveratrol had a decent benefit when the mice were obese and sedentary. The mice that were fed a lean diet and resveratrol lived significantly longer than other treated mice as well as those that had no healthy diet and no resveratrol. So resveratrol is not an excuse to be lazy or eat whatever you want." – Dr. David Andrew Sinclair

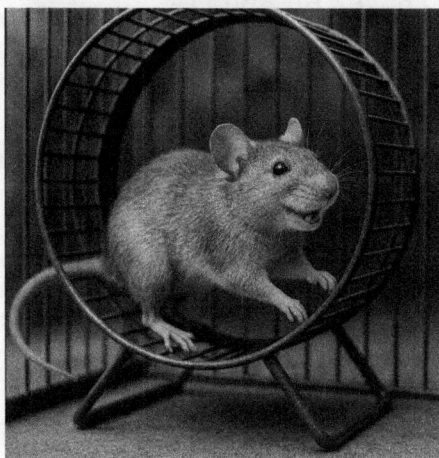

5.2.2: QUERCETIN, TRANS-PTEROSTILBENE, AND FISETIN
Cleaning Up the Junk and Protecting Cells

QUERCETIN

Think of quercetin (found in apples, onions, and red wine) like a street-cleaning crew. It sweeps away damaging particles, may reduce allergy symptoms, and has potential "senolytic" effects (helping the body clear out worn-out cells).

DIETARY SOURCES
Fruits & Vegetables: Apples, berries, grapes, citrus fruits, and leafy greens.
Other Foods: Onions, capers, and red wine.

SOLUBILITY AND BIOAVAILABILITY
Solubility: Quercetin is primarily water-soluble, but its absorption is somewhat limited.
Improving Absorption: Liposomal formulations or phytosome complexes have been developed to enhance bioavailability.

SYNERGY WITH OTHER SUBSTANCES: Taking quercetin alongside vitamin C can boost its antioxidant effects and improve overall absorption.

TRANS-PTEROLTILBENE

This is like resveratrol's close cousin, commonly found in blueberries. It's more easily absorbed than resveratrol, offering antioxidant and potential anti-inflammatory benefits for heart and brain health.

DIETARY SOURCES
Fruits: Blueberries (its primary natural source) and grapes.
Other Sources: It is less common in the typical diet, so supplementation is often recommended.

SOLUBILITY AND BIOAVAILABILITY
Solubility: Trans-Pterostilbene is fat-soluble, meaning its absorption is enhanced when taken with dietary fats.
Consuming it with a meal containing healthy fats (such as avocado or olive oil) can improve bioavailability.

FISETIN

Fisetin (from strawberries, apples, cucumbers) is emerging as another "senolytic" compound. By encouraging the removal of old or damaged cells, fisetin might help lower inflammation and support healthier aging overall.

DIETARY SOURCES
Fruits: Strawberries, apples, and persimmons.
Vegetables: Onions and cucumbers.

Other Sources: Certain teas also provide smaller amounts of fisetin.

SOLUBILITY AND BIOAVAILABILITY
Solubility: Fisetin is generally water-soluble.
Improving Absorption: Like quercetin, using enhanced formulations or combining with vitamin C may improve its uptake and efficacy.

BRYAN JOHNSON
Bryan Johnson is the tech guy who turned himself into a science project. **Bryan** made a fortune selling his company to PayPal, but at 45 he worried that bad joints and heart problems might run in his family. So he hired a team of doctors and scientists and began what he calls **"Blueprint."** Every day he swallows more than 100 pills, one of which is **200 mg of fisetin,** a plant compound scientists think may clear out "zombie" (senescent) cells.

After a year of blood tests and body scans, **Bryan** reported that his inflammation numbers went down and some doctors said his body now looks a few years younger than his birth certificate. He admits the plan is extreme, but it shows how targeted polyphenols can fit into a doctor-guided program.

"The discovery that we can program our existence and author our own lives has radically altered my life - transforming my identity, aspirations, and reason for existence." – Bryan Johnson

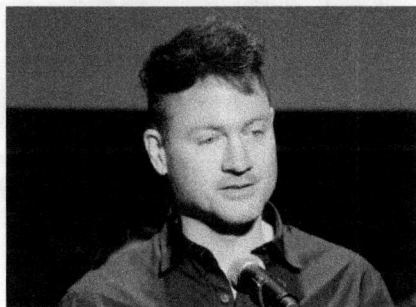

Bryan Johnson
Credit – Wikimedia Commons

DOSAGE AND SAFETY
Quercetin: Often 500–1,000 mg daily
Trans-Pterostilbene: Around 50–150 mg daily (some go higher)
Fisetin: 20–100 mg daily (human studies are ongoing, so these are rough guidelines)

They're typically considered safe at moderate doses. Excessive amounts could cause upset stomach or headaches. Taking quercetin with vitamin C can help your body use it more effectively. For pterostilbene, consuming it with healthy fats (like olive oil) might aid absorption.

In writing this book, I reread it several times for cohesion. I realized that it could be read in a linear sense, or it could be used as a reference for those who are passionate about gaining as much knowledge as possible about individual nutritional supplements and general health. Passion is a great driver for all of us. My friend **Bill Medley** was a *multi-platinum* recording artist with the #1 most played song of the 20th century on American Radio with his smash hit *"You've Lost That Lovin' Feelin,"* along with **Bobby Hatfield** as the **Righteous Brothers. Bill** said:

"Passion: It's what separates a singer from an entertainer. I hope I have passion for my music, my family, and my friends until they start shoveling dirt on my face."

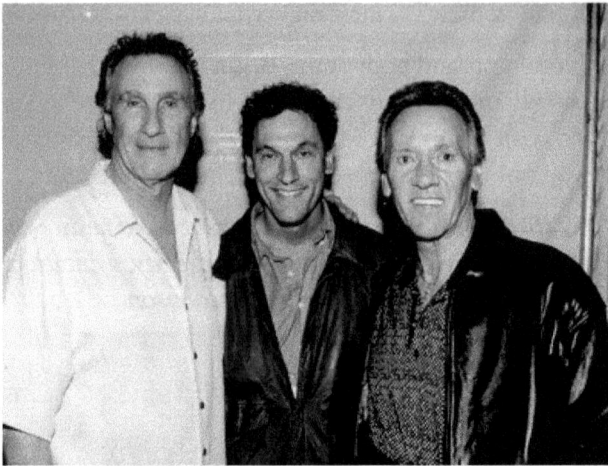

Tad Sisler With the Righteous Brothers
Source – Sisler Private Collection

5.2.3: COMBINING POLYPHENOLS EFFECTIVELY

Pairing polyphenols (like resveratrol and quercetin) can boost how well your body absorbs and uses them. Sometimes, adding other compounds (like glucosamine for joints) or essential fatty acids can give you even more benefits.

AVOID OVER-SUPPLEMENTATION

More isn't always better. A "balanced" dose can help the body's natural stress-response systems function well. If you pile on too many polyphenols, you might reduce your body's own protective responses.

QUALITY MATTERS

Look for reputable brands that test for purity. Low-quality supplements might not even contain the amounts they promise. Whole foods—like blueberries or red grapes—naturally have a mix of nutrients that work together, so don't forget to include them in your diet.

RAY KURZWEIL

Futurist and Inventor **Ray Kurzweil** developed an excellent piano keyboard which I used on my gigs for many years. **Ray** lost his dad to a heart attack at 58. This was a wake-up call for him, so he started a doctor-supervised supplement stack built around Resveratrol 100 mg & Quercetin 500 mg for artery health; **Ray** began publishing his blood-vessel scores and they vastly improved. He also has written books on longevity and age-reversal research, pointing to a future where we can revitalize our bodies on every level.

"Biology is a software process. Our bodies are made up of trillions of cells, each governed by this process. You and I are walking around with outdated software running in our bodies, which evolved in a very different era." -Ray Kurzweil

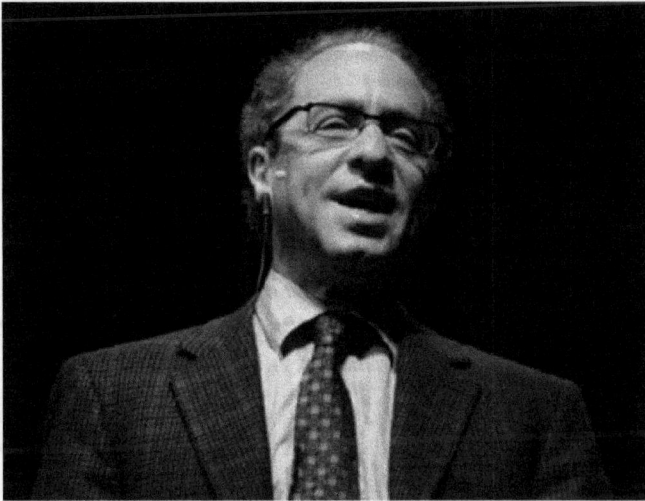

Ray Kurzweil
Credit – Wikimedia Commons

5.2.4: STRUCTURAL SUPPORT COMPOUNDS FOR JOINT AND SKIN HEALTH

HYALURONIC ACID

Think of hyaluronic acid as your body's internal lotion. It helps lubricate joints and keeps skin looking plump. People commonly take **100–200 mg** per day, sometimes more for bigger skin or joint concerns.

DIETARY SOURCES: Bone broth and animal tissues contain hyaluronic acid, although supplementation is often necessary for therapeutic benefits.

SYNERGY WITH OTHER SUBSTANCES: Combining hyaluronic acid with antioxidants and collagen-supporting nutrients (such as vitamin C) can often promote skin elasticity and joint health.

GLUCOSAMINE AND CHONDROITIN

If your cartilage is like a cushion between bones, glucosamine and chondroitin act like a repair team. They help maintain that cushion, so your joints can move smoothly. Typical doses:

Glucosamine: 1,500 mg daily

Chondroitin: 800–1,200 mg daily

Both are widely used to support people with osteoarthritis or those who feel joint stiffness. They're often paired with omega-3 fatty acids to help reduce inflammation.

DIETARY SOURCES: These compounds are naturally found in shellfish (for glucosamine) and animal cartilage, though effective dosages are typically not achieved through diet alone.

SOLUBILITY: Both compounds are water-soluble; eating them can enhance absorption and minimize digestive discomfort.

SYNERGY WITH OTHER SUBSTANCES: Combining these joint-support compounds with anti-inflammatory polyphenols or omega-3 fatty acids can offer synergistic effects, helping to reduce joint inflammation and improve overall mobility. Time can have debilitating effects on your joints. Supplementing may help your body to avoid pain and deterioration. Even television's famous *"Six-Million-Dollar-Man"* **Lee Majors** had trouble (which is ironic, considering that the show was based upon a man whose body parts were replaced by artificial parts!). **Majors** said:

"I figured my body always would be able to repair itself. I think all of us believe that — until you begin to age and get hit with deteriorating joints."

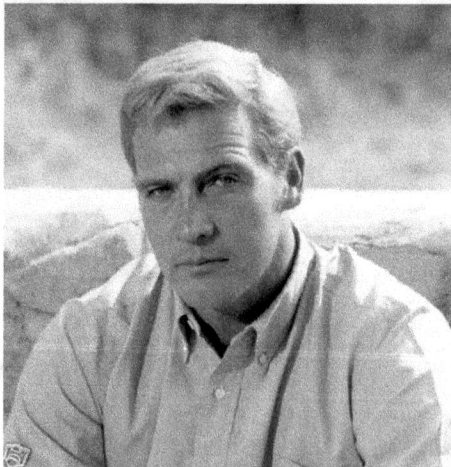

Lee Majors
Credit – Flickr/cowgirl196577/creativecommons.org

SECTION THREE
NOOTROPICS AND COGNITIVE ENHANCERS

5.3.1: N-ACETYL CYSTEINE (NAC), SAM-e, L-THEANINE, AND ACETYL L-CARNITINE (ALCAR)
Brain & Body Boosters for Mood, Calm, and Energy

N-ACETYL CYSTEINE (NAC)

NAC is like a special cleanup crew for your cells. It helps the body produce glutathione, a major antioxidant that tackles toxins and protects organs. People usually take **600–1,200 mg** per day (sometimes more, under guidance). It can slightly upset your stomach if you jump in at a high dose right away.

SAM-e

SAM-e is critical for mood, joint health, and helping your body with "methylation," a process that affects everything from brain chemicals to detox. Typical doses range from **400–1,600 mg**. It can interact with antidepressants, so be cautious if you're on those.

L-THEANINE

L-Theanine, found in green tea, helps you relax without making you drowsy. Many people take **100–200 mg** to mellow out. It's famous for pairing with caffeine to create a "calm focus" (less jittery than caffeine alone).

TIM FERRISS

Author Tim Ferriss wrote *The 4-Hour Workweek* and loves testing weird ideas on himself. When long writing days made him shaky from too much coffee, he tried adding **about 200 mg of L-theanine to his brew**. The theanine calmed the "coffee nerves," so he could type for hours feeling alert **and** relaxed—so much so that Tim still recommends the combo to fans who want energy "without the crash."

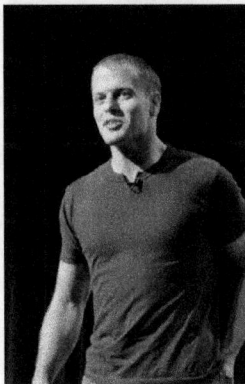

Tim Ferriss
Credit – Wikimedia Commons

ACETYL L-CARNITINE (ALCAR)

Acetyl L-Carnitine helps shuttle fatty acids into your cell's power plants, increasing energy output. That can translate into clearer thinking and possibly better workout endurance. People take **500–2,000 mg**. It's often paired with alpha-lipoic acid (ALA) for a 1-2 punch on energy and antioxidant support.

Many alternatives exist besides caffeine and nicotine to help us to be alert and present with positive energy. Olympic track star **Ashton Eaton** said:

"You're just constantly battling this thing that is telling you, 'I don't think I can do it.' I think we all have it. When you're fresh and alert, you can easily put those doubts down. But when you're tired, they easily come up to the surface."

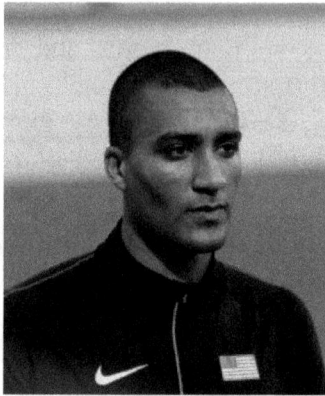

Ashton Eaton
Credit – Wikimedia Commons

It's as much a mental exercise as a physical challenge to stay alert and present. If you stay focused on the prize, you'll be just fine.

5.3.2: CHOLINE COMPOUNDS: PHOSPHATIDYLCHOLINE, alpha-GPC
BOOSTING BRAIN SIGNALS

Choline is necessary for making acetylcholine, a key neurotransmitter for learning and memory.

PHOSPHATIDYLCHOLINE: Often derived from soy or eggs, helps build healthy cell membranes (especially in the brain and liver).

ALPHA-GPC: A highly absorbable choline source that crosses the blood-brain barrier quickly, potentially improving focus and mental clarity.

SUGGESTED DAILY DOSAGE AND MAXIMUM DOSAGE
Phosphatidylcholine: 1,200–1,800 mg daily
Alpha-GPC: 300–600 mg daily

SOLUBILITY:

Phosphatidylcholine: It is amphiphilic (both water- and fat-soluble), which means it can integrate well with cell membranes and be absorbed effectively when taken with fats.

Alpha-GPC: Water-soluble, making it easy for the body to absorb and transport in the bloodstream.

SYNERGY AND COMPLEMENTARY SUBSTANCES:

Both compounds work well with omega-3 fatty acids and antioxidants, further supporting brain health and cellular integrity. They may also be used with B-vitamins to optimize energy metabolism and cognitive performance.

DRUG INTERACTIONS:
It's important to check for interactions—SAM-e and other compounds that affect neurotransmitter levels, for example, should be used cautiously. Some cholinergic or cholinesterase inhibitors might interact with these choline compounds.

DR. ANDREW HUBERMAN

As a brain scientist at *Stanford*, **Dr. Huberman** has to read piles of research papers. **Huberman** intimated that he first swallows **300 mg of alpha-GPC with an espresso**. He says it switches his mind into "laser-focus mode" for four to six hours. On his podcast Q&As he also explains how **phosphatidylcholine keeps brain-cell membranes healthy and boosts acetylcholine, the memory chemical**—so he adds PC on heavy workdays. **Huberman** jokes that the combo feels like "new RAM" for his brain, letting him teach class without mental fog.

Whatever we can do to increase our brain power should benefit us greatly.

"Brain power improves by brain use, just as our bodily strength grows with exercise. And there is no doubt that a large proportion of the female population, from school days to late middle age, now have very complicated lives indeed." – A. N. Wilson

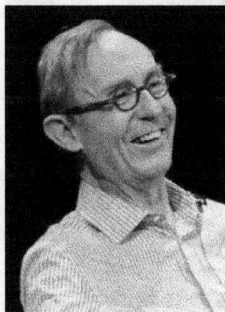

A.N. Wilson
Credit – Wikimedia Commons

OVERDOSE POTENTIAL

Both phosphatidylcholine and alpha-GPC are generally safe when taken within recommended dosages, but taking excessive amounts could lead to mild gastrointestinal upset or other minor side effects.

5.3.3: ATHLETIC PERFORMANCE COMPOUNDS: BETA-ALANINE AND CREATINE

Great things happen in our lives by chance or by design. We work out and build our bodies to peak performance through design, and then we discover new elements of ourselves through chance or serendipity in the process. Nobody understood that more than my friend, *multi-platinum* artist **Sergio Mendes**, an icon of Latin popular music.

There's a word in the English language that I like, "Serendipity"; it's the story of my life." – Sergio Mendes

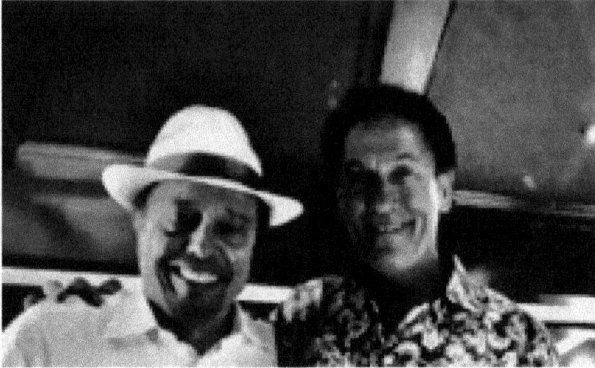

Sergio Mendes and Tad Sisler
Source – Sisler Private Collection

BETA-ALANINE

Think of your muscles like a race car engine that overheats with intense exercise. Beta-alanine increases carnosine in muscles, which helps control acid build-up so you can train a bit longer. Doses range from **3–6 grams** a day. Some people get a harmless tingling sensation known as "paresthesia," which can be reduced by splitting up the doses.

BIOAVAILABILITY: Beta-alanine is water-soluble and is typically absorbed through the digestive tract. It can be taken on an empty stomach or with a meal, although some athletes prefer to combine it with carbohydrates to enhance absorption.

DIETARY SOURCES: Beta-alanine is not abundant in most foods. However, it is present in small amounts in meat and poultry. Because the nutritional levels are low, supplementation is a popular option for athletes.

SYNERGY WITH OTHER SUBSTANCES:

Beta-alanine works well with creatine (discussed below) to support endurance and power. It may also be paired with carbohydrates to optimize absorption and reduce side effects like tingling.

DRUG INTERACTIONS AND OVERDOSE POTENTIAL:

While beta-alanine is generally safe, it is important to check for interactions if you are taking other supplements or medications. Over-supplementation can lead to temporary skin tingling, but it is not typically dangerous.

CREATINE

Creatine is like a fast charger for your muscles, boosting short, explosive movements—such as sprints or heavy lifting. A common schedule is to "load" with **20 grams per day** (split into 4 doses) for 5–7 days, then maintain with **3–5 grams daily**.

BIOAVAILABILITY: Creatine is water-soluble and is absorbed efficiently in the small intestine. It is often taken in powder form mixed with water or a sports drink, which helps it dissolve well.

DIETARY SOURCES: Creatine can be found in red meat and seafood, though the amounts in food are usually lower than those used for supplementation. Athletes often choose creatine supplements to meet their higher energy demands.

SYNERGY WITH OTHER SUBSTANCES:

Creatine can be taken with carbohydrates or protein to improve muscle uptake. It is often combined with beta-alanine to support power and endurance during exercise.

DRUG INTERACTIONS AND OVERDOSE POTENTIAL:

Creatine is generally safe; however, those with kidney issues or taking certain medications should consult a healthcare professional before use. Overuse beyond the recommended dosage might cause mild gastrointestinal discomfort.

MICHAEL JOHNSON

Back in the 1990s, **Michael Johnson** was the fastest man on earth, but he still hunted for an edge before the *1996 Atlanta Olympics*. Reporters said he "swore by" **creatine powder** to reload his muscles between explosive starts out of the blocks. The result? He zoomed to two gold medals and a world record in the 200-meter dash. **Johnson** later explained that the supplement, plus lots of water and good food along with visualizing, helped him blast off without cramping.

"One of the main techniques I used was focusing on the goal and visualising myself competing in the race before the race started."
— Michael Johnson

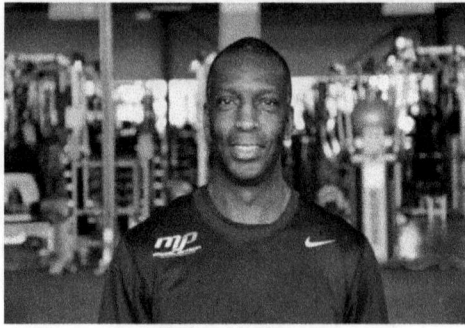

Michael Johnson
Credit – Wikimedia Commons

5.3.4: EYE HEALTH: LUTEIN AND ZEAXANTHIN

From their natural roles in filtering harmful light and fighting oxidative stress to their optimal dosages and ways to boost absorption— these compounds contribute to maintaining and enhancing eye health for a lifetime of clear, vibrant vision.

Built-In Sunglasses for Your Retina

Lutein and zeaxanthin help filter harmful blue light and support the macula, the part of your eye that gives you sharp, detailed vision. They also have antioxidant qualities to protect against age-related eye problems (like macular degeneration).

ROBERT KARLSSON

Robert Karlsson, a tall Swedish golfer on the *PGA TOUR* Champions, noticed that green slopes looked fuzzy as he got older. After testing his eyes with a special scanner, he began taking an eye vitamin that delivers about 10 mg of lutein and 10 mg of zeaxanthin each day (he swallows it with lunch so the healthy fat helps absorption).

Just three months later **Robert** told reporters, *"My test results are much better—I can read the greens and track the ball in the air way more clearly. The game is fun again!"*

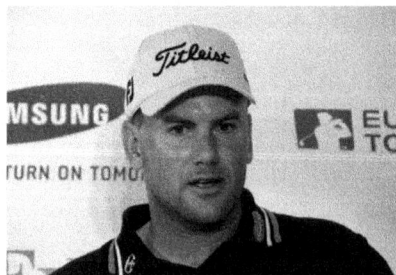

Robert Karlsson
Credit – Wikimedia Commons/Pgjansson/ https://commons.wikimedia.org/wiki/File:Robert_Karlsson.jpg

DOSAGE AND OVERDOSE POTENTIAL: Often found in supplements that combine **10 mg of lutein** with **2 mg of zeaxanthin** daily. Best absorbed with some dietary fat. Extremely high intakes might lead to harmless side effects like a slight yellowing of the skin (carotenodermia), which is rare and reversible once intake is reduced.

BIOAVALABILITY: Since lutein and zeaxanthin are fat-soluble, they require dietary fats for optimal absorption. This means that eating healthy fats—such as avocado, olive oil, or nuts—can enhance their uptake into the bloodstream. Many supplements are now formulated in oil-based carriers to boost bioavailability further, ensuring that your body can make the most of these beneficial compounds.

DIETARY SOURCES: These compounds are found naturally in a variety of foods. Lutein is abundant in dark leafy greens like spinach, kale, broccoli, and egg yolks. Zeaxanthin is found in foods like corn, orange peppers, and some leafy greens. Eating a colorful, balanced diet rich in these vegetables and fruits is one of the best ways to support eye health naturally.

SOLUBILITY WITH OTHER SUBSTANCES: Lutein and zeaxanthin are oil-soluble, so they are best taken with a fat-containing meal or in a supplement formulated with an oil base. They also work synergistically with other antioxidants such as vitamin C, E, and omega-3 fatty acids, further supporting eye health by reducing inflammation and enhancing overall cellular protection.

My father, **Maynard**, and sister, **Suzanne**, had two detached retinas in each of their eyes. My father's happened in the day when traditional surgery was required to repair the retina. My sister had one surgery traditionally, and by the time her other retina detached, she had laser surgery. So, when I was experiencing eye problems in 2016, I went immediately to an ophthalmologist who misdiagnosed me. Within months, I had a catastrophic detachment that permanently damaged one eye. A skilled surgeon saved my eye, but my eyesight will forever be distorted in one eye. He took the time to laser the other eye so that when it detached later, I could retain full vision in that eye. My uncle Ted, a wonderful man and skilled dentist, lost his eyesight in his seventies. Believe me, when you don't have your eyesight, you realize the miracle we experience every day just by being able to see. I highly recommend being good to your eyes in any way you can, including supplementation, assuming your doctor agrees.

"The reasons why images are so primal and people immediately relate to it is that we are exquisitely engineered to interpret information that is arrayed in two dimensions. That's our eyesight. That's how our eye-brain system

works. So it immediately feels to us when we look at an image like we have extended our senses." – Carolyn Porco

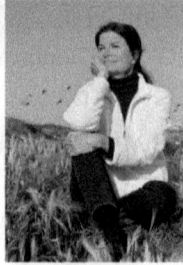

Carolyn Porco
Credit – Christopher Michel/Wikimedia Commons

5.3.5: ADAPTOGENIC NOOTROPICS: BACOPA, LION'S MANE REVISITED

Bacopa and Lion's Mane support memory, stress resilience, and nerve health, contributing to a holistic approach to cognitive enhancement and longevity.

JIM KWIK

Jim Kwik is the brain coach who trains superheroes! As a kid, Jim had a head injury that left him the "slow" student. Determined to fix it, he grew up studying how the brain learns. Today, before teaching memory tricks to movie stars, Jim drinks a smoothie that includes Lion's Mane for neuron growth and Bacopa for sharper recall. He tells audiences the combo helps him remember dozens of names at live events and keeps stage fright low because his thoughts stay clear.

BACOPA MONNIERI

Think of Bacopa as a library organizer for your brain, helping improve memory recall and easing stress. Its active components are called "bacosides." Many people take **300–450 mg** of standardized extract daily, noticing benefits in a few weeks.

CLASSIFICATION: Bacopa monnieri is an adaptogenic herb used in traditional Ayurvedic medicine for centuries. It is classified as a nootropic because of its ability to enhance cognitive function and support stress resilience.

BIOAVALABILITY: Bacopa is typically consumed in extract form. It is water-soluble and is best absorbed with a meal including some fat to aid in overall nutrient uptake.

DIETARY SOURCES: Bacopa is not commonly found in everyday foods, but it is widely available as a standardized supplement extract. Traditional forms include powders and capsules.

SYNERGY WITH OTHER SUBSTANCES: Bacopa often works well in combination with other adaptogens, such as ashwagandha or Rhodiola, and antioxidants that help protect against oxidative stress. It may also be taken with omega-3 fatty acids to support overall brain health.

LION'S MANE (Hericium erinaceus)

Lion's Mane mushroom can stimulate nerve growth factor (NGF), helping maintain and possibly regenerate nerve cells. People usually consume **500–3,000 mg** as an extract. It's often combined with other nootropics for an overall brain boost.

CLASSIFICATION: Lion's Mane is a medicinal mushroom categorized as a functional food and nootropic. It is known for its potential to support nerve regeneration and enhance cognitive function.

BIOAVAILABILITY: Lion's Mane is typically available as a water-soluble extract or powder. Taking it with food can improve absorption and reduce the chance of stomach upset.

DIETARY SOURCES: Although you can eat Lion's Mane mushrooms when fresh, most therapeutic benefits are obtained from concentrated supplements, such as extracts or powders, which provide a more consistent dose of its active compounds.

SYNERGY WITH OTHER SUBSTANCES: Lion's Mane can be combined with other nootropics or adaptogens to enhance cognitive function. It works well with compounds that reduce inflammation and oxidative stress, such as curcumin or omega-3 fatty acids, providing a holistic approach to brain health.

"Time moves in one direction, memory in another." – William Gibson

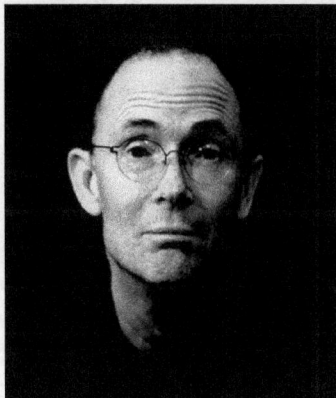

William Gibson
Credit – Fred Armitage/Wikimedia Commons

5.3.6: SAFETY AND ETHICAL CONSIDERATIONS

Before adding a bunch of nootropics or supplements, do your homework. The supplement world isn't always tightly regulated, so look for trusted brands and consider speaking with a doctor or specialist—especially if you have any medical conditions or take medications. Don't get hooked on overblown "smart drug" promises; progress often comes from a balanced approach that includes good sleep, a nutritious diet, and regular exercise.

5.3.7: LEGAL STATUS OF NOOTROPICS

Nootropics, such as NAC, SAM-e, L-theanine, ALCAR, choline compounds, beta-alanine, creatine, lutein, zeaxanthin, and adaptogenic herbs like bacopa, aim to enhance cognitive function. Their legal status varies by country and substance, impacting availability and use. Always verify local regulations and consult a healthcare provider before starting nootropics, especially if on medications.

United States: Most nootropics in this chapter (e.g., NAC, L-theanine, creatine) are classified as dietary supplements under the Dietary Supplement Health and Education Act (DSHEA), available over the counter. However, some, like modafinil (for narcolepsy), require prescriptions, and psilocybin is a Schedule I controlled substance, illegal outside research settings (Mind Lab Pro). A 2025 review notes unauthorized ingredients in some nootropic supplements, urging caution (PubMed).

European Union: Regulations are stricter, with piracetam requiring prescriptions in some countries and banned in others. Natural nootropics like L-theanine and bacopa are generally available as supplements, but synthetic compounds face tighter controls (Earth Secret).

Other Regions: In Canada, Australia, and the UK, natural nootropics are typically legal, but synthetic ones like racetams may require prescriptions or be restricted. Globally, regulations evolve, with 2025 updates tightening oversight of unapproved substances (Nootropics Expert).

Safety Tips: Purchase from reputable brands with third-party testing (e.g., USP, NSF) to avoid contaminants or unauthorized ingredients. Check labels for certifications and consult a doctor to ensure compatibility with your health needs.

NEXT UP

With these supplements and nutrients in mind, we'll move into the realm of healthy fats, oils, and essential fatty acids, which can further support your heart, brain, and overall well-being. Keeping your body balanced is like tuning a piano—you might do one thing at a time, but ultimately, you want every key to play in harmony.

Before I continue, I have a personal request for you, my reader…
PLEASE MAKE A DIFFERENCE WITH YOUR BOOK REVIEW
Unlock the Power of Kindness

"Sharing our gifts helps others shine bright."

My father's example as an exemplary healer guided my perception of medicine and health. I was lucky to have great teachers and mentors who helped me grow and pushed me to learn more about enhancing the human condition. Now, I want to help others find their own way towards health and longevity, too.

Would you help someone just like you—excited about getting on the right track but not sure where to start learning how to master health and longevity?

My mission is to educate as many people as possible about new and upcoming age reversal discoveries leading us all towards longer, healthier lives.

But to reach more people, I need your help.

Most people choose books based on reviews. So, I'm asking you to help another by leaving a review.

It doesn't cost anything and takes less than a minute, but it could change someone's journey. Your review could help…

- …one more person find their way to healthy habits.
- …one more child know there's a possibility of loving grandparents longer.
- …one more person gain confidence to adopt a new lifestyle.
- …one more dream of a better life come true.

If you purchased my book on Amazon, please go into your "Orders" section of your Amazon account and leave your review. It will mean the world to me!

If you love helping others, you're my kind of person. Thank you from the bottom of my heart! **Tad Sisler**

CHAPTER SIX

BENEFICIAL OILS AND ESSENTIAL FATTY ACIDS

Not all fats are created equal! In fact, some can be the fountain of youth for your cells – if you know which ones to choose. When most people hear the word **fat**, they picture greasy fries or a doctor's warning. But the right kinds of fat behave more like tiny repair crews and delivery trucks, carrying nutrients where they're needed and putting out the little fires of inflammation that smolder inside us every day. In this chapter we'll meet the star players—omega-3s and a few other special oils—and learn how to invite them onto our plates without turning the kitchen into a chemistry lab.

"There's a great metaphor that one of my doctors uses: If a fish is swimming in a dirty tank and it gets sick, do you take it to the vet and amputate the fin? No, you clean the water. So, I cleaned up my system. By eating organic raw greens, nuts and healthy fats, I am flooding my body with enzymes, vitamins and oxygen." – Kris Carr

SECTION ONE: OMEGA-3 POWERHOUSES

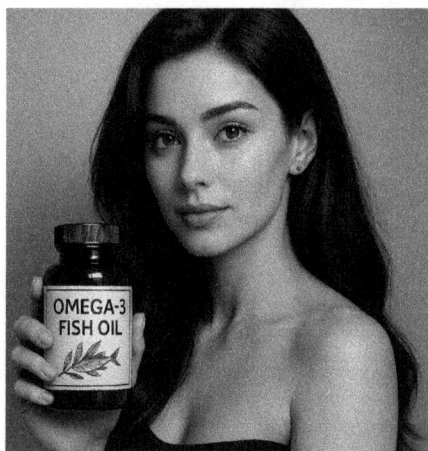

6.I.I: FISH OIL (EPA/DHA), KRILL OIL

Close your eyes and imagine millions of microscopic superheroes swimming through your blood. Their capes are labeled **EPA** and **DHA**, and they come from the oils of cold-water fish such as salmon, sardines, and mackerel. Once inside you, they calm angry tissues, keep artery walls flexible, and polish the gears in your brain so thoughts glide instead of grind.

Some people swallow these heroes in ordinary **fish-oil capsules**; others prefer **krill-oil soft-gels** harvested from shrimp-like creatures in Antarctica. Krill brings an extra bodyguard called **astaxanthin**—a red pigment that shields the fragile omega-3s from damage and may help your own cells stay strong.

DAILY GAME PLAN

• General health: 250–500 mg of combined EPA + DHA

• Heavy hitters (high triglycerides, joint flare-ups): up to 2 g, but clear it with your doctor first.

Take the capsules with a meal that contains some fat—think eggs, avocado toast, or yogurt—so the oil doesn't just float past your gut unused.

TOM BRADY

Legendary *NFL* Quarterback **Tom Brady** spent two decades dodging 300-pound linemen. To keep the swelling in his knees and elbows low, he added an **omega-3 fish-oil capsule to his daily TB12 routine** and called the fatty acids "natural anti-inflammatories." Reporters noted that he even launched his own TB12 brand of fish-oil pills for fans who wanted the same edge. **Brady** says the extra EPA & DHA, plus lots of salmon and sardines, helped him recover faster after games so he could throw perfect spirals the following week.

"You have to believe in your process. You have to believe in the things that you are doing to help the team win. I think you have to take the good with the bad." – Tom Brady

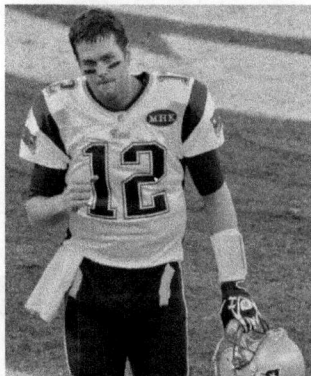

Tom Brady
Credit - Wikimedia Commons

QUALITY CONCERNS: HEAVY METAL CONTAMINATION

In my book **"Stay Healthy, Stay Youthful: The Science of Living to 150"**, I go into detail about how you can test yourself for heavy metals in your body. When using fish oil, avoid contaminants like mercury or heavy metals. Choose brands that have third-party testing or certifications (e.g., IFOS, USP) to ensure purity and quality. Reputable krill oil brands should also provide information on their testing for purity and sustainability.

DIETARY SOURCES:

Fish Oil Sources: Salmon, sardines, mackerel, anchovies (at least two servings of fatty fish per week if not supplementing).

Krill Oil Source: Antarctic krill. Since it's hard to eat krill directly, krill oil is usually taken as a supplement.

SOLUBILITY: Both fish oil and krill oil are **oil-soluble**. It's best to take them with a meal containing some healthy fat. This can help your body absorb the beneficial fats more effectively.

SYNERGY WITH OTHER SUBSTANCES: Fat-containing meals: Taking fish oil or krill oil with meals that include dietary fats helps with absorption.

Antioxidants: Pairing with antioxidant-rich foods (fruits and vegetables) can further support overall health and reduce oxidative stress.

OVERDOSE POTENTIAL: While **omega-3 overdose** is uncommon, very high doses (well above 3 grams daily) could increase the risk of bleeding or affect blood clotting. If you're on blood thinners or have a bleeding disorder, always check with a healthcare provider before taking high-dose fish or krill oil.

Storage: Keep your fish oil or krill oil supplements in a cool, dark place. Heat and light can damage the delicate oils.

Side Effects: You may experience mild stomach upset, fishy aftertaste, or burping. Enteric-coated or "burp-less" formulations can help with this.

Sustainability: Look for brands that harvest fish or krill responsibly to protect marine ecosystems.

"Omega-3 fatty acids are essential nutrients that we must get from our diets because our bodies cannot make them; they are crucial for early brain development, and there is much evidence that they promote cardiovascular health and cognitive function." – Dr. Joel Fuhrman

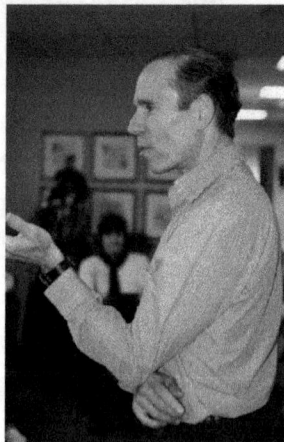

Joel Furhman
Credit - Khürt Williams / Wikipedia / creativecommons.org

6.1.2: PLANT-BASED OMEGA-3 (FLAX, ALGAL OIL)

If you're a vegetarian, I have great news for you! Whether you are vegetarian, vegan, or simply looking to add more plant-based nutrients, you can enjoy the benefits of these critical omega-3 sources for better heart, brain, and overall health.

My old friend **Herb Jeffries** was the first African-American singing cowboy movie star in the 1930s. He had an amazing musical career in the 1940s and 1950s, with huge hits like *"Flamingo"* with **Duke Ellington** which sold 14 million copies. **Herb** lived to the ripe old age of 100, largely because he emphasized his general health throughout his life, and he was a delightful person to know. Although he wasn't a vegetarian, he was a strong believer in supplements. **Herb Jeffries** also had a great sense of humor. He said:

"Most people come to this world by stork. I came by Flamingo, and Duke Ellington delivered me!"

As a human being, **Herb** was one of the kindest, most giving men I've ever met. God bless **Herb Jeffries** in Heaven!

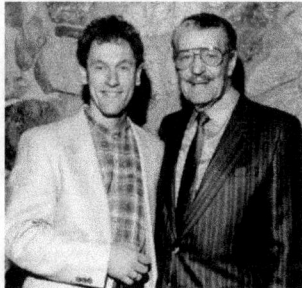

Tad Sisler with Herb Jeffries
Source – Sisler Private Collection

FLAXSEED OIL

Imagine your body is like a well-watered garden, where everything needs the proper nourishment to grow strong. Flaxseed oil is like an exceptional plant food for your garden—it's packed with a type of healthy fat called ALA, which can help support your heart and brain. Even though your body can't use all of it ideally (it has to change ALA into other forms), flaxseed oil is still a great way to plant "good seeds" for better health!

FLAXSEED OIL HIGH IN ALA, WHICH CAN CONVERT TO EPA/DHA (LIMITED EFFICIENCY)

Why ALA matters: ALA (alpha-linolenic acid) is an essential omega-3 fatty acid in flaxseed, chia seeds, and walnuts. Your body uses it to create EPA (eicosapentaenoic acid) and DHA (docosahexaenoic acid).

Limited conversion: The human body often converts only a small percentage of ALA into EPA and DHA. Genetics, diet, and nutrient levels (e.g., zinc, vitamin B6) can influence how well this conversion works.

DIETARY SOURCES:
Flaxseed oil, ground flaxseed, chia seeds, walnuts, hemp seeds.

SUGGESTED DAILY DOSAGE: Around 1–2 tablespoons (about 7–14 grams) of **flaxseed oil** per day can provide a good dose of ALA for general health. Some people may use more under professional guidance, but watch for total calorie intake.

Maximum dosage: There's no strict "upper limit" for flaxseed oil, but taking more than 2–3 tablespoons daily could lead to digestive upset or excessive calorie intake.

SOLUBILITY: Best when taken with meals containing some dietary fat.

SYNERGY WITH OTHER SUBSTANCES
Pair with antioxidants (e.g., vitamin E) or antioxidant-rich foods (berries, vegetables) to protect the oil from oxidation inside your body.

ALGAL OIL
Now imagine the ocean as a giant underwater forest full of tiny plants called algae. Algal oil comes from these mini sea plants and gives your body a direct form of a healthy fat called DHA—no extra steps needed! That makes it super handy for people who don't eat fish. It's like getting a VIP pass to the best nutrients for your brain, heart, and eyes without having to munch on seafood.

ALGAL OIL OFFERS DIRECT DHA FOR VEGANS
It's a plant-based source of **DHA** and often EPA, making it perfect for vegans and vegetarians who want to boost their omega-3 intake without fish.

DIETARY SOURCES: Mostly found as supplements. Certain algae-based foods (spirulina, chlorella) contain other nutrients but may not be as high in DHA/EPA unless produced explicitly for that purpose.

SUGGESTED DAILY DOSAGE: Many algal oil supplements provide **200–300 mg** of DHA (sometimes combined with EPA) per capsule. Taking 1–2 capsules daily can help meet basic needs.

Maximum dosage: Generally, up to about **1,000 mg** (1 g) of combined DHA/EPA per day is considered safe for most people, but always check with a healthcare provider if you go higher.

SOLUBILITY: Oil-soluble, similar to fish oil. Best with meals containing healthy fats. Take algal oil with a meal and add **some fat** (avocado, nuts, olive oil) to help absorption.

VENUS WILLIAMS

After an autoimmune illness, tennis legend **Venus Williams** went all-in on plant nutrition and created her own shake brand. Every scoop of the shake she drinks daily contains **DHA omega-3 from algal oil,** so she gets a steady dose without touching fish. **Venus** says the drink helped her bounce back to tournament shape and keeps her mind sharp for split-second shots on court.

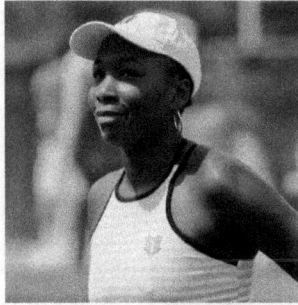

Venus Williams
Credit – Wikimedia Commons

STORE PROPERLY to avoid rancidity: Omega-3 oils (from flax or algae) can go "bad" (rancid) if exposed to heat, light, or air.

Storage tips: Keep bottles in a **cool, dark** place (a refrigerator is ideal). Make sure containers are sealed tightly to limit air exposure. Check expiration dates and sniff for any "off" or foul odor.

Rancid oil risks: Consuming rancid oil won't provide the same health benefits and may even cause digestive upset or inflammation.

BALANCE RATIO OF OMEGA-3 TO OMEGA-6 FOR OPTIMAL HEALTH: Omega-6 fats (in many vegetable oils and processed foods) can promote inflammation if eaten excessively. Omega-3 fats (from flaxseed, algae, fish, etc.) help counteract this effect.

Recommended ratio: Many experts suggest aiming for a ratio of around **4:1** (omega-6 to omega-3) or even **2:1** for optimal benefits. Typical Western diets can be **10:1** or higher.

PRACTICAL TIPS: Use **olive oil** or **avocado oil** instead of refined vegetable oils. Include omega-3 sources daily (e.g., flaxseed oil, algae-based supplements). Be mindful of processed snacks and fried foods, which can be high in omega-6.

OVERDOSE POTENTIAL: Actual "overdose" on plant-based omega-3s is rare. However, taking extremely high doses (far above recommended amounts) could cause digestive issues or interact poorly with blood thinners.

Pair with a Healthy Diet: For best results, combine omega-3 supplements with a balanced diet rich in whole foods, fruits, veggies, and moderate amounts of healthy fats. If you have underlying health conditions or take medications like

blood thinners, talk to a healthcare provider before starting high-dose omega-3 supplements. Pair any Omega-3 oils with meals to enhance absorption. One of my nutritionist friends tells me that Omega-3's are probably the most important supplement you can take for overall health. A recent study by the **Mayo Clinic** noted: *"There's strong evidence that omega-3 fatty acids can significantly reduce blood triglyceride levels."*

6.1.3: OMEGA-3 TO OMEGA-6 RATIOS

Omega-3 and Omega-6 fatty acids are essential fats your body can't produce, so you need them from food or supplements. Balancing their intake is crucial for reducing inflammation, which is linked to chronic diseases like heart disease, arthritis, and cancer, supporting longevity.

WHY THE RATIO MATTERS

Modern Western diets often have an Omega-6 to Omega-3 ratio of 15:1 or higher, far from the ancestral 1:1 to 2:1. High Omega-6 intake, from oils like corn, soybean, and sunflower, promotes inflammation, while Omega-3s, found in fatty fish, flaxseeds, and walnuts, reduce it. A 2025 meta-analysis of 32 studies (n=1,200) found that ratios closer to 4:1 lower inflammatory markers like CRP by 15%. Imbalanced ratios may increase risks of cardiovascular disease and cognitive decline.

IDEAL RATIO

Experts suggest aiming for a 1:1 to 4:1 Omega-6 to Omega-3 ratio, though achieving this requires dietary changes due to high Omega-6 prevalence in processed foods. A 2024 review notes that ratios below 4:1 correlate with reduced mortality risk.

HOW TO IMPROVE YOUR RATIO

Increase Omega-3 Intake: Eat fatty fish (salmon, mackerel, sardines) twice weekly, use flaxseed or algal oil, or consider high-quality Omega-3 supplements (EPA/DHA, 500–1000 mg/day) after consulting your doctor.

Reduce Omega-6 Intake: Limit processed foods, fast foods, and oils high in Omega-6 (corn, soybean, sunflower). Opt for olive or avocado oil for cooking.

Balance Your Diet: Choose grass-fed meats and wild-caught fish, which have better fatty acid profiles. Include nuts like walnuts (high Omega-3) and limit seeds high in Omega-6 (e.g., sunflower seeds).

Practical Tips:

Check food labels for Omega-3 content and avoid high Omega-6 oils.

Use olive oil for dressings and low-heat cooking to maintain balance.

If supplementing, choose third-party tested Omega-3 products (e.g., USP, NSF) to ensure purity.

Monitor your diet with apps like MyFitnessPal to track fatty acid intake.

SECTION TWO: OTHER NOTABLE OILS (EVENING PRIMROSE, BLACK SEED, MCT)

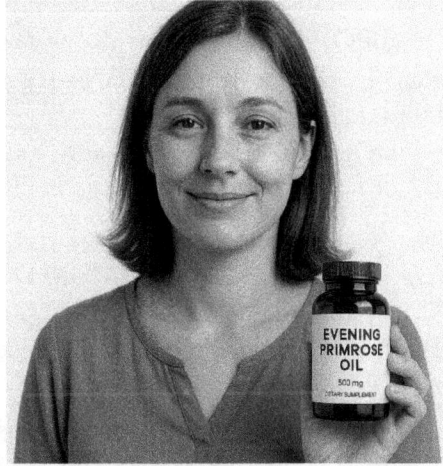

6.2.1: EVENING PRIMROSE OIL AND BORAGE OIL

Evening Primrose Oil and **Borage Oil** can provide valuable GLA for skin health and hormonal balance. They may ease eczema, help with PMS symptoms, and support general well-being.

EVENING PRIMROSE OIL

Imagine your skin and body as a group of friends who sometimes don't get along—there can be arguments (inflammation) or up-and-down feelings (hormones). Evening Primrose Oil works like a peacemaker! It has a special helper called **GLA** that can calm these arguments and help the friends (your cells) work together more smoothly. Some people notice smoother skin and fewer "bad moods" when they take it regularly.

BORAGE OIL

Picture a set of puzzle pieces that fit perfectly to make your skin glow and your body feel balanced. Borage Oil has a high amount of **GLA**, which is like that missing puzzle piece your body needs to stay comfortable—especially if you have itchy or flaky skin. It can also help settle hormonal roller coasters so everything feels more balanced.

THESE OILS CONTAIN GLA (Gamma-Linolenic Acid)

What is GLA? GLA is an omega-6 fatty acid the body converts into substances that help reduce inflammation.

Why it's helpful:

Skin: Supports moisture and elasticity, potentially helping with conditions like eczema or dryness.

Hormonal Balance: GLA may help ease menstrual-related symptoms by supporting healthy hormone levels.

DIETARY SOURCES

Evening Primrose Oil (EPO): Extracted from the evening primrose plant's seeds. You won't typically eat this plant directly—it's mainly found as a supplement (soft gels or liquid).

Borage Oil: Comes from borage seeds and is also commonly taken as a supplement in capsules or liquid form. Borage oil generally has a **higher GLA content** than evening primrose oil.

SUGGESTED DAILY DOSAGE AND MAXIMUM DOSAGE

Evening Primrose Oil: Typical daily doses range from **1,000 to 3,000 mg** (1–3 grams). Many EPO supplements specify the amount of GLA per capsule. **320–480 mg of GLA** per day is standard for general health.

Borage Oil is often used in lower quantities because it has a higher percentage of GLA. Dosages can range from **500 mg to 1,500 mg** per day.

Maximum dosage: There's no hard-and-fast "upper limit," but exceeding **3–4 grams** of these oils daily could cause digestive upset or other mild side effects. Always consult a healthcare provider if you're considering high doses.

OIL-SOLUBLE: Both EPO and borage oil are oil-soluble. It's best to take them with a meal containing some healthy fats to improve absorption and minimize stomach discomfort.

SYNERGY WITH OTHER SUBSTANCES: Pairing with a small amount of dietary fat (like avocado, nuts, or a meal) can help absorption. Including antioxidants (such as vitamin E or C) can help protect these oils from oxidation in the body.

SOME EVIDENCE FOR EASING ECZEMA, PMS SYMPTOMS

Skin Conditions (Eczema/Atopic Dermatitis): Research suggests that GLA may help reduce the dryness, itching, and overall irritation associated with eczema.

PMS/Hormonal Support: Many people report that EPO or borage Oil helps ease mood swings, breast tenderness, or cramping associated with PMS or perimenopause.

HEIDI KLUM

Fun fact: my granddaughter **Makalya Phillips** went on *America's Got Talent* at the age of 15 and was given the coveted *Golden Buzzer* by supermodel **Heidi Klum! Makayla** went on to the semifinals, and then made it to the top ten on *American Idol* two years later. **Heidi** became **Makayla's** good friend, and we appreciate her support that launched **Makayla's** career.

Heidi spends long hours under bright lights that leave her face dry and itchy. Before bed she smooths on a night serum whose star ingredient is **evening primrose oil**. **Heidi** says the oil "nourishes and smooths" her skin overnight; by morning the tight, flaky feeling is gone and she's ready for the next photo shoot.

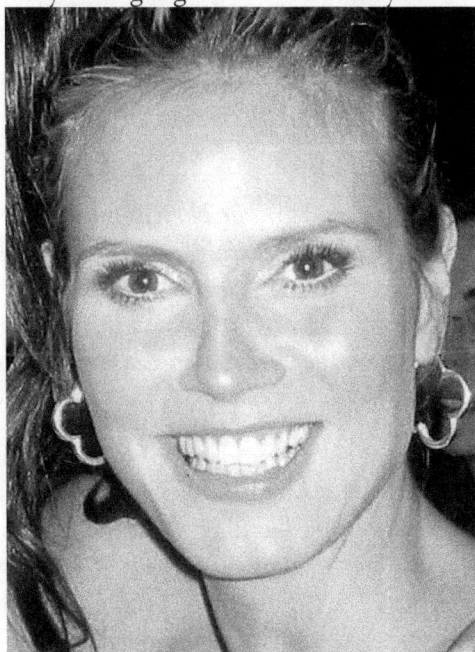

Heidi Klum
Credit – Wikimedia Commons

POTENTIAL MILD GI UPSET OR INTERACTIONS WITH SEIZURE MEDS

Gastrointestinal Issues: Taking these oils on an empty stomach could lead to mild nausea or stomach discomfort. If so, you could start with a lower dose and slowly increase it.

Medication Interactions: Some evidence suggests that **GLA-rich oils** might lower the threshold for seizures in people on certain seizure medications. Anyone taking anti-seizure drugs should consult a healthcare provider before using evening primrose or borage oil.

CHECK FOR REPUTABLE SOURCES TO AVOID RANCID OILS

GLA-containing oils can spoil (become rancid) if they're old or stored improperly. Rancid oils can lose their health benefits and may even be harmful.

Choose supplements labeled **cold-pressed** or **expeller-pressed**. Look for certifications like **USP** or **NSF** for quality assurance. Store in a **cool, dark** place—some people even refrigerate these oils to extend shelf life.

OVERDOSE POTENTIAL: Actual overdose is unlikely, but very high intakes (above 3–4 grams daily) may increase the risk of diarrhea, bloating, or other GI discomfort. If you have a **bleeding disorder** or take **blood-thinning medication**, talk with a healthcare provider before starting high-dose GLA.

Combined with a Healthy Lifestyle, Omega-3 fatty acids, a balanced diet, and adequate hydration can further support skin and hormone health.

Consistency is Key: Noticeable improvements in skin or hormonal symptoms often take **several weeks** of consistent use.

"Eczema, you've made me cry at night because my whole body gets itchy, and it burns so much... Unfortunately, you came into my life without asking. You were genetically passed down to me. You've showed me how life is rough, and you're an obstacle I've learned to overcome." –
Samantha Loya, in "An Open Letter to Eczema

6.2.2: BLACK SEED OIL (NIGELLA SATIVA)

Black seed oil (*nigella sativa*) has a rich history in Middle Eastern and South Asian cultures. It is backed by modern studies highlighting its antioxidant and anti-inflammatory powers—largely credited to thymoquinone. Middle-Eastern grandmothers swear that **black seed oil** is "a remedy for everything but death." Science hasn't proven that, but the oil's main compound, **thymoquinone**, is a talented antioxidant and inflammation-tamer. A teaspoon drizzled into hummus or swallowed straight can support balanced immunity and steady blood sugar. Start small—the flavor is bold and a tablespoon may upset tender stomachs.

MIGHT BENEFIT SKIN AND HAIR

Think of your skin and hair as plants that need the proper nutrients to grow strong. Black seed oil has helpful compounds that can be like fertilizer for your skin and hair, making them healthier and happier.

DIETARY SOURCES: In addition to the oil itself, black seeds can be found in spice mixes like *Kalonji* and certain flatbreads or curries. However, the most concentrated form is the oil extracted directly from the seeds.

CONTAINS THYMOQUINONE - STUDIED FOR ANTIOXIDANT AND ANTI-INFLAMMATORY PROPERTIES

Thymoquinone is like the "star player" in black seed oil. Research shows it has strong antioxidant properties (it helps defend cells from damage) and anti-inflammatory effects (it helps reduce excessive swelling in the body). The Prophet **Mohammed** is quoted to have said:

"There is healing in Black Seed for all diseases except death."

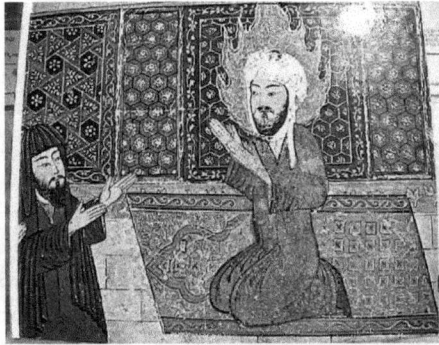

Mohammed Greeting Ambassadors from Medina

OVERHYPED CLAIMS - RELY ON PEER-REVIEWED DATA

Because black seed oil has so many traditional and folk uses, some claims online make it sound like a magical cure-all. It's important not to believe everything you read on the internet. Look for studies in scientific journals (peer-reviewed research) rather than just testimonials. Reliable data helps us separate fact from fiction and use black seed oil safely and effectively.

Safety & Side Effects: Most people tolerate black seed oil well in moderate amounts. However, if you take too much, you might experience an upset stomach, nausea, or other mild issues. Always start with small amounts to see how your body reacts.

SOLUBILITY: Since it's an oil, black seed oil mixes well with other fats but not with water. You can drizzle it into foods or combine it with a healthy source of fat (like olive oil) in a salad dressing for easier consumption.

SYNERGY WITH OTHER SUBSTANCES

With Food: Taking black seed oil with meals can help your body absorb it better and may reduce the chance of stomach upset.

Pairing with Other Healthy Fats: Mixing black seed oil into meals that contain good fats (avocado, olive oil, nuts) can help its beneficial compounds absorb more smoothly.

OVERDOSE POTENTIAL

Possible Side Effects: While there's no widely reported "toxic overdose" level for black seed oil, extremely high amounts can lead to digestive distress, kidney or liver strain, or allergic reactions in rare cases.

Safe Moderation: Stick to the recommended doses, and if you develop any adverse effects (like stomach pain or rash), reduce the amount or stop taking it and consult a healthcare provider.

Pregnancy & Children: If you're pregnant, breastfeeding, or considering giving black seed oil to children, it's crucial to get professional guidance first.

Medication Interactions: Black seed oil may interact with certain medications (such as those that affect blood clotting or blood pressure). Always consult a healthcare professional if you're on prescription meds.

6.2.3: MCT OIL (MEDIUM-CHAIN TRIGLYCERIDES)

MCT oil is a special type of fat that provides quick energy, making it especially popular for people on keto diets or athletes seeking a fast fuel source. It also supports weight management and mental clarity. Imagine tossing dry twigs onto a campfire; they catch fast and burn hot. That's how **medium-chain triglycerides** behave in your body. Unlike longer fats, MCTs skip the usual digestive line and head straight to the liver, where they're converted into ketones—jet fuel for muscles and brains running on low carbs.

Begin with one teaspoon in coffee or a smoothie. Too much too soon can turn your gut into a water slide, so inch up to a tablespoon only after your stomach gives the thumbs-up.

MIGHT HELP YOU WITH WEIGHT CONTROL: Think of your body as a car's engine. Sometimes, adding MCT oil is like giving your engine fuel that might help it run more efficiently so you don't overfill the tank with extra weight.

WORKS WELL WITH LOW-CARB DIETS: If you've heard of the "keto" diet, it's like a unique road your body travels to burn fat. MCT oil helps keep that road clear and smooth, giving you quick energy when you eat fewer carbs.

RAPIDLY ABSORBED FOR QUICK ENERGY; POPULAR IN KETOGENIC DIETS: MCTs (Medium-Chain Triglycerides) are shorter fat chains than most foods. Because they're shorter, the body can break them down faster. This provides a quick energy source, making them a favorite among people following a ketogenic (keto) diet.

DIETARY SOURCES:

Coconut Oil: Roughly 50–60% MCTs (it also contains other types of fat).
Palm Kernel Oil: Another natural source of MCTs.
Dairy Products: Butter, cheese, and milk (especially goat's milk) contain smaller amounts of MCTs. However, many people use bottled or powdered MCT oil because it's a more concentrated source.

HOW TO USE

- Blend it into coffee or tea (popular in "Bulletproof" or "Keto" coffee).
- Add to smoothies, salad dressings, or protein shakes.
- Drizzle it over cooked vegetables. (Its low smoke point makes it unsuitable for high-heat frying.)

MAY SUPPORT WEIGHT MANAGEMENT AND MENTAL CLARITY

Weight Management: Some studies suggest MCT oil can help slightly boost metabolism. It promotes a feeling of fullness, so people on weight-loss journeys sometimes find it helpful. **Remember,** it's still a fat with calories, so portion control matters.

Mental Clarity: MCTs provide an alternative energy source to glucose, especially on a low-carb diet. The brain can run on ketones derived from MCTs, potentially enhancing focus and mental sharpness in some individuals.

HALLE BERRY

When Oscar-winning actress **Halle Berry** trains for her intense movie fight scenes, she skips sugary energy drinks and adds a spoonful of **MCT oil to her morning coffee**. She says the oil gives her a steady "brain-fuel" boost so she can power through long stunt rehearsals without the mid-morning slump. Think of it like pouring premium gasoline into a sports car so it can zoom all day without sputtering. And, although **Halle** is gorgeous, she knows that there's more to good looks than just a pretty face.

"Beauty is not just physical." – Halle Berry

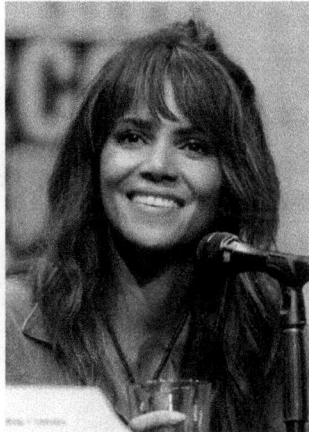

Halle Berry
Credit – Wikimedia Commons

START WITH SMALL DOSES TO GAUGE TOLERANCE

Low/Moderate Intake: Daily 1–2 teaspoons (5–10 mL).

Typical Usage Range: 1–2 tablespoons (15–30 mL) split across meals or at one time if tolerated.

Maximum Dosage: There is no strict universal maximum, but exceeding 3–4 tablespoons per day can increase the risk of digestive upset or unnecessary extra calories. Always listen to your body and check with a healthcare professional if you are uncertain.

SOLUBILITY: MCT oil is a fat and does not mix well with water. You'll want to blend it into foods or beverages with fats or use an emulsifier to mix it into liquids.

SYNERGY WITH OTHER SUBSTANCES: Adding MCT oil to meals can help minimize digestive issues. It's also a great addition to smoothies or protein shakes.

Ketogenic Diet: MCT oil is especially popular in low-carb or ketogenic diets to maintain energy and support ketone production.

OVERDOSE POTENTIAL

No Known "Toxic" Level: There's no established toxic overdose of MCT oil, but too much fat—and fat—can lead to digestive distress and excess calorie intake. Moderation is key.

Listen to Your Body: If you experience bloating, cramps, or diarrhea, reduce the amount or stop taking it until you consult a healthcare professional.

Allergies: Rare, but if you're allergic to coconut or palm-related products, proceed cautiously.

Pregnancy & Children: Generally recognized as safe, but always discuss with a doctor if pregnant or planning to give it to a child.

Combining with Medicines: MCT oil may interact with certain medications (especially for cholesterol or diabetes); consult a healthcare provider if you're on any prescriptions.

If you're attempting to lose weight and having a hard time, maybe with a ketogenic diet or another avenue to weight loss, don't lose faith. Anything worth fighting for is not going to be easy. My friend, **Bo Bice**, was a finalist on **American Idol** and went on to have a great career as a rock star. **Bo** said:

"Just practice hard and stay grounded. Treat people like you want to be treated and work hard."

Use the Golden Rule in life, never give up, and you're bound to succeed.

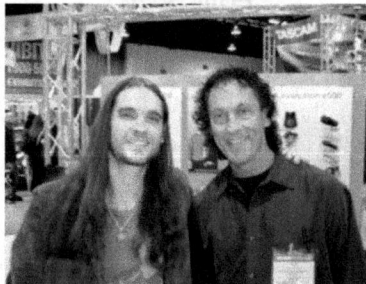

Bo Bice and Tad Sisler
Source – Sisler Private Collection

6.2.4: OIL STABILITY AND STORAGE

I mention storage and rancidity in other parts of this book. This section contains overall guidelines for proper storage of oils. Storing oils properly preserves their health benefits and prevents oxidation, which can produce harmful compounds. Oils high in polyunsaturated fats, like flaxseed or fish oil, are especially prone to spoilage, while monounsaturated (e.g., olive oil) and saturated (e.g., coconut oil) oils are more stable.

WHAT MAKES OIL UNSTABLE

Oxidation occurs when oils are exposed to heat, light, oxygen, or time, breaking down fats into free radicals and off-flavors. A 2025 study found that oxidized oils increase oxidative stress, linked to aging and disease. Polyunsaturated oils have multiple double bonds, making them less stable than monounsaturated (fewer double bonds) or saturated oils.

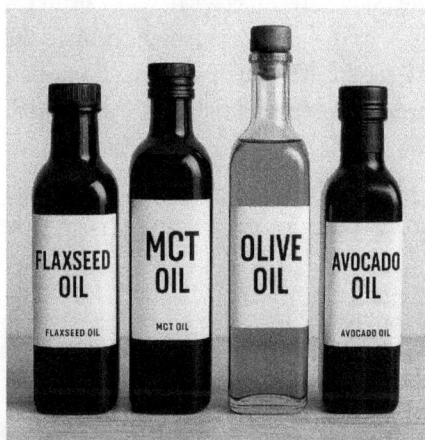

HOW TO STORE OILS PROPERLY

Keep Cool: Store oils in a cool (below 75°F), dark place, away from stoves or sunlight.

Use Dark Bottles: Dark glass or opaque containers protect oils from light exposure.

Seal Tightly: Close lids securely to limit oxygen exposure.

Refrigerate Delicate Oils: Store flaxseed, fish, or krill oil in the fridge to extend shelf life.

Check Expiry Dates: Use oils within their shelf life (typically 6–12 months) and discard if rancid.

SIGNS OF RANCIDITY

Smell: Rancid oils may smell like paint, crayons, or fish.

Taste: Bitter or off flavors indicate spoilage.

Appearance: Cloudiness or sediment may suggest oxidation, though not always.

PRACTICAL TIPS

Buy oils in small quantities to use within a few months.

Use stable oils (avocado, coconut) for high-heat cooking; save flaxseed or fish oil for dressings or low-heat uses.

Avoid reusing oils for frying, as repeated heating accelerates oxidation.

Choose brands with third-party testing to ensure quality and freshness.

SECTION THREE: PRACTICAL INTEGRATION OF HEALTHY FATS

6.3.I: COOKING VS. SUPPLEMENTATION

My **Robin** cooked with Canola and other Vegetable oils for years, because she was taught her delicious recipes by her grandmother, who also cooked in the same manner. Recently, she switched to cooking with Avocado oil and was delighted to find the same results with a healthier oil. **Robin's** other grandmother was Italian, and she generously used olive oil, which is also super-healthy. When integrating healthy fats into your diet, match the right oil to the proper cooking method. Flaxseed and fish oils are best enjoyed cold to preserve their delicate, beneficial fatty acids. Meanwhile, avocado and coconut oils stand up to higher cooking temperatures.

COLD USE (Flaxseed) vs. HIGH-HEAT COOKING (Avocado, Coconut)

FLAXSEED OIL

Why Cold? Flaxseed oil has a low smoke point, so it breaks down quickly under heat. High temperatures can destroy its beneficial omega-3 fatty acids and create harmful byproducts.

Suggested Uses: Drizzle it on salads, blend it into smoothies, or use it as a finishing oil on roasted veggies (after they've cooled slightly) to preserve its nutrients.

AVOCADO OIL

High-Heat Hero: Avocado oil has one of the highest smoke points among cooking oils, often exceeding 500°F (260°C). This makes it ideal for frying, sautéing, or roasting without breaking down and creating unwanted compounds.

Nutritional Profile: Rich in monounsaturated fats (similar to olive oil), plus vitamin E for antioxidant benefits.

COCONUT OIL

Stable Saturated Fats: Coconut oil is high in saturated fat, which remains more stable at higher temperatures than many polyunsaturated fats. It has a moderate to high smoke point (350–400°F or 175–205°C).

Flavor Profile: It imparts a subtle coconut taste and is suitable for Asian-inspired dishes or baking.

COOKING WITH FISH OIL IS NOT RECOMMENDED DUE TO OXIDATION:
Fish oil has a high amount of omega-3 fatty acids and prone to oxidation when exposed to heat. Oxidation can produce off-flavors and potentially harmful compounds.

BEST PRACTICE
Supplement Form: Most people take fish oil as a capsule or liquid added to cold foods.

Direct Dietary Sources: For cooking and eating fish, opt for fresh or lightly cooked salmon, mackerel, sardines, or other fatty fish to get intact omega-3s without the risk of damaging them.

TOO MUCH OF ANY OIL CAN ADD EXCESS CALORIES
Calorie Density: All oils are calorie-rich, at about 120 calories per tablespoon. Even healthy oils can contribute to weight gain if consumed in excess.

Moderation and Variety: Using different oils for different purposes—like flaxseed in dressings and avocado for sautéing—can help you enjoy the full range of benefits without adding unnecessary calories.

ROTATING DIFFERENT OILS CAN PROVIDE BENEFITS
Each oil has unique profile of fatty acids, antioxidants, and vitamins. Using different oils expands the range of nutrients you're getting.

Sample Rotation:

Olive Oil is perfect for low- to medium-heat cooking, salads, and drizzling. It is rich in polyphenols and monounsaturated fats.

Avocado Oil: High smoke point for roasting or sautéing; also a good source of monounsaturated fats.

Coconut Oil: Stable saturated fats for specific baking or medium-heat cooking; unique flavor.

Flaxseed Oil: Best used cold, high in alpha-linolenic acid (an omega-3).

Sesame Oil (toasted variety) adds a nutty flavor to Asian dishes and contains lignans, which have antioxidant properties.

Watch Cooking Temperatures: Even with rotating oils, monitor smoke points. Overheating can destroy beneficial compounds and create harmful byproducts.

Combine With Whole Foods: Healthy fats shine brightest when paired with nutrient-dense ingredients like dark leafy greens, lean proteins, colorful vegetables, and whole grains.

Check Quality & Freshness: When possible, opt for cold-pressed or extra-virgin varieties. Store oils properly to maintain their nutrient content and flavor.

MIND YOUR SERVING SIZES: Healthy or not, oils are calorie-dense. Measure what you use to avoid unintended calorie spikes.

My dear friend, *Academy-Award-winning* actress **Cloris Leachman** became more aware of healthy eating as she aged. She learned to eliminate unhealthy oils as part of her regimen. **Cloris** said:

"When I decided to become vegetarian, I had to learn how to 'recook', if you will. For example, I used to put red wine in a big pot with the meat that I'd cooked in fat, and it was, of course, delicious. When I gave up meat, I wondered what I would make. That turned out to be vegetables, really organic and fresh."

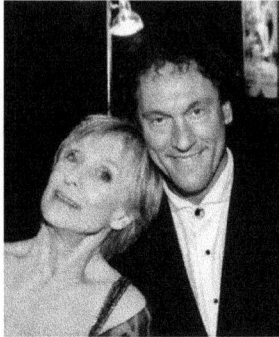

Cloris Leachman and Tad Sisler
Source: Tad Sisler's Personal Collection

6.3.2: SAFETY AND STORAGE

STORE OILS IN COOL, DARK PLACES TO DELAY OXIDATION
FRESH, UNREFINED OILS MAXIMIZE NUTRIENT CONTENT

Over time, oils can oxidize, go rancid, or lose their beneficial nutrients. Always check expiration dates and store in a cool, dark place. Unrefined, cold-pressed, or "extra virgin" oils often retain more antioxidants and natural flavors than heavily processed ones. Look for terms like "cold-pressed," "unrefined," or "virgin" on labels. Avoid oils that smell or taste "off," as rancid oil can be harmful.

• Store oils in dark glass, away from heat. Rancid oil smells like old paint—when in doubt, throw it out.

• Fat-soluble vitamins A, D, E, and K ride best with a little oil. Add olive oil to steamed carrots and your body grabs more beta-carotene.

• Balance the fat ratio: aim for four parts omega-6 (corn, soy) to one part omega-3. Swapping a handful of walnuts for chips is an easy win.

Remember, every tablespoon of oil packs about 120 calories. Pour thoughtfully, listen to your body, and let these friendly fats do their quiet, powerful work—keeping your heart pumping, your joints gliding, and your brain sparking with ideas well into the decades ahead.

CHECK EXPIRATION DATES - RANCID OILS PRODUCE HARMFUL BYPRODUCTS: Just like any perishable product, oils have a shelf life. While it may be tempting to ignore expiration dates, consuming rancid oils can lead to unwanted health consequences. Oxidized oils can produce free radicals and other compounds that may trigger inflammation or gastrointestinal distress. Always verify the "best by" or "use by" date, and perform a quick smell and taste check before using an oil—if it smells "off" (chemical or paint-like) or tastes bitter, it's likely rancid and should be discarded.

BEN GREENFIELD

Fitness coach and podcaster **Ben Greenfield** warned followers that "taking a **bad fish oil is worse than taking none at all**." He admitted cheap capsules once gave him fishy burps and belly bloating—classic signs of spoiled oil. After switching to a higher-quality product stored in the fridge, the burps stopped and his stomach felt normal again. Now he tells athletes to ditch any bottle that smells off.

DARK GLASS BOTTLES HELP REDUCE LIGHT EXPOSURE

Packaging matters. Light accelerates the breakdown of fats, especially those rich in polyunsaturated fatty acids (PUFAs). Dark glass bottles or other opaque containers act as shields, limiting how much UV and visible light can penetrate the oil. Look for oils bottled in dark amber or tinted containers for maximum freshness and potency. These help maintain the oil's stability by preventing early oxidation, further extending the product's shelf life.

"Polynesian women are known for their long hair, glowing skin, and thick nails. And that comes from the local diet, which is mostly plant based with a little bit of fish and a lot of natural fats and oils." – Nikki Reed

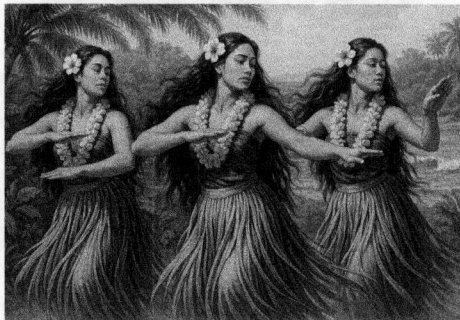

MONITOR YOUR BODY'S RESPONSE TO CHANGES IN FATS

Everyone's body reacts differently to dietary changes, including introducing new oils or removing certain fats. Pay attention to signs like digestive comfort, energy levels, skin and hair health, and mood. If you notice any adverse symptoms—such as persistent bloating, breakouts, or fatigue—consider adjusting your consumption or switching to a different type of oil. As always, seeking personalized guidance from a healthcare provider or nutritionist can help ensure you use the right fats for your unique needs.

We've tackled macronutrients and popular supplements – now let's turn to powerful micro-warriors: probiotics and the world of digestive support.

CHAPTER SEVEN
PROBIOTICS AND DIGESTIVE ALLIES

"I believe the best way to activate genius within the immune system is by ingesting certain superherbs and superfoods, taking probiotics and cultured foods, minimizing toxic food exposure by eating pure organic raw-living foods, and making appropriate healthy lifestyle improvements.
- David Wolfe

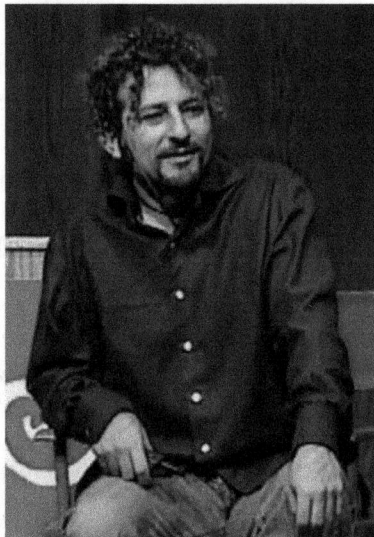

David Wolfe
Credit – Wikimedia Commons

Your gut contains trillions of microorganisms – many beneficial, some less so. Could harnessing them be the key to vibrant health? Some health gurus swear that gut health is the key to overall health. Inflammation and disease can begin in the gut, and a healthy microbiome is an important key to optimum health

SECTION ONE: UNDERSTANDING THE MICROBIOME

7.1.1: WHY GUT HEALTH MATTERS

Picture your digestive tract as a humming, twenty–four-hour city. Trillions of microscopic citizens—bacteria, yeasts, even the occasional virus—buzz around doing their jobs. When the good citizens outnumber the bad, the streets stay clean, traffic flows, and everyone feels safe. In practical terms that means you digest food smoothly, absorb vitamins with ease, wake up with steady energy, and even enjoy a brighter mood. That's no exaggeration: certain gut bugs actually make serotonin, the "feel-good" chemical most people associate with the brain.

But a city needs more than friendly neighbors. It also needs garbage collectors, road crews, and peacekeepers. **Digestive enzymes** slice food into bite-sized pieces; **fiber** keeps waste moving like cars on an uncongested highway; soothing herbs act like park rangers who calm hot tempers in a crowd. Together these allies prevent traffic jams—better known as bloating, gas, or constipation—and they keep harmful invaders from seizing control.

When the balance tips the wrong way—a condition called **dysbiosis**—the whole metropolis struggles. Harmful microbes throw trash in the streets, triggering inflammation. You may feel foggy, exhausted, or mysteriously achy. Some people even slide toward autoimmune trouble because their confused immune "police force" starts arresting innocent bystanders. The good news? Restoring balance usually starts with small, doable steps: cleaner food, lower stress, and targeted probiotics.

CASE STUDY

Christina, a 35-year-old teacher with long-standing IBS, began a doctor-recommended probiotic. Within weeks her cramps eased and her frantic dashes to the restroom nearly vanished. Right bugs, huge payoff.

FOOD SENSITIVITIES MAY BE TIED TO MICROBIOME IMBALANCES: Many people who experience uncomfortable reactions to certain foods—like dairy or gluten—may not have a classic allergy but a sensitivity. An imbalanced microbiome can sometimes contribute to these sensitivities by compromising the gut lining (leading to a "leaky gut"). When the gut barrier is weakened, partially digested food particles can trigger an immune response, resulting in bloating, rashes, or other inflammatory symptoms. You can often find relief from food sensitivities by improving gut flora and healing the digestive tract.

PROBIOTICS ARE NOT A CURE-ALL; DIET AND LIFESTYLE REMAIN IMPORTANT: Even though probiotics play a crucial role in restoring balance within the gut, they can't work miracles on their own. A diet rich in whole foods—mainly vegetables, fruits, and whole grains—provides the nutrients and fibers that "feed" beneficial bacteria. Managing stress, getting plenty of sleep, and staying physically active are equally vital. Think of probiotics as valuable team members, but they still need a supportive environment to do their jobs effectively. Without proper diet and lifestyle choices, even the best probiotic supplement may fail to deliver lasting health benefits.

So, when someone says, *"listen to your gut"* or *"go with your gut feeling,"* they may not just be talking about your instincts! Quoting again the words of the great **Deepak Chopra:**

> *"There are receptors to these molecules in your immune system, in your gut and in your heart. So when you say, 'I have a gut feeling' or 'my heart is sad' or 'I am bursting with joy,' you're not speaking metaphorically. You're speaking literally."*

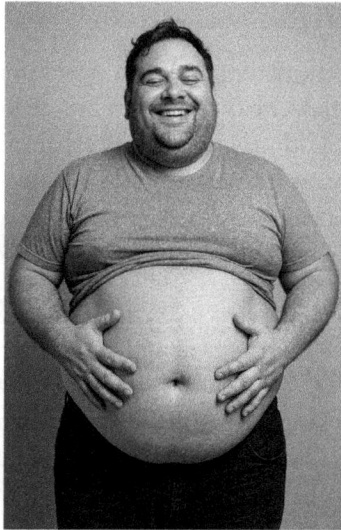

7.1.2: KEY PROBIOTIC STRAINS (LACTOBACILLUS, BIFIDOBACTERIUM)

LACTOBACILLUS

Imagine you have a tiny superhero living in your gut who loves to eat harmful germs for breakfast. That's what Lactobacillus is like! It's a friendly kind of bacteria that helps break down foods—especially dairy—so your tummy can handle them better. Some types, like *Lactobacillus acidophilus*, can even help people who have trouble digesting milk feel less bloated. Think of Lactobacillus as a helper that keeps your stomach and intestines peaceful and happy.

DIFFERENT STRAINS OFFER DIFFERENT BENEFITS
(e.g., Lactobacillus acidophilus for Lactose Intolerance)

Not all probiotics are the same—just like different sports teams have players with specialized skills. For instance:

• *Lactobacillus acidophilus* is known to help digest lactose (the sugar in milk).
• *Lactobacillus rhamnosus* is often studied to support gut health and reduce diarrhea risk.
• *Lactobacillus reuteri* has been linked to oral health benefits and some anti-inflammatory effects.

DIETARY SOURCES: Fermented foods like yogurt, kefir, sauerkraut, kimchi, and kombucha often contain Lactobacillus strains. *L. acidophilus* is specifically common in many commercially available yogurts.

SUGGESTED DAILY DOSAGE: Probiotic supplements typically range from I billion to 50 billion CFUs (colony-forming units) per serving. Doses of I–10 billion CFUs per day are commonly cited for Lactobacillus acidophilus, which is used to support lactose intolerance.

MAXIMUM DOSAGE / OVERDOSE POTENTIAL: Large amounts are considered safe for most healthy adults, with some high-dose supplements reaching 100 billion CFUs or more. "Overdose" in the traditional sense is rare; however, extremely high doses can sometimes cause bloating or discomfort.

SOLUBILITY: Probiotics are live organisms, not typically classified by water- or fat-soluble in the same way as vitamins. They're delivered in capsules or as powders. Some are micro-encapsulated to survive stomach acid, but the concept of "oil-soluble" vs. "water-soluble" doesn't strictly apply.

SYNERGY WITH OTHER SUBSTANCES: Often taken with **prebiotics** (fibers like inulin, fructooligosaccharides/FOS) that help feed and grow the good bacteria. There is no specific "must-take-with-food" rule, but many manufacturers suggest taking probiotics with a meal to improve survival through an acidic stomach.

BIFIDOBACTERIUM

Picture a busy construction crew working inside your belly daily, building strong walls to keep out harmful invaders. That's what Bifidobacterium does, especially in your colon (the last part of your digestive system). Bifidobacterium helps keep bad germs from taking over and ensures your immune system (the body's defense team) stays alert. Bifidobacterium enables you to feel your best from the inside out by supporting healthy digestion and a strong gut lining.

MODULATES IMMUNITY IN THE COLON: Bifidobacterium is like a guardian for your large intestine, helping maintain the gut barrier and moderating immune responses. Key benefits include:
• Protection against harmful bacteria.
• Improved bowel regularity.
• Support for overall immune health.

DIETARY SOURCES: These are mainly found in fermented foods, such as certain yogurts labeled specifically with Bifidobacterium (for example, *Bifidobacterium Animalis* in some brands), fermented soy products, and certain probiotic-fortified dairy.

SUGGESTED DAILY DOSAGE: Common supplements range between I billion to 20 billion CFUs of Bifidobacterium species. Some gut health regimens suggest up to 10 billion CFUs daily for immune or digestive support.

MAXIMUM DOSAGE / OVERDOSE POTENTIAL: Similar to Lactobacillus, high doses (up to 50–100 billion CFUs) have been used in some clinical studies with minimal side effects, although gas or mild digestive upset may occur.

SOLUBILITY AND SYNERGY: Like Lactobacillus, Bifidobacterium does best when it has fibers (prebiotics) to feed on. Pairing with a balanced diet that includes fruits, vegetables, and whole grains will enhance its effectiveness.

RESEARCH STUDY:
Preliminary research often indicates that multi-strain formulations can be more effective than single-strain supplements for some conditions, such as IBS (Irritable Bowel Syndrome). Having multiple players on the team (different strains) can address multiple symptoms or issues at once. However, single strains can still be effective for specific problems—always check if the chosen strain matches your health goal.

Practical Tip: If you're exploring probiotics for IBS relief, look for products that specify which strains they include and at what CFU count. Consult a healthcare professional for personalized advice.

CFU COUNTS (Colony-Forming Units) MATTER, BUT BIGGER ISN'T ALWAYS BETTER

The CFU count tells you how many live microbes are in each dose. While "higher" often sounds more potent, it's not always necessary: The effectiveness of a probiotic depends on the specific strain and the individual's gut environment. A very high CFU supplement might not offer additional benefits if your body doesn't need or can't accommodate that many.

OPTIMAL RANGE

A typical maintenance dose might be between 1–10 billion CFUs. Certain conditions, such as severe gut imbalances, may benefit from 20+ billion CFUs. Start low, observe your body's response, and adjust if necessary.

SIDE EFFECTS: While generally safe, too high a CFU count for some people can cause bloating, gas, or mild digestive upset. Reducing the dose often fixes these issues.

REFRIGERATION OR SHELF-STABLE FORMS DEPEND ON THE STRAIN

Some probiotic strains need cooler temperatures to stay alive (like ice cream that melts if left out too long). Others are more robust and can remain shelf-stable at room temperature:

Lactobacillus acidophilus often requires refrigeration to maintain potency. Newer technology (like freeze-drying or micro-encapsulation) can stabilize certain strains without refrigeration.

STORAGE TIPS: Always follow the label instructions. Check expiration dates carefully, as CFU counts can drop over time if they are not stored properly. People with heavily weakened immune systems or serious illnesses should consult a doctor before using high-dose probiotics.

BEST WAY TO TAKE PROBIOTICS: These are often recommended with meals to protect bacteria from stomach acid. Combining with prebiotics (bananas, onions, garlic, chicory root, or specialized fiber supplements) can help the friendly bacteria thrive.

Everyone's microbiome is unique. What works best for one person might not work as well for another. Although I do not endorse anyone, nor am I a paid spokesperson, I take an excellent probiotic product from *Seed Health*. Always check with a healthcare professional regarding specific health concerns, allergies, or conditions.

In short, probiotics are like good neighbors in your gut community: they help keep things clean, orderly, and healthy. By choosing the correct strain and dosage for your needs—and keeping them in a supportive environment (with the proper diet and storage conditions)—you can help ensure these friendly microbes thrive.

Quoting again the words of my friend **Suzanne Somers**:

"When your body absorbs toxins, it stores them in fat, which is why fiber and probiotics are strategic weapons for weight loss. Fiber keeps your colon healthy and reduces your body's absorption of toxins."

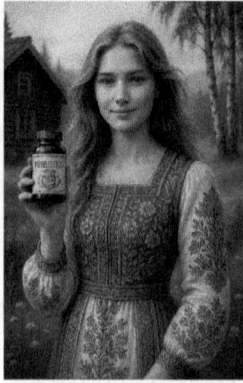

7.1.3: SPORE-BASED PROBIOTICS AND YEASTS

Spore-based probiotics and friendly yeasts like *Saccharomyces boulardii* play important roles in keeping the gut healthy. They're like sturdy explorers and friendly bakers who help your gut stay balanced, strong, and ready to protect you—no matter where your travels take you.

SPORE-BASED PROBIOTICS

Imagine you have tiny, helpful "seed" friends that can live in your body. These seeds are called spore-based probiotics. Like seeds that can survive a long, cold winter in the ground, these probiotic "seeds" can stay safe in your stomach's acidic environment, then grow and help your intestines. Once they reach your gut, they help keep the peace between all the other bacteria. This can help you digest food better and keep your tummy feeling good.

BENEFICIAL YEASTS

Think of beneficial yeasts—like **Saccharomyces boulardii**—as the friendly "bread bakers" inside your body. As bakers work in the kitchen to make the dough rise, these yeasts can help balance the "bad" yeasts and other unwanted germs in your gut. They pitch in to keep everything running smoothly so your body isn't overwhelmed by the wrong kind of yeast. You'll likely stay healthy and avoid tummy troubles when everything is balanced.

On a side note, amazing discoveries in human longevity center around yeast! It appears that we can learn much from the biogenome of yeast as it applies to human aging. I address this in my book **Stay Healthy, Stay Youthful: The Science of Living to 150.**

"Simple genome engineering of bacteria and yeast is just the beginning of the rise of the true biohackers. This is a community of several thousand people, with skill sets ranging from self-taught software hackers to biology postdocs who are impatient with the structure of traditional lab work." – Ryan Bethencourt

---

BACILLUS STRAINS CAN HANDLE STOMACH ACID

Bacillus strains (like *Bacillus clausii*, *Bacillus subtilis*, and *Bacillus coagulans*) are unique because they form a protective shell (spore) that allows them to make it through the acidic "moat" of your stomach. Once in your intestines, they can help crowd out harmful bacteria, support digestion, and assist with regular bowel movements.

DIETARY SOURCES: These spores are naturally found in soil; trace amounts may be present on unwashed fruits and vegetables. However, most people get them from dietary supplements rather than food.

DAILY DOSAGE: A typical daily dose is about 1–10 billion CFUs (colony-forming units). Many supplement brands offer capsules in this range.

Maximum Dosage: There isn't a strict "maximum" for Bacillus-based probiotics, but taking over 50 billion CFUs daily can sometimes cause mild bloating or gas. Lower the dosage and talk to a healthcare professional if you notice discomfort.

WATER-SOLUBLE: Probiotics are generally considered water-soluble, though the spore form is relatively stable in many environments.

SYNERGY WITH OTHER SUBSTANCES: To give probiotics the best chance to thrive, it can be helpful to take spore-based probiotics with a meal or alongside prebiotics (like fiber from fruits, vegetables, or supplements such as inulin).

OVERDOSE POTENTIAL: True "overdose" is unlikely. However, extremely high doses may lead to temporary digestive upset.

HELPS FIGHT OFF PATHOGENIC YEASTS

Saccharomyces boulardii (often shortened to "*S. boulardii*") is a friendly yeast that can "outcompete" harmful yeasts. It's primarily known for helping with diarrhea, balancing gut flora, and reducing the risk of inevitable digestive upsets.

DIETARY SOURCES: Unlike some bacteria found in fermented foods, *S. boulardii* is mostly obtained from supplements. It was originally isolated from tropical fruits like lychee, but it won't commonly be found in everyday foods.

SUGGESTED DAILY DOSAGE: 5–10 billion CFUs per day are often recommended. Some people take it as a short course when traveling or dealing with specific gut issues.

Maximum Dosage: Higher doses, like 20–50 billion CFUs daily, have been used in research settings, typically without significant problems. Still, it's best to start low and increase gradually.

SOLUBILITY: *S. boulardii* is generally stable as a powder or capsule that dissolves in water.

SYNERGY WITH OTHER SUBSTANCES: Taking it with a meal or alongside other friendly bacteria (like Lactobacillus or spore-based probiotics) might help support a balanced gut environment.

OVERDOSE POTENTIAL: Overdosing is rare. Very high amounts might cause minor digestive upset or gas.

DR. MICHAEL MOSLEY

Dr. Mosley, the BBC presenter behind the show *"Trust Me, I'm a Doctor,"* often reports from crowded summer festivals and overseas shoots. After one unpleasant bout of "festival tummy," (sometimes called *Montezuma's Revenge*) he started warning viewers about food-borne bugs. In his gut-health column he calls **S. boulardii "the perfect festival probiotic,"** because it survives heat, crowds out bad germs, and keeps you out of the porta-loo. So, remember to take some along if you're going to the next *Burning Man* or *Coachella!*

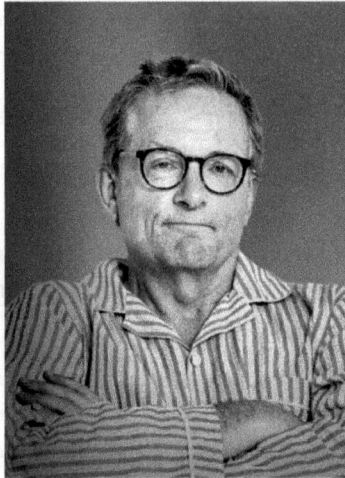

Dr. Michael Mosley

Credit - YouTube /Does Australia have a sleep problem? | Australia's Sleep Revolution with Dr Michael Mosley /creativecommons.org

SOME SPORE-BASED FORMULAS MAY BE BENEFICIAL FOR SMALL INTESTINE COLONIZATION

Many probiotics work best in the large intestine, but some Bacillus spores might also help in the small intestine. This can be particularly useful if you have digestion or nutrient absorption issues.

Complementing Other Probiotics: Since spore-based probiotics are hardy, they can pair well with other strains like Lactobacillus and Bifidobacterium, creating a more comprehensive "team effort" throughout the gut.

QUALITY CONTROL AND THIRD-PARTY TESTING REMAIN IMPORTANT

Not all probiotic or yeast supplements are created equal. Some might contain fewer live cultures than advertised or be contaminated. Choose products that undergo third-party testing for potency (to ensure they have the advertised CFU count) and purity (to ensure no harmful contaminants). Certificates from organizations like NSF International, USP, or ConsumerLab can be good signs of quality.

STORAGE: Check if your spore-based or yeast probiotics require refrigeration. Many spore-based products are shelf-stable, but it is usually best to store them in a cool, dry place.

POSSIBLE SIDE EFFECTS: Mild gas or bloating can occur when first taking probiotics or *S. boulardii*. Usually, this goes away as your body adjusts. If severe discomfort or allergic reactions happen, discontinue and consult a healthcare professional. People with weakened immune systems or those on certain medications should check with a doctor before starting high-dose probiotics.

"Weird stuff, for me, is not that weird. I guess if it were other people, they'd think it was weird. I eat nutritional yeast. And sometimes I take clay shots to help pull toxins out of my body. I eat weird L.A. food, so I guess that's probably weird in other people's eyes." – Stephanie Beatriz

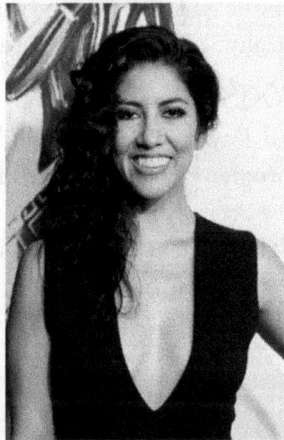

Stephanie Beatriz
Credit – Wikimedia Commons

7.1.4: POSTBIOTICS

Postbiotics are bioactive compounds produced by probiotics during fermentation, offering health benefits without live bacteria. These include short-chain fatty acids (SCFAs), bacteriocins, and other metabolites that support gut health and immunity. A 2025 review in *Gut* highlights their role in reducing inflammation and strengthening the gut barrier, potentially aiding longevity (*Gut*).

TYPES OF POSTBIOTICS

Short-Chain Fatty Acids (SCFAs): Butyrate, acetate, and propionate, from fiber fermentation, support colon health and may reduce colorectal cancer risk (*Nature Reviews Gastroenterology & Hepatology*).

Bacteriocins: Antimicrobial peptides that inhibit harmful bacteria, enhancing gut balance.

Exopolysaccharides: Sugars that act as prebiotics, feeding beneficial bacteria.

Cell Wall Fragments: Stimulate immune responses, boosting defense against pathogens.

BENEFITS

Immune Support: Postbiotics enhance immunity without risks of live bacteria, suitable for immunocompromised individuals.

Gut Health: They improve gut barrier function and reduce inflammation, potentially easing IBS or leaky gut.

Safety: Lack of live organisms lowers infection or antibiotic resistance risks.

SOURCES AND USAGE

Find postbiotics in fermented foods like yogurt, sauerkraut, and kimchi, or as supplements. Choose products specifying postbiotic types and concentrations, verified by third-party testing (e.g., USP, NSF). Consult a healthcare provider before supplementing, especially with health conditions.

7.1.5: GUT-BRAIN AXIS

In my book **The Unlimited Power of Your Mind and Body: How to Live Longer Naturally by Reprogramming Your Mind, Body, and Genes for Strength and Vitality,** I delve deeper into the gut-brain axis. The gut-brain axis is a communication network between your gut and brain, influencing mood and cognition via neural, hormonal, and immune pathways. A 2025 *Microbiome* study shows gut bacteria affect mental health, reducing depression and anxiety risks (*Microbiome*).

MECHANISMS

Vagus Nerve: Connects gut and brain, transmitting mood-regulating signals.

Neurotransmitters: Gut bacteria produce serotonin, dopamine, and GABA, impacting mood and cognition.

Immune System: Gut microbes regulate inflammation, linked to brain health and neurodegenerative diseases.

Hormones: Stress hormones like cortisol alter gut microbiota, affecting mental well-being.

IMPACT ON MENTAL HEALTH

Depression and Anxiety: Gut dysbiosis is linked to higher mental health risks; probiotics and prebiotics may improve symptoms.

Cognitive Health: A balanced microbiome supports memory and may lower Alzheimer's risk.

PRACTICAL TIPS

Diet: Eat fiber-rich foods (fruits, vegetables, whole grains) and fermented products (yogurt, kefir) to support gut bacteria.

Probiotics and Prebiotics: Consider supplements or foods to enhance gut health.

Stress Management: Use meditation or yoga to reduce stress, benefiting the gut-brain axis.

Consult Professionals: Work with healthcare providers for tailored gut health strategies, especially for mental health concerns.

SECTION TWO:
PREBIOTICS AND FIBERS

7.2.1: INULIN, FOS, GOS

Inulin, FOS, and GOS are special treats for the good microbes in your intestines. They're found naturally in certain plants (onions, garlic, chicory root) and dairy sources (for GOS) and are available as supplements. Friendly microbes can't thrive on air alone; they need dinner. **Inulin, FOS, and GOS** are special plant fibers the human body can't digest, so they cruise down to the large intestine intact, where good bacteria throw a feast. Onions, garlic, chicory root, and even lentils are naturally rich sources, but you can also sprinkle a measured powder into a smoothie.

Begin with **two or three grams—about half a teaspoon**—because hungry bacteria produce gas while they eat. Give your gut a week or two to adjust, then rise gradually to five or even ten grams if you like. The payoff is worth it: better regularity, calmer digestion, and a stronger immune shield.

EXCESS CAN LEAD TO BLOATING IN SENSITIVE INDIVIDUALS

As good bacteria feast on inulin, FOS, and GOS, they produce gases as a natural byproduct. Some people's digestive systems are more sensitive to these gases, which can lead to bloating or mild discomfort.

MANAGING SIDE EFFECTS:

Start Low: Introduce these fibers slowly, at a low dose, to allow your gut time to adjust.

Split Doses: Instead of taking one large dose, spread smaller doses throughout the day.

MAXIMUM DOSAGE: Some people may tolerate doses up to **15–20 grams** daily, but going too high too quickly can cause uncomfortable bloating or gas.

OVERDOSE POTENTIAL: There's no actual "toxic" overdose, but excessive amounts can lead to digestive distress (bloating, cramps, diarrhea).

SOLUBILITY: Inulin, FOS, and GOS are **water-soluble** fibers. They dissolve quickly in water or other liquids, often found in powdered supplements you can stir into drinks.

SYNERGY WITH OTHER SUBSTANCES

With Probiotics: These prebiotics can be beneficial if you also take probiotics (like *Lactobacillus* or spore-based strains). The probiotics benefit from having a ready food supply, enhancing their survival and activity in your gut.

With Meals: Taking prebiotic supplements with meals can lessen the chance of stomach upset and help slow absorption, potentially reducing bloating.

POSSIBLE CONCERNS:

Digestive Upset: Gas, bloating, or loose stools may occur if you take a dose that is too high or start too quickly.

Allergies: These are rare, but if you notice a rash or severe discomfort, discontinue use and consult a healthcare professional.

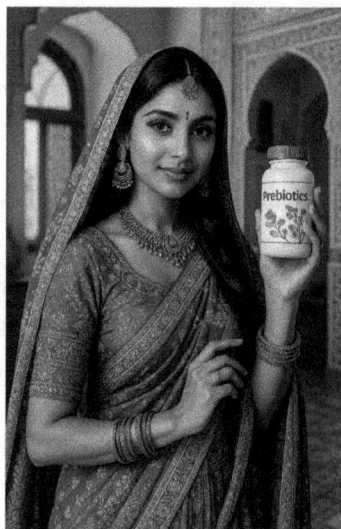

WHO MIGHT WANT TO BE CAUTIOUS?

People with IBS (Irritable Bowel Syndrome) or other sensitive stomach conditions might need to introduce prebiotics more carefully. Some people following low-FODMAP diets temporarily reduce inulin, FOS, and GOS intake to manage symptoms.

"If you're suffering from gut-induced depression, how do you reset your gut microbiome to steer you back to a healthy mental state? The key is to increase probiotics and prebiotics in your diet. Probiotics are live bacteria that convey health benefits when eaten. Probiotic-rich foods contain beneficial bacteria that help your body." – Uma Naidoo

7.2.2: PSYLLIUM HUSK, RED YEAST RICE, GLUCOMANNAN

PSYLLIUM HUSK

Psyllium Husk works like a gentle street sweeper. Mix one rounded teaspoon (about five grams) into a tall glass of water and it forms a gel that traps extra cholesterol and escorts waste out of town.

DIETARY SOURCES: Psyllium comes from the seeds of the Plantago ovata plant. It's usually sold as a powder or in capsules rather than in everyday foods. However, certain high-fiber cereals and fiber supplements list psyllium husk as an ingredient.

MAXIMUM DOSAGE: Under medical supervision, up to **20-25 grams** per day can be used, but higher amounts can cause bloating or discomfort. Always drink plenty of water to help it move through your system.

OVERDOSE POTENTIAL: It's hard to "overdose" on fiber, but too much could cause bloating, gas, or even blockages if you don't drink enough water.

SOLUBILITY: Psyllium husk is **water-soluble** (it absorbs water and becomes gel-like). It's best taken with a large glass of water, about 8 ounces or more, to prevent clumping in your throat or stomach. People looking to manage cholesterol might take it alongside a meal, especially if it has some dietary fat to help bind extra cholesterol.

Psyllium can help with regularity (reducing constipation or diarrhea) and support cholesterol management by trapping cholesterol in its gel-like fiber so your body removes it rather than absorbing it.

RED YEAST RICE

Picture rice grains that have been painted red by a friendly fungus. These grains turn into a superhero for your heart. **Red Yeast Rice** is fermented rice naturally laced with mild statin-like compounds. One or two 600-mg capsules at dinner can nudge LDL cholesterol downward, but because it behaves like medication, loop your doctor in before you start.

DIETARY SOURCES: Red yeast rice is formed by fermenting rice with a specific yeast (*Monascus purpureus*). It's not typically found in everyday foods, but you can buy it in capsules or tablets. In some Asian cuisines, it's used as a coloring agent or flavor enhancer.

MAXIMUM DOSAGE: There's no officially established "maximum," but experts often advise not going much over **2,400 mg per day** without medical supervision due to potential side effects similar to prescription cholesterol-lowering drugs.

OVERDOSE POTENTIAL: Taking too much red yeast rice might increase the risk of side effects like muscle pain or liver issues—similar to what happens with certain cholesterol medications. It's best to check with a healthcare provider if you plan on taking larger doses or have existing health conditions.

SOLUBILITY?: Red yeast rice isn't typically categorized by water or oil solubility for everyday use; it's generally taken in capsule or tablet form. Some practitioners recommend taking it with meals with some healthy fat or alongside **CoQ10** (coenzyme Q10) because red yeast rice can reduce CoQ10 levels in the body.

Besides helping manage cholesterol, red yeast rice may also offer anti-inflammatory benefits and support healthy blood sugar and blood pressure, but results can vary from person to person. Ensure your red yeast rice supplement is tested for purity (to avoid contaminants).

"I mean, when you've had a problem in your past, whether it's attributed directly to high cholesterol or not, you want to lower your cholesterol. You want to eat healthy. You want to feel healthy. You want to have a little more energy." – Mike Ditka

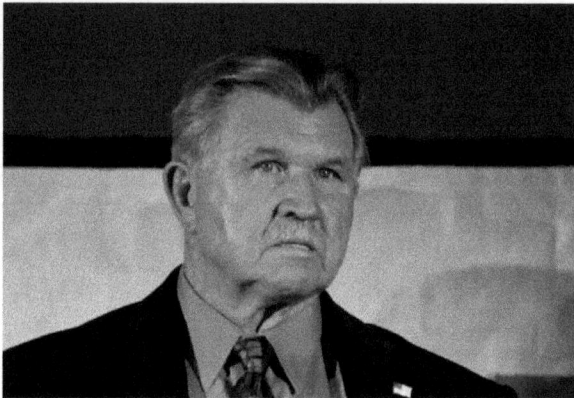

Mike Ditka
Credit – WEBN-TV/Flickr/creativecommons.org

GLUCOMANNAN

Glucomannan is the ultimate sponge, soaking up fifty times its weight in water. Two grams in a big glass before meals helps you feel pleasantly full and blunts blood-sugar spikes. Forget the water, though, and you'll feel like you swallowed a brick—so hydrate!

DIETARY SOURCES: Glucomannan is extracted from the roots of the **konjac** plant, and it is commonly used in some Asian foods (like shirataki noodles).

MAXIMUM DOSAGE: Do not exceed **4-5 grams** daily. Taking too much can increase the risk of stomach discomfort or blockages if you don't drink enough water.

OVERDOSE POTENTIAL: If not enough water is consumed, overusing glucomannan can lead to choking or blockages in the digestive tract. Otherwise, it's generally considered safe within recommended amounts.

AMANDA SEYFRIED

While filming in New York, movie star **Amanda Seyfried** found a restaurant that served *Miracle Noodles*—shirataki strands made from the konjac plant. They're almost all water and **glucomannan fiber**, so they fill you up without many calories. A *People* magazine story says **Amanda** happily ordered the dish for dinner, calling it her guilt-free way to stay satisfied between long days on set.

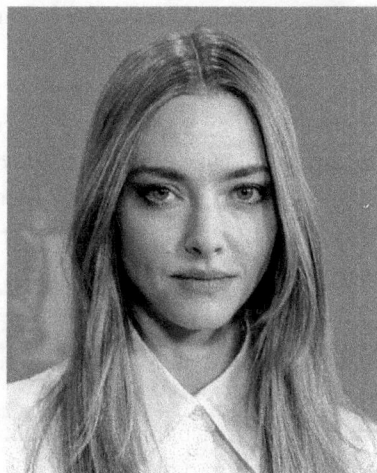

Amanda Seyfried
Credit – Wikimedia Commons

SOLUBILITY: Glucomannan is **water-soluble** and can absorb up to 50 times its weight in water. Always take glucomannan with plenty of water—at least 8 ounces. This helps the fiber expand safely in your stomach rather than in your throat. If weight management is your goal, some people find taking it shortly before a meal helps them feel full sooner.

Some research shows glucomannan may help control blood sugar if you have type 2 diabetes. Because it slows down the quickness of food's removal from your stomach, it may prevent blood sugar spikes after a meal.

MUST DRINK ADEQUATE WATER to prevent choking or blockages: Because psyllium and glucomannan swell up when they absorb water, staying hydrated is very important. Think of these fibers like little sponges; without enough water, they can get stuck in places you don't want them to, potentially causing discomfort or blockages.

7.2.3: FERMENTED FOODS VS. SUPPLEMENTS

FERMENTED FOODS

Imagine little helpers swimming around in your stomach, ensuring your food is well-digested, and your body gets the energy it needs. Fermented foods—like sauerkraut, kimchi, and kefir—are packed with these friendly "good guy" germs called probiotics. These probiotics help keep your tummy happy, strengthen your immune system, and boost your mood. Plus, these foods often come with extra vitamins and minerals made during fermentation, like hidden treasures waiting to support your health.

SUPPLEMENTS

Now, picture you're building a sports team, and you can pick the players you need for a big game. Supplements are kind of like that. They let you choose specific strains of probiotics—particular "good guy" germs that experts think are the strongest for your needs. They also tell you exactly how many of these microbes you're taking in, almost like having players lined up in neat rows. This can be super handy if you need special help, like focusing on your tummy troubles or allergies, and you want to take them anywhere you go.

FERMENTED FOODS- PROBIOTIC STRAINS PLUS NUTRIENTS

Main Benefits: These foods contain diverse probiotic bacteria that help balance your gut. They're also naturally rich in vitamins, minerals, and enzymes—nutrients your body can use for energy and repair.

Real-Life Examples: Sauerkraut (fermented cabbage), kimchi (spicy, seasoned cabbage and veggies), and kefir (cultured dairy) have all been eaten for hundreds of years in different cultures. Whole foods contain fiber and other compounds that can further support digestion and overall health.

SUPPLEMENTS TARGET SPECIFIC STRAINS:

If you need help with a particular health issue—like bloating or immune support—supplements let you pick the exact probiotic strains that studies have shown to help.

Dosage Control: Supplements often list the number of live bacteria in Colony-Forming Units (CFUs) on the label so you know how much you're taking.

Convenience: They're easy to pack and swallow, and they come in capsules, powders, or even gummies.

COMBINING BOTH IS OFTEN IDEAL

Best of Both Worlds: Fermented foods give you a broad range of good bacteria plus nutrients, while supplements give you precise strains and dosages.

You might enjoy fermented foods most days and use a supplement if you need a little extra support (e.g. when traveling, after taking antibiotics, or during stressful times).

WATCH SODIUM LEVELS IN SOME FERMENTED PRODUCTS

Foods like kimchi, sauerkraut, and pickles can contain high levels of salt, used both for flavor and for preservation. If you're watching your sodium intake, look for low-sodium versions or rinse some brine before eating. Also, pay attention to portion sizes to keep salt in check.

"In nineteenth-century Russia, sauerkraut was valued more than caviar." –
Mark Kurlansky

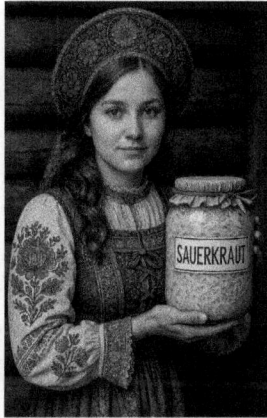

SECTION THREE: ENZYMES AND DIGESTIVE AIDS
7.3.1: DIGESTIVE ENZYMES (BROMELAIN, PAPAIN, ETC.)

Heavy steak sitting like a rock? **Bromelain** from pineapple and **papain** from papaya act as molecular scissors, trimming long protein chains into smaller links your body can absorb. A capsule supplying 500–1,000 mg of either enzyme with a protein-rich meal often erases that post-dinner bloat.

DIETARY SOURCES:

Bromelain is naturally found in the stem and juice of pineapples.
Papain is found in papaya fruit and leaves' latex (milky sap).

SUGGESTED DAILY DOSAGE:

Bromelain: Often recommended in a range of **500 mg to 2,000 mg** per day, usually split into 2–3 doses.

Papain: Common supplements can range from **25 to 150 mg** per serving; total daily amounts can vary, but staying under a few hundred milligrams per day is typical.

MAXIMUM DOSAGE: There is no universally agreed-upon "official" maximum for these enzymes, but extremely high amounts (in the thousands of milligrams) may lead to side effects like stomach upset. Following product labels and talking with a healthcare professional is always wise.

SOLUBILITY: Both bromelain and papain are **water-soluble** enzymes, meaning they dissolve in water-based fluids like digestive juices. Taking them **with or right before a meal** can help digest the food in your stomach.

Some people combine digestive enzymes with **probiotics** or **fiber supplements** for overall gut health. Since digestive enzymes dissolve well in water, make sure to drink water when taking them.

OVERDOSE POTENTIAL: Overdosing is uncommon but can happen if you take very high doses for a long time. Side effects may include diarrhea, nausea, or skin rashes. If you notice anything unusual, stop use and consult a healthcare provider.

JILLIAN MICHAELS

On her blog, celebrity trainer and fitness coach **Jillian Michaels** admits big, protein-heavy meals used to leave her feeling "bloated and blah." She began carrying a broad-spectrum digestive-enzyme tablet that lists **bromelain and papain** right on the label. **Jillian** tells readers that these two fruit enzymes *"help break down the protein in your food so you don't puff up like a balloon"* and recommends taking them right before eating. After a few weeks she noticed far less belly-bloat and now calls enzymes one of her top de-bloat tools.

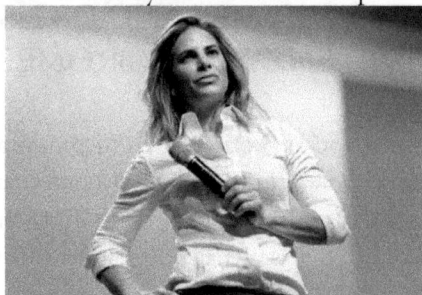

Jillian Michaels
Credit – Flickr / creativecommons.org

MAY RELIEVE BLOATING OR INDIGESTION: Because bromelain and papain speed up the breakdown of proteins, they may **lessen the workload on your stomach**, potentially reducing bloating or that heavy, uncomfortable feeling after meals. Results vary from person to person, so while some feel immediate relief, others may notice only a small benefit—or none at all.

ALLERGY POTENTIAL: If someone is allergic to pineapple or papaya, they may also react to bromelain or papain. Common allergic reactions can include itching, rash, and swelling. People with allergies should be cautious and talk to a healthcare professional before using these enzymes.

QUALITY AND DOSAGE VARY WIDELY: Supplement brands may differ in **purity, concentration,** and **enzyme potency** (look for units like GDUs or activity levels on the label). To ensure you get a trustworthy product, look for **certifications** like GMP (Good Manufacturing Practices) or third-party testing.

When I was a small boy, my mother would exercise every day in front of the television to **Jack LaLanne.** He was a big believer in the power of exercise, especially when it comes to speeding up digestion. He must have done something right, because he lived healthy to the ripe old age of 96. Exercise, in addition to a healthy diet and the addition of digestive enzymes, can do a lot to boost your general health.

"Yes, exercise is the catalyst. That's what makes everything happen: your digestion, your elimination, your sex life, your skin, hair, everything about you depends on circulation. And how do you increase circulation?"
– Jack LaLanne

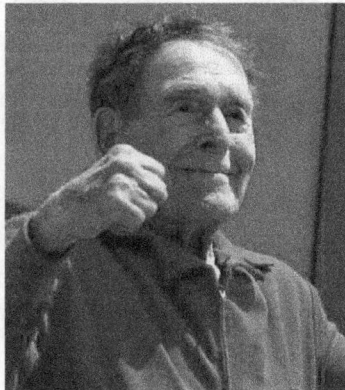

Jack LaLanne
Credit – Wikimedia Commons

OTHER ENZYMES FOR DIGESTION:
Amylase: Helps break down carbohydrates (like starches and sugars).
Lipase: Helps break down fats.
Protease: A general term for enzymes breaking down proteins (bromelain and papain are types of proteases).

Lactase: Assists in breaking down lactose, the sugar in dairy products.

If you have trouble digesting different types of nutrients, including a blend of these enzymes in supplements can offer more **comprehensive** digestive support.

7.3.2: BETAINE HCl AND APPLE CIDER VINEGAR

BETAINE HCl

Imagine your stomach is like a big swimming pool; the acid inside it is the water. If there isn't enough water, you can't swim properly. In the same way, if your stomach doesn't have enough acid, it can't break down your food well. Betaine HCl acts like a "refill" for that pool, adding more acid so your stomach can do its job, which might help some people digest proteins more efficiently.

APPLE CIDER VINEGAR

Think of apple cider vinegar as a sour juice made from apples. If your stomach is feeling a bit sluggish, a small amount of this tangy liquid might wake it up—like a jolt of energy—to help break down food better. Some people say it helps them with mild heartburn or indigestion, but it's always good to be cautious because vinegar is strong and can bother your stomach or teeth if you use too much.

INCREASES STOMACH ACIDITY FOR BETTER PROTEIN BREAKDOWN

Betaine HCl provides additional hydrochloric acid (HCl) to the stomach, helping to lower the pH and enhance protein digestion.

Apple Cider Vinegar (ACV): This contains acetic acid, a weaker acid that may still help raise stomach acidity slightly.

DIETARY SOURCES

Betaine HCl: Commonly found in supplement form; naturally, betaine can be found in beets, spinach, and whole grains, though not as hydrochloride.

Apple Cider Vinegar is gleaned from fermented apples. It can be used in salad dressings and marinades or diluted in water.

SUGGESTED DAILY DOSAGE

Betaine HCl: It is often recommended to take **650 mg to 2,000 mg** per meal, sometimes with digestive enzymes or pepsin. The exact dose varies widely depending on an individual's needs.

Apple Cider Vinegar: A common approach is **to take 1–2 tablespoons** diluted in a large glass of water once or twice a day, usually before or with meals.

MAXIMUM DOSAGE

Betaine HCl: Using more than **5,000–6,000 mg per day** can increase the risk of gastric irritation. It's best to use the minimal effective dose.

Apple Cider Vinegar: Consuming large amounts (more than a few tablespoons per day undiluted) can irritate the throat, erode tooth enamel, and upset your stomach. Always dilute it.

SOLUBILITY

Betaine HCl: Generally considered **water-soluble**, mixing with the watery environment of the stomach.

Apple Cider Vinegar is also **water-soluble** (acetic acid dissolves well in water).

SYNERGY WITH OTHER SUBSTANCES

Betaine HCl: Commonly taken with **protein-containing meals** to aid digestion. Some supplements combine it with **pepsin** (a digestive enzyme) for enhanced effect.

Apple Cider Vinegar: It is often taken **before or with meals**—diluted in water—to help with digestion. Combining it with ginger or honey can make it more palatable.

"I make a wonderful cure-all called Four Thieves, just like my mum did. It's cider vinegar, 36 cloves of garlic, and four herbs, representing four looters of plague victims' homes in 1665 who had their sentences reduced from burning at the stake to hanging for explaining the recipe that kept them from catching the plague." – Paul O'Grady

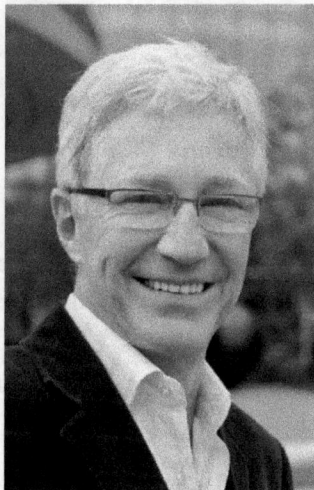

Paul O'Grady
Credit – Wikimedia Commons

OVERDOSE POTENTIAL

Betaine HCl: Too much can lead to **acid reflux, heartburn, or stomach irritation**. People with ulcers or gastritis should seek medical advice before use.

Apple Cider Vinegar: Excessive use may cause **throat irritation**, damage to tooth enamel, or upset stomach. Always dilute.

MAY HELP WITH ACID REFLUX

Acid reflux often happens when acid travels back up the esophagus. Some believe adding acid (through Betaine HCl or ACV) can improve the closure of the valve at the top of the stomach. Others argue it may worsen symptoms if too much acid is present. Everyone's digestive system is unique, so results vary.

VICTORIA BECKHAM

Fashion icon and former *Spice Girl* **Victoria Beckham** posted on Instagram that she felt lighter and had steadier digestion after morning ACV shots. She drinks **two tablespoons of raw apple-cider vinegar** in water first thing every day, then repeats the ritual before meals on busy workdays to "support digestion and balance blood sugar." Fashion magazines like *Vogue* regularly list ACV as her top wellness habit.

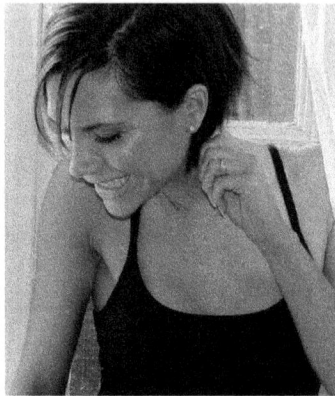

Victoria Beckham
Credit – Flickr / creativecommons.org

OVERUSE CAN LEAD TO G.I. IRRITATION

Taking **too many tablets** of Betaine HCl or drinking **too much ACV** can irritate the lining of the stomach and esophagus. Symptoms might include **burning, pain, or nausea.**

MEDICAL SUPERVISION RECOMMENDED IF YOU SUSPECT LOW STOMACH ACID

Get Tested: If you suspect you have low stomach acid (hypochlorhydria), consult a healthcare professional. They might perform specific tests to confirm. Supplementing with acids when not needed can cause or worsen reflux and damage tissues.

SUPER BEETS

Many "super beets" supplements, including gummies, boast incredible health benefits, including the presence of betaine HCl. Beets (Beta vulgaris) are a nutrient-dense vegetable, providing multiple health benefits from their high content of vitamins, minerals, antioxidants, and nitrates. Here are the main benefits:

SUPPORTS HEART HEALTH: Beets are rich in dietary nitrates, which help dilate blood vessels, improve blood circulation and lower blood pressure. Studies show that regular beet consumption can reduce the risk of cardiovascular diseases, like heart attacks and strokes.

ENHANCES ATHLETIC PERFORMANCE: The nitrates in beets improve oxygen use and endurance by increasing nitric oxide levels, which enhances blood flow to muscles. Many athletes use beet juice as a natural performance enhancer to increase stamina and reduce fatigue.

IMPROVES BRAIN FUNCTION: Increased blood flow from nitrates benefits brain health by enhancing cognitive function and shortening the risk of neurodegenerative diseases like dementia. As mentioned, beets contain betaine, which helps reduce homocysteine levels, lowering the risk of cognitive decline.

SUPPORTS DETOXIFICATION AND LIVER HEALTH: Beets contain betalains, powerful antioxidants that help the liver detoxify harmful substances and support liver function. They assist in breaking down toxins and improving bile production, which aids digestion.

AIDS DIGESTION AND GUT HEALTH: Beets are high in fiber, promoting healthy digestion, preventing constipation, and feeding beneficial gut bacteria. The natural prebiotics in beets help maintain a balanced gut microbiome.

REDUCES INFLAMMATION: In my book **"Stay Healthy, Stay Youthful: The Science of Living to 150,"** I outline the evidence that inflammation may be the most serious problem your body deals with when it comes to health and longevity. Betalains and other antioxidants in beets help lower inflammation, slowing the risk of chronic diseases like arthritis, heart disease, and cancer. Beets may help decrease markers of inflammation such as C-reactive protein (CRP).

SUPPORTS HEALTHY BLOOD SUGAR LEVELS: Beets have a moderate glycemic index but contain fiber, helping slow down sugar absorption and preventing spikes in blood glucose. Research suggests that beets may improve insulin sensitivity.

PROMOTES HEALTHY SKIN AND ANTI-AGING: Beets contain antioxidants, including vitamin C and betalains, helping to protect skin from damage from free radicals. They also support collagen production, which keeps skin firm and youthful.

MAY HELP PREVENT CANCER: In some studies, betalains in beets have shown potential in reducing cancer cell growth. Beets contain antioxidants that protect cells from DNA damage and oxidative stress.

SUGGESTED DAILY DOSAGE

Raw Beets: 1 small to medium beet (~100-150 grams) daily.
Beet Juice: 1/2 to 1 cup (120–240 ml) per day is commonly recommended for heart and performance benefits.
Beet Powder: 1-2 teaspoons (about 4-8 grams) daily.
Beet Supplements (Capsules/Tablets): Follow manufacturer recommendations, usually around 500-1000 mg daily.
Note: High intake can cause "beeturia" (pink or red urine) and may not be suitable for those with kidney stones due to oxalates.

SYNERGY WITH OTHER SUBSTANCES

Beets work well when combined with other nutrients and compounds for enhanced health effects:

Beets + Citrus (Vitamin C) → Boosts iron absorption from beets, helping prevent anemia.

Beets + Ginger/Turmeric → Enhances anti-inflammatory benefits.

Beets + Dark Leafy Greens (Spinach, Kale) → Increases nitrate and folate intake for improved heart and brain function.

Beets + Black Pepper (Piperine) → Improves the absorption of betalains and other antioxidants.

Beets + Coconut Water → Enhances hydration and electrolyte balance for better athletic performance.

Beets + Garlic → Combined vasodilation effect for more potent blood pressure-lowering benefits.

Beets + Apple Cider Vinegar → Supports digestion and liver detoxification.

"With their earthly flavor and lovely color, beets are a welcome addition to any winter dish. They are inexpensive, versatile and hearty, and you can even eat beet greens to reduce food waste." – Natalie Rizzo, today.com

COCONUT WATER is celebrated for it's rich electrolyte content. It's great for hydration especially after exercise, containing potassium, magnesium, sodium, and calcium. Coconut water supports muscle function, it's low in calories and fat, rich in nutrients, helps regulate blood sugar, supports heart health, prevents kidney stones and has antioxidant properties. On a recent trip to St. Lucia, our Caribbean tour guide told us that his father used coconut water to cure "all ailments!" He said that whenever he was sick as a child, he was given coconut water, and he swore he felt better very soon after drinking it.

7.3.3: PRACTICAL INTEGRATION FOR DIGESTIVE WELLNESS

Start small: add one new helper, give it two weeks, and keep notes. Fiber demands water, so aim for eight to ten cups daily. Remember, supplements are teammates, not saviors; sleep, stress control, and real food are the stadium they play in.

A sample day might look like this:
Breakfast – Greek yogurt with berries and chia; cup of green tea.
Lunch – Big salad with apple-cider-vinegar dressing, grilled chicken, and a psyllium-spiked smoothie.
Snack – Carrot sticks with hummus.
Dinner – Salmon, roasted veggies, and a scoop of sauerkraut.
Evening – Probiotic capsule if you skipped fermented foods, glass of water before bed.

Track how you feel—energy, mood, bathroom visits—and adjust. Your gut is as unique as your fingerprint, but once its citizens live in harmony, the rest of your body tends to follow suit.

HYDRATION IS NECESSARY FOR FIBER-BASED SUPPLEMENTS

Fiber—especially **soluble** varieties like psyllium husk, glucomannan, or inulin— absorbs water and swells, helping to move waste through your intestines. However, if you don't drink enough water, fiber can dry and compact, leading to constipation or discomfort. Keep these tips in mind:
Some health gurus advise drinking a minimum of **8–10 cups (64–80 ounces)** water each day, adjusting for climate and activity level.
Timing: When you take a fiber supplement, drink an entire glass of water (8 ounces) immediately afterward to help it travel smoothly through your digestive tract.
Gradual Increase: If you're new to higher fiber intake, start small and slowly build up to avoid gas, bloating, or cramping.

QUICK TAKEAWAYS
• Good bugs = better digestion, immunity, and mood.
• Feed them with prebiotic fibers and fermented foods.
• Use enzymes or acid boosters when heavy meals fight back.
• Water and patience turn small tweaks into lifelong habits.
• Take care of your inner city and it will take care of you—today, tomorrow, and decades down the road.

We've explored internal health, but what about specialized compounds pushing the boundaries of age-defying science? Let's find out next.

CHAPTER EIGHT
ADVANCED AND EMERGING LONGEVITY COMPOUNDS

C ould the secret to age reversal lie in molecules like NMN, senolytics, or even repurposed pharmaceuticals? Science is racing to find out. I've explored the following compounds in greater depth in my book "Stay Healthy, Stay Youthful: The Science of Living to 150."

"I would like to recapture that freshness of vision which is characteristic of extreme youth when all the world is new to it." – Henri Matisse

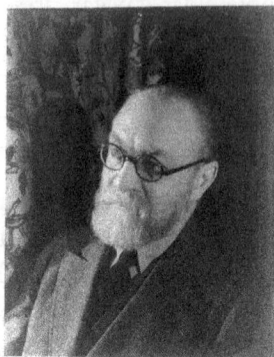

Henri Matisse

Imagine actually reversing your age, going back to youthful energy and health! It's not as far-fetched as you might imagine, and new discoveries on the horizon will be opening up a new world to human longevity. Let's look at the most promising compounds:

SECTION ONE: NAD+ BOOSTERS AND SENOLYTICS
8.1.1: NAD+ PRECURSORS (NMN, NR)

NMN (Nicotinamide Mononucleotide)
Imagine your body's cells are like tiny factories that make energy. These factories need a "power switch" to keep the lights on. NMN acts like a key that turns up that power switch by helping your cells make **NAD+** (a crucial energy molecule). When there's enough NAD+, the cells in your body can work more efficiently, possibly allowing you to feel more energetic and supporting healthy aging.

NR (Nicotinamide Riboside)
Think of NR as a close cousin to NMN—another type of "key" for your body's energy system. By taking NR, you also boost your **NAD+** levels, which may help your cells function better, much like giving your phone's battery a steady charge so it doesn't run out in the middle of the day. Some people believe

NR might support metabolism and even help with exercise endurance as they get older.

ELEVATE NAD+ FOR ENHANCED MITOCHONDRIAL FUNCTION

NAD+ is essential for the tiny power plants in your cells, known as mitochondria. NAD+ levels naturally decline as we age, potentially leading to less efficient energy production and cellular repair. **NMN** and **NR** convert into NAD+ in the body, potentially helping to restore or maintain higher NAD+ levels, thus supporting mitochondrial health.

Higher NAD+ may improve **energy**, cellular repair, and overall metabolism.

SOME ANIMAL STUDIES SHOW IMPROVED METABOLIC HEALTH, EXERCISE TOLERANCE

In rodents, supplementing with NAD+ precursors (NMN or NR) often leads to **better endurance** during exercise tests, improved insulin sensitivity, and may help **protect against age-related weight gain**.

While these findings are encouraging, human studies are still evolving. Some early human trials suggest mild improvements in metabolic markers and exercise performance, but more data is needed to confirm long-term benefits.

TONY ROBBINS

One of my favorite longevity books (besides my own) is **LIFE FORCE**, co-authored by motivational icon **Tony Robbins**. In the book, he describes adding NMN to his morning routine after reading mouse studies showing dramatic stamina gains. The book—and a follow-up article summarizing his regimen—call NMN a "key part" of the stack that helps him chase the vitality of someone decades younger. When Tony bounds onto a huge stage, his mission is pumping up thousands of people. To keep that fire burning, he swallows an NMN pill with breakfast, lifts weights, and eats lots of colorful food. He says the combo makes him feel like his body's batteries stay charged all day, not just during the show.

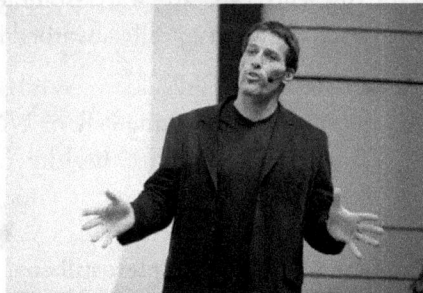

Tony Robbins
Credit – Wikimedia Commons

HUMAN DATA GROWING BUT STILL NOT DEFINITIVE ON LONG-TERM SAFETY

Short-term use of NMN and NR in humans appears **generally safe** and well-tolerated, with mild side effects like nausea or flushing in some cases. The long-term effects—over years or decades—are less established. Ongoing clinical trials aim to uncover more about **safety** and **optimal dosing**. If you're considering high-dose or long-term use, consult a healthcare provider to weigh potential benefits and risks.

SYNERGY WITH DIET AND EXERCISE

A nutrient-rich diet and regular exercise help naturally maintain healthier NAD+ levels. Combining NMN or NR with consistent **physical activity** and a **balanced diet** of veggies, fruits, and lean proteins may enhance potential benefits.

Exercise and good nutrition support **cellular health** and **stress resilience**. Adding NAD+ precursors could give your cells an additional nudge toward optimal function.

DIETARY SOURCES

NAD+ Precursors in Foods: Trace amounts of NR and other NAD+ precursors can be found in **milk** and **some fish** (like sardines), but these are typically too small to significantly boost NAD+ alone.

Supplement Form: NMN and NR are commonly consumed as **powder** or **capsules**.

SUGGESTED DAILY DOSAGE / MAXIMUM DOSAGE

Typical Ranges: NMN: Often in the range of **250 mg to 1,000 mg** per day. NR: Often in the range of **300 mg to 1,000 mg** per day.
Maximum Dosage: There is no universally agreed-upon "maximum" because long-term human data is limited. Many experts suggest staying within **1,000 mg** daily unless advised otherwise by a healthcare professional.

SOLUBILITY: Both NMN and NR are **water-soluble**. They dissolve in water-based fluids in your body and are typically absorbed in the digestive tract.

SYNERGY WITH OTHER SUBSTANCES: While there's no absolute rule, some anecdotal reports suggest that taking **NR** or **NMN with meals** may reduce stomach upset. Combining these with **healthy fats** might help if a supplement also includes forms of vitamin B3, but it's not strictly necessary.
Synergistic Nutrients: Some people combine NAD+ precursors with **resveratrol** (a compound in red wine) or **pterostilbene**, believing they may further support cellular health. Adequate **vitamin B levels** also support overall NAD+ metabolism.

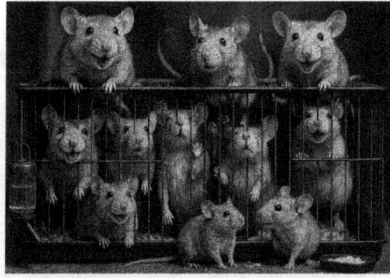

"A group of mice that were put on NMN late in life are getting very old. In fact, only seven out of the original forty mice are still alive, but they are all healthy and still moving happily around the cage. The number of mice alive that didn't get the NMN? Zero." – Dr. David Sinclair

OVERDOSE POTENTIAL:

There are no well-documented cases of severe toxicity in humans. Extremely high doses could theoretically cause **liver stress** or digestive discomfort, but more research is needed. If you notice unusual symptoms like persistent nausea, headaches, or fatigue, consider reducing the dose or discontinuing it and consulting a healthcare professional.

8.1.2: SENOLYTICS (FISETIN, DASATINIB, AND QUERCETIN)

CLEARING SENESCENT (ZOMBIE) CELLS THAT ACCUMULATE WITH AGE

Senolytics (Fisetin, Dasatinib, and Quercetin) target "zombie" cells—older, malfunctioning cells that can linger in tissues and contribute to inflammation and aging. By helping the body remove these cellular stragglers, senolytics may support healthier aging processes.

FISETIN (A "berry" special helper)

Imagine your body is like a garden and sometimes weeds—called "zombie cells"—start to take over. Fisetin, found in strawberries and other fruits, is like a friendly gardener who helps clear those pesky weeds. Doing this may help keep your body's "garden" healthier, allowing your cells and tissues to stay vibrant for a longer time.

DIETARY SOURCES: Predominantly found in strawberries (the richest food source), apples, persimmons, onions, and cucumbers.

SUGGESTED DOSAGE: Human data is limited, but studies often use 100–500 mg daily in supplement form. Some experimental "senolytic protocols" involve higher intermittent doses (e.g., 20 mg/kg body weight for a few days).
Maximum Dosage: There is no established maximum. Safety data in humans at very high doses are lacking, so caution is advised.

SOLUBILITY: Fisetin is poorly water-soluble and can be better absorbed with dietary fat or a meal. Some formulations use unique complexes or absorption enhancers (e.g., piperine).

SYNERGY WITH OTHER SUBSTANCES: Often combined with Quercetin or other polyphenols. Taking it with a fat-containing meal may enhance its bioavailability.

OVERDOSE POTENTIAL: While fisetin appears relatively safe at moderate doses, its long-term safety at high doses is unknown. Toxicity studies in humans are still scarce.

DASATINIB (The professional cleanup crew)

Think of Dasatinib as a specialized cleaning team that only shows up when there's a big mess to clear. Originally used to help treat certain blood cancers, scientists are now exploring how it might help remove old, unhealthy "zombie cells" from our bodies. By packing these worn-out cells, Dasatinib could help keep our tissues working better, like a freshly cleaned classroom where everyone can learn without distractions.

DIETARY SOURCES: Dasatinib is a prescription medication, not a naturally occurring compound in foods.

SUGGESTED DOSAGE: Dasatinib is not typically recommended as a daily supplement. In research for senolytic effects, off-label "D+Q" (Dasatinib + Quercetin) protocols have used doses around 50–100 mg of Dasatinib daily for one or two days per month, but this is strictly under clinical supervision.

Maximum Dosage: Medically speaking, this is a potent tyrosine kinase inhibitor with well-defined dosages in oncology. It should only be used under a physician's guidance outside of cancer treatment.

SOLUBILITY: Dasatinib is slightly more water-soluble than the average flavonoid but is still best absorbed with food.

SYNERGY WITH OTHER SUBSTANCES: Commonly paired with Quercetin in research studies to enhance senolytic effects ("D+Q protocol").

OVERDOSE POTENTIAL: Yes—Dasatinib is a prescription drug with known side effects. Overdosing can lead to serious complications, so it is not advisable to self-experiment.

QUERCETIN (The apple-and-onion defender)

Quercetin is a natural compound in apples, onions, and other colorful fruits and veggies. Picture it as a friendly guard in shining armor, patrolling your body for troublemakers. It fights off bad molecules called "free radicals" and teams up with other compounds to tackle those pesky zombie cells. Keeping these cells under control helps your body stay healthier, like a neighborhood watch that keeps your whole community safe.

DIETARY SOURCES: Apples, onions, grapes, berries, kale, broccoli, and many other colorful fruits and vegetables.

SUGGESTED DOSAGE: Common supplement dosages range from 250 to 1,000 mg per day. Some protocols in senolytic research use it intermittently with Dasatinib.

Maximum Dosage: There is no officially established upper limit; however, very high doses (2,000 mg or more daily) should be approached cautiously and under professional supervision.

SOLUBILITY: Quercetin is poorly water-soluble. It can be better absorbed with meals or a small amount of healthy dietary fat. Formulations like quercetin phytosome or Quercetin combined with bromelain can also improve absorption.

SYNERGY WITH OTHER SUBSTANCES: Often paired with Dasatinib for senolytic purposes. It is also regularly combined with vitamin C or bromelain for better absorption and enhanced antioxidant activity.

OVERDOSE POTENTIAL: Quercetin appears to be relatively safe at moderate doses. However, high-dose long-term data are limited, so caution is warranted.

EARLY RODENT STUDIES SHOW LIFESPAN EXTENSION AND IMPROVED TISSUE FUNCTION

In animal research, these compounds have been associated with delaying age-related diseases and extending a healthy lifespan. Rodents given senolytics have shown enhanced physical function, reduced inflammation, and sometimes increased overall lifespan. However, translating these findings from rodents to humans is an ongoing study area.

RESEARCH ANECDOTE

Scientists at aging conferences often share unpublished data suggesting that senolytics may improve markers of cellular health in humans. Anecdotal reports from small pilot studies and case reports generate excitement, though much of this information has yet to go through extensive peer review or long-term trials.

SELF-EXPERIMENTATION IS RISKY; CONSULT PROFESSIONALS

Individual Variability: Genetics, medical history, and other factors can affect how one responds to these compounds.

Drug Interactions: Senolytics, especially prescription drugs like Dasatinib, may interact with other medications.

Side Effects and Monitoring: Blood tests or medical evaluations might be needed to check for potential liver or kidney stress, nutrient imbalances, or other issues.

SAFETY PROFILE NOT FULLY ESTABLISHED FOR LARGE-SCALE USE

Limited Human Trials: Most data come from in vitro (test tube) or animal studies. Human studies are small and short-term.

Unknown Long-Term Effects: We lack comprehensive data on possible risks when used over months or years.

Regulatory Status: Fisetin and Quercetin are available as dietary supplements but are not approved treatments for any age-related condition. Dasatinib is a prescription drug approved only for certain cancers.

I believe that we all strive for longevity to have more time to experience life, to see our loved one's lives come into fruition, to accomplish more, to stay with our family and friends for as long as possible. Within that reality is the realization that everything we experience will not be always positive, because that's how life works. Nobody knows this better than my friend **Tony Kaye**, legendary **David Bowie** keyboardist and founding member of the band **"Yes"**. **Tony** said:

"Everything that happens is meant to be. It's meant to happen like that. But sometimes you don't know at the time that it's meant to be a disaster."

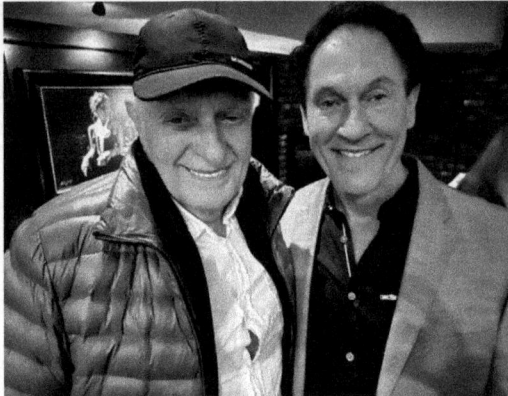

Tony Kaye and Tad Sisler
Source – Sisler Private Collection

No matter what life throws at us, we are breathing, and if we are breathing, I believe there is a reason why we are here. If you strive to live life to its fullest and prioritize love and family, you should be generally happy. These supplements along with new discoveries should give us an edge on extending our lifespans and healthspans.

8.1.3: OTHER POTENTIAL LONGEVITY AGENTS (RAPAMYCIN, METFORMIN)

RAPAMYCIN (The "Traffic Light" for Cell Growth)

Imagine a busy road in your body where cells are zooming around, growing and dividing. Rapamycin acts like a smart traffic light that can slow down this busy traffic when necessary. By telling cells to take a break, it may help them live longer and stay healthier, like cars that avoid crashes by following well-timed signals. Scientists have seen that animals taking rapamycin often live longer and have fewer age-related problems.

RAPAMYCIN TARGETS mTOR
SHOWN TO EXTEND LIFESPAN IN ANIMALS

Rapamycin blocks mTOR (mechanistic Target of Rapamycin), a protein involved in cell growth and metabolism. When mTOR activity is reduced, cells shift into "maintenance mode," which may slow aging processes. Research in mice, flies, and other organisms often shows lifespan extension and improved markers of health.

DIETARY SOURCES: There are no traditional "food" sources of rapamycin. It was initially discovered from a bacterium on Easter Island. Rapamycin is not available as a supplement; it's a pharmaceutical drug.

SUGGESTED DAILY DOSAGE AND MAXIMUM DOSAGE:

For Clinical Use: Rapamycin is usually prescribed to organ transplant patients to prevent rejection or investigated off-label in lower doses for potential anti-aging effects.

Anti-Aging Context: In preliminary research settings, doses often range from 1–6 mg once weekly or biweekly, but no standard anti-aging protocol exists yet.

Maximum Dosage: Because it's a potent immunosuppressant, higher doses can increase infection risk and other side effects. The dose must be individualized and closely monitored by a physician.

SOLUBILITY: Rapamycin is **poorly water-soluble**, so formulations often come as tablets or capsules designed to improve absorption.

SYNERGY WITH OTHER SUBSTANCES: Rapamycin is prescription-only and should be taken exactly as directed. Some physicians explore combining it with other compounds (e.g., metformin) to maximize longevity effects, but this is highly experimental.

OVERDOSE POTENTIAL: Yes. Rapamycin is a powerful drug that affects the immune system. Overdosing can lead to severe immunosuppression, mouth sores, poor wound healing, and other complications. Medical guidance is critical. Since it weakens immune responses, there's a higher chance of infections. It may also affect cholesterol levels and wound healing.

Prescription-Only: In most countries, it's illegal to obtain rapamycin without a prescription.

Early-Stage Anti-Aging Use: We do not have large-scale, long-term human trials confirming its safety or efficacy for general longevity.

"Does rapamycin suppress aging and extend lifespan by preventing diseases, or does it prevent diseases by slowing aging?
Actually, both reflect the same process."
— Mikhail V. Blagosklonny, quoted in NIH article

METFORMIN (The "Sugar Manager")

Think of metformin as a friendly coach in your body that helps keep your blood sugar levels on track. It reminds your cells not to let too much sugar pile up in your bloodstream. Originally used to help people with diabetes, scientists now wonder if it can also slow down aging. Early studies show that people on metformin sometimes age more gracefully and avoid some health troubles like a wise coach making sure everyone on the team is in top shape.

METFORMIN (A DIABETES DRUG) STUDIED FOR ANTI-AGING EFFECTS IN TAME TRIALS

Metformin improves how the body handles blood sugar and insulin, reducing inflammation and oxidative stress. Researchers hypothesize these effects may slow the aging process.

TAME (Targeting Aging with Metformin): This ongoing trial aims to see if metformin can delay age-related diseases (like heart disease, cancer, and dementia).

DIETARY SOURCES: Metformin is not found in foods—it's a synthetic medication initially derived from a compound in the French lilac plant (Galega officinalis). You cannot obtain it naturally through diet.

SUGGESTED DAILY DOSAGE AND MAXIMUM DOSAGE

Standard Use (Diabetes): Ranges from 500 mg to 2,000 mg per day, usually split into doses.

Anti-Aging Context: There is no officially established "anti-aging" dosage. Longevity researchers sometimes explore the lower end (e.g., 500–1,500 mg/day).

Cautions: Dosing should be tailored to kidney function and overall health. Always under physician guidance.

SOLUBILITY: Metformin is **water-soluble**. It's generally taken with meals to reduce stomach upset.

SAM ALTMAN

News outlets say *OpenAI* chief **Sam Altman** takes the diabetes drug **metformin** even though he isn't diabetic. He hopes it will "slow aging" while he eats well, exercises, and sleeps enough. **Sam** flies all over the world to talk about AI. Before take-off he pops a tiny metformin pill—like a secret battery booster—so his energy stays steady and his blood sugar doesn't bounce around. He still eats veggies and works out, but he's curious whether the pill will help him stay sharp for decades. Scientists remind him big studies are still in progress, so **Sam** treats it as an experiment, not a magic cure.

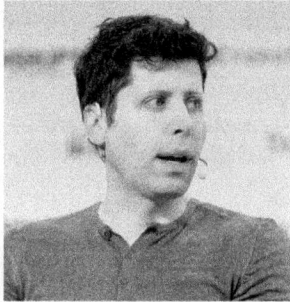

Sam Altman
Credit – Wikimedia Commons

SYNERGY WITH OTHER SUBSTANCES: It's typically taken with food to minimize gastrointestinal side effects. Some longevity researchers explore combining metformin with other compounds (e.g., rapamycin, supplements) but robust data on synergy are lacking.

OVERDOSE POTENTIAL: Yes. Taking too much metformin can lead to a serious condition called lactic acidosis, which can be life-threatening. Proper medical supervision is essential.

Side Effects: Commonly includes stomach upset, diarrhea, and vitamin B12 deficiency over the long term. Regular monitoring can help manage these issues.

Prescription-Only: Similar to rapamycin, metformin typically requires a doctor's prescription in most countries.

Ongoing Research: While some observational studies show people on metformin may live longer or have fewer age-related diseases, the TAME trial is expected to provide more definitive data.

Self-Experimentation is Risky: These drugs can have significant side effects, and they're not officially approved for "anti-aging" usage. Always consult a qualified healthcare provider. Both rapamycin and metformin are at the forefront of longevity research. While early data are compelling, large-scale, long-term human studies are still underway to confirm their benefits, ideal doses, and safety profiles. Although it is generally considered a diabetes drug, some believe that it also has cancer-thwarting potential.

"Metformin may have already saved more people from cancer deaths than any drug in history." – Lewis Cantley, director of the Meyer Cancer Center at Weill Cornell Medical College

8.1.4: AMPK ACTIVATOR SUPPLEMENTS

Supplements mentioned here are also highlighted in other sections.

AMPK (Adenosine Monophosphate-Activated Protein Kinase)

Imagine your body is a busy city, and energy is like the cars driving around to deliver supplies. AMPK is the traffic cop who directs these cars. When traffic is smooth, cells get the energy they need, and everything works well. But sometimes, there isn't enough energy, or there's a big traffic jam. That's when AMPK steps in and tells your cells to make more energy or save the energy they already have. AMPK activator supplements are like special instructions that remind the traffic cop to keep things running smoothly. They help your body manage weight, improve how cells work, and can even copy some of the good things that happen when you eat less or exercise more.

Known as the "metabolic master switch," AMPK helps maintain cellular energy balance by boosting energy production (catabolism) and reducing energy consumption (anabolism).

Proper AMPK function supports healthy metabolism, weight management, and overall cellular health. It's also been studied for its potential role in longevity, as it can mimic some benefits of calorie restriction and exercise.

DR. PETER ATTIA

On his podcast *The Drive*, longevity expert **Dr. Peter Attia** shares that he takes **berberine** (an AMPK booster) for metabolic health and discusses research showing it can mimic some benefits of exercise on energy use.

Over weeks he sees steadier energy lines and slightly lower cholesterol, so he keeps the pill in his routine—while reminding listeners that healthy food and workouts still matter.

ACTIVATING AMPK: HEALTH BENEFITS

Improved Metabolic Health: AMPK activation can enhance how the body processes sugars and fats, helping maintain balanced blood sugar and cholesterol levels—and reducing the potential risk of type 2 diabetes, metabolic syndrome, and related issues.

Weight Management: When AMPK is "turned on," it prompts the body to turn to using stored fat for energy. It could potentially support healthy weight loss or maintenance alongside diet and exercise.

Enhanced Cellular Function: AMPK helps cells clean up and recycle old or damaged parts, improving overall cell efficiency. It may benefit longevity and slow down specific age-related declines.

Mimics Effects of Calorie Restriction & Exercise: Both fasting (or eating fewer calories) and exercise naturally boost AMPK. Supplements that activate AMPK may offer some of those same benefits. Individuals see potential improvements in energy levels, metabolic health, and cellular resilience.

DIETARY SOURCES

There isn't a single "AMPK supplement" derived from one plant or vitamin, although I have seen "AMPK ACTIVATOR" supplements on the market. Several known compounds can activate AMPK. Here are some you might find in supplement blends:

Berberine (from barberry, goldenseal, or Oregon grape root)

Resveratrol (found in grapes, red wine, and some berries)

EGCG (Epigallocatechin Gallate) (from green tea)

Alpha-lipoic acid (ALA) (found in small amounts in spinach, broccoli, and organ meats)

Curcumin (from turmeric) – mild AMPK activation in some studies

While these are found naturally in foods, many people use concentrated supplements for a stronger AMPK effect.

SUGGESTED DAILY DOSAGE AND MAXIMUM DOSAGE

No Universal AMPK Dose: Because "AMPK activator" is a broad category, the dosages depend on which compound you're taking.

Berberine: Often taken in 500 mg doses 2–3 times daily (1,000–1,500 mg total).

Resveratrol: Typical supplement doses range from 100–500 mg daily.

EGCG: Could range from 200–400 mg daily.

ALA: Commonly 300–600 mg daily.

Maximum Dosage: Safe upper limits vary by compound. For instance, berberine shouldn't exceed ~2,000 mg/day in most guidelines. Exceeding recommended doses can lead to digestive distress or other side effects. Always check reputable sources or consult a healthcare provider.

SOLUBILITY

Berberine: Moderately water-soluble but can still be challenging to absorb; often recommended with a meal or in divided doses.

Resveratrol: Not very water-soluble; some prefer "micronized" or specialized formulations to enhance absorption.

EGCG: Water-soluble (it's a green tea extract), but taking it with meals may reduce stomach upset.

ALA: Somewhat water-soluble but also functions in both fat and water environments. Typically taken on an empty stomach for best absorption.

Because each compound has different absorption characteristics, following product instructions is important.

SYNERGY WITH OTHER SUBSTANCES

Many AMPK activator supplements include additional ingredients to enhance bioavailability or complementary effects:

Piperine (Black Pepper Extract): Often used with curcumin or resveratrol to boost absorption.

Healthy Fats: Fat-soluble ingredients may absorb better with a small amount of fat in a meal.

Synergistic Blends: You'll sometimes see berberine combined with alpha-lipoic acid or resveratrol for multi-faceted metabolic support.

OVERDOSE POTENTIAL

Potential for Overuse: While generally safe at recommended dosages, too much of any AMPK-activating compound can lead to gastrointestinal distress, interference with medications, or, in the case of berberine, possible liver enzyme modulation.

Medication Interactions: This is especially true for berberine, which can affect how the liver processes certain drugs.

Medical Supervision: People with diabetes, liver conditions, or chronic illnesses should consult a professional before use.

Lifestyle Matters: While supplements can support AMPK activity, exercise, and eating a balanced diet remain key factors in metabolic health. Stay positive, and enjoy each moment as much as you can. My old friend, iconic entertainer **Trini Lopez** had a string of hits, selling millions of records, and he was a favorite of **President John F. Kennedy**. **Trini** said:

"Everything is attitude. It's very important to always like what you're doing."

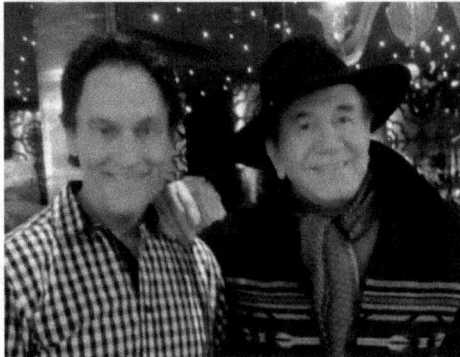

Tad Sisler with Trini Lopez
Source – Sisler Private Collection

Research Is Ongoing: Although many studies show promise, large-scale clinical trials are still underway to confirm the long-term benefits of AMPK activators for longevity.

Quality & Purity: Look for reputable brands that perform third-party testing to make sure the supplement meets quality standards. As you work towards a healthier lifestyle, remember that your attitudes and emotions can be another factor in your overall health. For instance, it's been said that anger is an acid that eats its own container.

8.1.5: CURRENT CLINICAL TRIALS

Clinical trials are critical for validating the safety and efficacy of longevity compounds like NAD+ precursors, senolytics, rapamycin, metformin, and AMPK activators. As of May 2025, numerous studies are exploring their potential to extend healthspan and combat age-related diseases. While early results are promising, many trials are ongoing, and consulting a healthcare provider is essential before use. In my book **Stay Healthy, Stay Youthful: The Science of Living to 150: Cutting-Edge Longevity Science for Reversing Aging and Living a Healthier, Longer Life**, I go into great detail about these and other exciting developments in longevity research.

NAD+ PRECURSORS

Nicotinamide Mononucleotide (NMN): A 2024 phase II trial (n=80, ages 60–75) showed NMN (500 mg/day for 12 weeks) improved muscle strength and insulin sensitivity in older adults. A 2025 trial is investigating NMN's effects on cardiovascular health, with results expected in 2026.

Nicotinamide Riboside (NR): The 2023 NADPARK trial (n=30) found NR (1000 mg/day) increased brain NAD+ levels and reduced Parkinson's symptoms after 30 days. A 2025 phase III trial is testing NR for cognitive decline in mild cognitive impairment.

SENOLYTICS

Dasatinib and Quercetin: The SToMP-AD trial (2025, n=200) is evaluating this combination for Alzheimer's disease, aiming to reduce senescent cell burden and slow cognitive decline. Early data suggest improved biomarkers after 12 weeks.

Fisetin: A 2024 trial (n=60, ages 65+) reported fisetin (20 mg/kg for 2 days monthly) reduced senescent cells and improved physical function in frail elderly. Further trials are exploring osteoarthritis benefits.

RAPAMYCIN

The 2023 PEARL trial in dogs (n=50) showed rapamycin extended healthspan by improving immune function. Human trials in 2025 are testing low-dose rapamycin (5 mg/week) for skin aging and immune modulation, with interim results indicating reduced inflammatory markers.

METFORMIN

The TAME trial, launched in 2024 (n=3,000, ages 65–79), is assessing metformin's ability to delay age-related diseases like diabetes and dementia. Interim data from 2025 suggest improved metabolic markers, with full results expected by 2027.

AMPK ACTIVATORS

Compounds like AICAR are in preclinical stages, with a 2024 mouse study showing enhanced muscle endurance and reduced inflammation. Human phase I trials are planned for 2026 to evaluate safety and efficacy in aging populations.

SECTION TWO: PEPTIDES, GENE THERAPIES, AND PLASMA APPROACHES

8.2.1: PEPTIDE THERAPIES (e.g. EPITHALON, THYMOSIN) AND POLYAMINES (SPERMIDINE)

WHAT ON EARTH IS A PEPTIDE?

Picture a tiny string of beads. Each bead is an amino acid; the whole string is a peptide. In nature, peptides act like text messages between cells: "Grow." "Repair." "Fight germs." Scientists can now copy—or slightly tweak—those messages in the lab. Two of the buzziest names are **Epithalon** and **Thymosin**.

EPITHALON (A "Timekeeper" for Your Cells)

Every time a cell divides, the protective tips on its DNA—called telomeres—get a little shorter, like frayed shoelaces. Early animal studies hint that Epithalon might slow that fraying. Fans call it a "time-keeper." Reality check: human trials are tiny, doses vary, and most countries treat Epithalon as a prescription-only research drug. If you ever see it for sale online, remember: quality is a roll of the dice and legality is murky.

THYMOSIN (Your Immune System's "Drill Sergeant")

Your thymus gland trains T-cells, the soldiers that spot viruses and rogue cells. Thymosin peptides (alpha-I or beta-4) act like refresher courses for those troops. Doctors sometimes use them in very specific immune disorders or wound care, but the leap to "anti-aging tonic" is still experimental. Again, injections under medical supervision are the norm; grocery-store gummies are pure fantasy.

DIETARY SOURCES: Both peptides are lab-made; you can't munch kale and get Epithalon.

SUGGESTED DAILY DOSAGE: Biohackers trade protocols—10-20 days, a few milligrams—but science hasn't settled on a gold standard.

QUALITY ROULETTE: Reputable clinics test every vial; shady websites may ship salt water—or worse.

POLYAMINES: SPERMADINE (The Cell "Housekeeper")

Switching gears to something you can actually eat: **spermidine**, a polyamine found in wheat germ, aged cheese, soy, and mushrooms. Inside cells it nudges a clean-up process called autophagy—think spring-cleaning for worn-out parts. Early human data suggest 1–10 mg a day (food or supplement) looks safe and may support heart and brain health. It won't rewind decades overnight, but adding wheat-germ flakes to oatmeal is an easy, tasty experiment.

SOLUBILITY: Spermidine is water-soluble, making it relatively easy to absorb via diet or supplements.

SYNERGY WITH OTHER SUBSTANCES: Spermadine is often discussed alongside fasting protocols or calorie restriction mimetics because of its role in promoting autophagy—a "cellular cleanup" process. Rapamycin and Spermadine have been shown to work together to strengthen their overall effects.

"Messenger molecules – known as peptides, which were known to send and register information around the brain – are also in organs throughout your body, including your intestines, stomach, heart, liver, kidneys, and spine. These organs also send and register information." – Marcia Conner

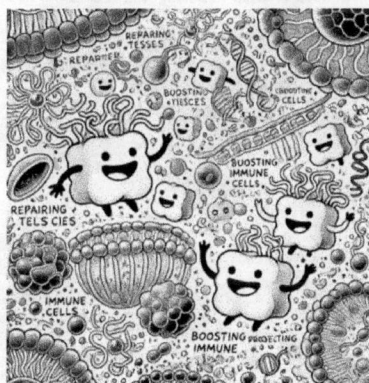

8.2.2: GENE EDITING (CRISPR) AND SiRNA

Although gene editing has really nothing to do with supplements, it's another amazing tool in the arsenal of new developments and possibilities in curing disease and promoting overall health. I go into much greater detail on this in my book **Stay Healthy, Stay Youthful: The Science of Living to 150.**

Imagine your DNA as a 3-billion-letter cookbook. A single misspelled word can ruin the recipe and cause disease. **CRISPR** is the spell-checker that can cut out the typo and paste in the right letter. **siRNA** is more like a sticky note that covers a bad sentence so it can't be read.

Where we are now: Doctors have used CRISPR to treat a handful of patients with sickle-cell disease and beta-thalassemia—promising but very controlled trials. No home kits, no over-the-counter sprays.

Why it matters for aging: Some scientists dream of editing age-accelerating genes or dialing down inflammation genes with siRNA. That's years—maybe decades—away, and every step raises big ethical questions: Who gets access? Could edits pass to future generations?

Bottom line: Follow the news, cheer the progress, but remember this is hospital-grade science, not a supplement aisle purchase.

Many people believed that strides like gene editing were never going to happen, but as time goes by, we are finding that this is just the tip of the iceberg in decoding the human genome. New, exciting discoveries are on the horizon. Never let anyone tell you it can't be done. A great example of someone who lives this admonition is my friend, *NBA* basketball legend **Earvin "Magic" Johnson.** **Magic** said:

> *"I tell people to look at me and understand that everybody first told me that I couldn't be a 6-foot, 9-inch point guard, and I proved them wrong. Then they told me I couldn't be a businessman and make money in urban America, and I proved them wrong. And they thought I couldn't win all these championships, and I proved them wrong there as well. To me, everything is wonderful. Life is wonderful."*

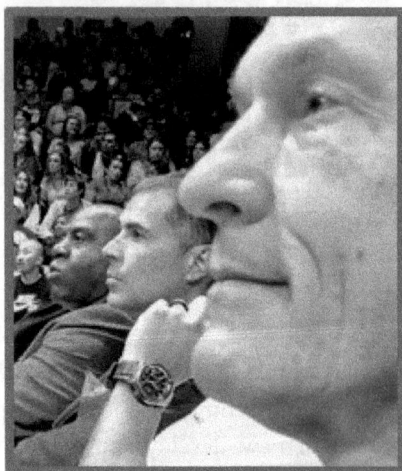

Tad Sisler on the L.A. Lakers Bench with Magic Johnson
Source – Sisler Private Collection

8.2.3: PLASMA EXCHANGE / APHERESIS

Think of your bloodstream as the water in a fish tank. Over time waste builds up. **Plasma exchange (apheresis)** siphons out the "old" liquid part of blood and replaces it with fresh donor plasma or a clean solution. Mouse studies where old and young blood were swapped sparked headlines about reversing aging. Human trials are tiny and mixed; the procedure is pricey and carries infection risks.

REMOVING PRO-AGING FACTORS FROM THE BLOOD

The core theory behind plasma exchange is that specific proteins and molecules in older blood may accelerate aging or worsen disease conditions. By filtering out a patient's plasma (the liquid part of our blood) and replacing it with fresh or specially treated plasma, doctors hope to reduce these harmful substances. Early studies suggest this might help improve overall health or slow age-related decline, though much more research is needed.

Some dedicated research groups and philanthropists are supporting trials examining how plasma exchange affects older individuals. For example, an organization might fund studies that recruit older adults with specific conditions, testing whether regular plasma exchange sessions help improve their energy levels, cognitive function, or other health markers.

STILL IN EXPERIMENTAL STAGES

Despite the excitement, plasma exchange for anti-aging is far from routine. Currently, it's considered highly experimental, with limited clinical evidence to prove its long-term safety and benefits. Most treatments still occur under strict research conditions or in specialized settings. As a result, it's not something a doctor would typically prescribe for everyday aging concerns.

"A healthy body means a healthy mind. You get your heart rate up, and you get the blood flowing through your body to your brain. Look at Albert Einstein. He rode a bicycle. He was also an early student of Jazzercise. You never saw Einstein lift his shirt, but he had a six-pack under there." – Steve Carell

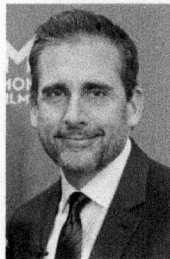

Steve Carell
Credit – Wikimedia Commons

WEIGH RISKS (e.g., Infection, Mismatch) IN ANY BLOOD-BASED PROCEDURE

Procedures involving blood carry inherent risks, including infection or reactions due to mismatched blood products. Plasma exchange also requires sterile conditions and careful monitoring to prevent complications like clotting problems or allergic reactions. Individuals exploring these treatments must work closely with medical professionals, ensuring that any potential benefits outweigh the known risks.

8.2.4: ETHICAL CONSIDERATIONS IN GENE THERAPIES

Gene editing technologies like CRISPR hold potential to treat age-related diseases and extend lifespan, but they raise significant ethical challenges. Addressing these ensures safe and fair use.

SAFETY CONCERNS

CRISPR's precision has improved, but off-target effects risk unintended genetic changes, potentially causing health issues. A 2025 *Nature Biotechnology* review emphasizes rigorous testing to minimize risks. Long-term studies are needed to confirm safety.

ACCESSIBILITY AND FAIRNESS

Gene therapies are costly, potentially limiting access to wealthy individuals. A 2025 WHO report calls for policies to ensure fair distribution, preventing health disparities. Subsidies and global collaboration are proposed solutions.

GERMLINE EDITING

Editing genes passed to future generations raises concerns about consent and ecological impacts on the gene pool. A 2025 *Nature Ethics* article advocates for a moratorium on germline editing until ethical frameworks are established.

ENHANCEMENT VS. THERAPY

Using gene editing to extend lifespan beyond normal limits blurs the line between therapy and enhancement. A 2025 *Science* debate questions whether aging is a disease, impacting regulatory approaches. Public input is crucial to define boundaries. It's inevitable that rogue laboratories or nations will ignore regulations, but still a framework must be in place.

REGULATORY OVERSIGHT

In 2025, the FDA and EMA have updated guidelines for gene therapies, requiring extensive safety data. A 2025 WEF consortium emphasizes transparency and public engagement to guide ethical development.

Balancing innovation with ethical oversight ensures gene therapies benefit humanity responsibly. Public dialogue and robust regulations are key to a fair future.

SECTION THREE: PRACTICAL CONSIDERATIONS AND RESPONSIBLE USE

8.3.1: REGULATORY AND ETHICAL DIMENSIONS

Regulation reality – Many peptides and gene tools are prescription-only or research-only. If a website sells them like candy, be skeptical.

Hype detector – A single mouse study does not equal a human breakthrough. Always look for peer-reviewed, placebo-controlled trials.

Doctor partnership – Blood tests, liver panels, and honest symptom logs keep experiments from becoming accidents.

Listen to the advice of professionals! They usually know what they're talking about. My old friend, legendary broadcaster **Larry King** once said:

"I remind myself every morning: Nothing I say this day will teach me anything. So, if I'm going to learn, I must do it by listening."

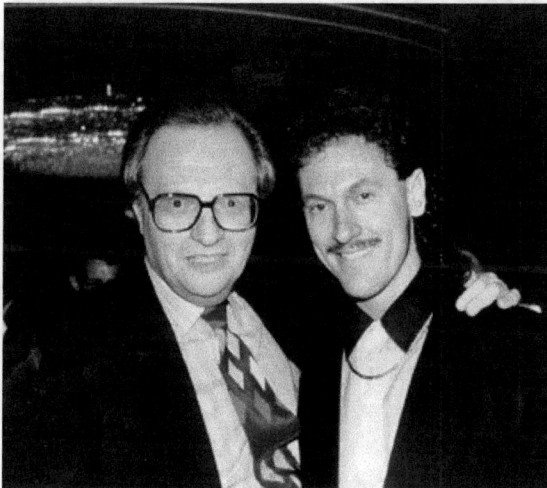

Larry King and Tad Sisler
Source – Sisler Personal Collection

8.3.2: LIFESTYLE INTEGRATION WITH EMERGING SCIENCE

COMPOUNDS ARE SUPPLEMENTS TO - NOT REPLACEMENTS FOR - DIET, EXERCISE, AND SLEEP

Even though they are promising, emerging longevity compounds cannot compensate for the foundational pillars of health. A balanced diet, consistent physical activity, and adequate rest are what you need the most. Think of these lifestyle habits as the "fuel" for your body—without them, even the best new compound can't perform at its full potential.

FASTING, CALORIC RESTRICTION, AND LOW-STRESS LIVING CAN AMPLIFY SUPPLEMENT BENEFITS

Research shows intermittent fasting or mild caloric restriction can trigger cellular repair mechanisms that improve metabolic health. When combined with stress-reduction techniques—like meditation or regular social interaction—these methods may enhance the effectiveness of supplements aimed at longevity.

PSYCHOLOGICAL ASPECTS (STRESS MANAGEMENT, COMMUNITY) ALSO IMPACT LONGEVITY

Chronic stress can undermine even the most carefully crafted supplement routine, leading to hormonal imbalances and a weakened immune system. Make time for hobbies, nurture your relationships, and seek help when you need it.

Life is easier when you have added stamina. Legendary punk singer **Wendy O. Williams** said:

"The important thing is to build up my cardiovascular system, so I have the stamina to do stunts. To me, stepping over the line, taking a chance and succeeding is the ultimate freedom, be it in rock and roll or when executing a really challenging routine."

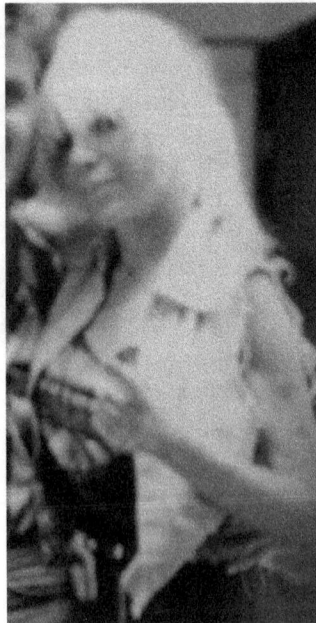

Wendy O. Williams
Credit – Wikimedia Commons

8.3.3: MONITORING AND FOLLOW-UP

REGULAR BLOOD TESTS (Lipids, Glucose, Hormone Levels) TO TRACK CHANGES

Get basic lab work—cholesterol, blood sugar, and key hormones—at least once a month when you first start a new supplement. The numbers show if the product is helping or causing trouble. Once things look steady, you can stretch the tests to every two or three months.

GENETIC TESTING OR EPIGENETIC MARKERS IF EXPLORING ADVANCED ROUTES

If you want to go deeper, you can run a DNA test to see your inherited risks, or an epigenetic test to see how your habits are turning genes on or off. Do this with a knowledgeable doctor so the results make sense and you don't worry over nothing. One checkup a year is plenty for most people.

DOCUMENT SIDE EFFECTS OR IMPROVEMENTS

Write down what you take each day, the dose, how you feel, how you sleep, and any workouts. After a few weeks you'll spot patterns—like, *"I sleep better on days I skip the late coffee,"* or *"That new pill gives me headaches."*

BE PREPARED TO ADJUST OR DISCONTINUE

Everybody's body is different. If you notice side effects—anything from mild stomach upset to something more serious—lower the dose or stop and talk to your doctor. The goal is to feel better, not worse, so stay flexible and listen to your body.

Now we'll bridge cultural wisdom with modern science, diving into how different global traditions have shaped our understanding of herbs, poultices, and more.

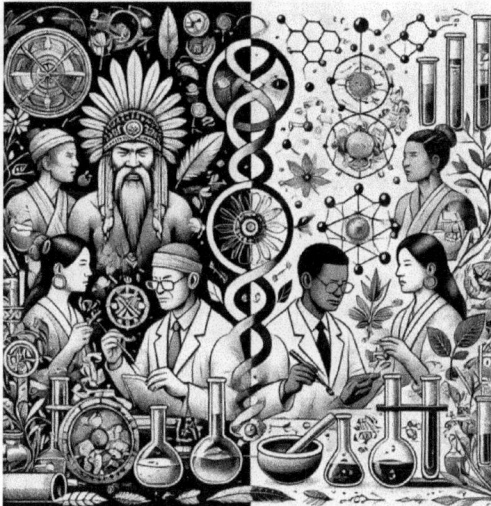

CHAPTER NINE
CULTURAL AND HISTORICAL PERSPECTIVES ON HEALTH AND LONGEVITY

From Traditional Chinese Medicine to Ayurvedic practices, many of today's top supplements trace back to ancient wisdom. Let's see how history informs modern approaches.

SECTION ONE: TRADITIONAL CHINESE MEDICINE (TCM) INSIGHTS
9.1.1: TCM HERBS
DANG GUI (Angelica sinensis)

Imagine you have a big, beautiful garden, and every day, you water it just enough so all the plants stay healthy and bright. Dang Gui is like special plant food that helps keep your "garden" (your body) well-watered and balanced—especially the parts that involve your blood. In TCM, people often use Dang Gui to help with blood circulation and to support women's health, such as easing menstrual discomfort. Think of it like a gentle teammate that allows your body's "blood river" to flow smoothly.

Why people take it: Women have used it for centuries to ease period cramps and balance iron after monthly blood loss. Older adults value it for warm hands and feet—signs that circulation is humming along.

Typical kitchen use: Grandparents slice 3–9 grams of the dried root—about the size of two almonds—drop it into chicken soup, and simmer for an hour. The broth tastes slightly sweet and earthy, like carrots mixed with celery.

Capsules for busy lives: A modern bottle often says "500 mg" per pill. Two pills with breakfast and dinner roughly equal a medium-strength tea.

How it behaves in the body: Its main chemicals dissolve in hot water, so soups, stews, and teas work well. Because it helps blood flow, very large amounts can thin blood too much. That's why TCM doctors cap single-herb doses around 15 grams a day.

Smart pairings: Practitioners often team Dang Gui with **Astragalus** (for energy) or a slice of fresh **ginger** (to warm the stomach). Eaten with food, it rarely upsets digestion.

When to be careful: If you bruise easily, have heavy periods, or already take aspirin, ask a doctor before adding Dang Gui. Too much could turn a paper cut into a long bleeder.

HUANG QIN (Scutellaria baicalensis)

Picture you're out playing on a warm day, and you come inside feeling overheated. Huang Qin is like a cool lemonade for your body. TCM practitioners use Huang Qin to help calm extra heat in the body and support your immune system. It's known for special substances (flavonoids) that can help with swelling and calmness inside the body. So, if your body is feeling "hot" or irritated, Huang Qin is often used to bring it back to a comfortable temperature.

Where it shines:
• Calming angry skin (eczema flare-ups, acne breakouts).
• Easing a hot, dry cough or irritated throat.
• Supporting the liver when spicy food or stress makes you feel inflamed inside.

How people brew it: Three to nine dried root slices—think french-fry size—simmered in a mug of water for 20 minutes. The tea tastes mildly bitter, like unsweetened cocoa. Adding a spoon of honey softens the edge.

Capsule math: One 500-mg capsule roughly equals half a teaspoon of powdered root. Two capsules, twice a day, copy the average tea dose.

Cooling but not freezing: Because it lowers "heat," taking more than 15 grams daily can make some folks feel cold, sluggish, or give them loose stools. People who already run chilly—cold hands, low appetite—should use smaller amounts or mix in warming herbs like **cinnamon twig**.

Fun science fact: Its star flavonoid, **baicalin**, has shown antioxidant power in lab tests, which modern researchers think explains the anti-redness effect.

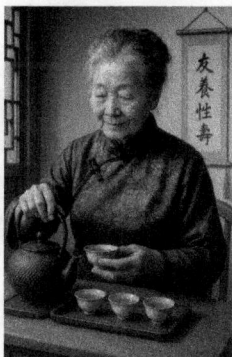

DAN SHEN (Salvia miltiorrhiza)

Imagine the roads in your city clogged with traffic—nobody can move, and everyone is getting upset. Dan Shen is like a traffic officer who helps clear up blockages so cars can move smoothly again. In TCM, Dan Shen promotes good blood flow, especially around the heart. It's often used to support cardiovascular health, like ensuring your heart and blood vessels have fewer "traffic jams" and more open roads.

Classic uses: Keeps tiny blood vessels around the heart and brain open and flexible. Breaks up old "traffic" (what TCM calls blood stasis) that can cause stabbing chest pain or lingering bruises.

Kitchen prep: Five to ten grams—about a tablespoon of broken root—boiled for 30 minutes makes a ruby-red tea. Some folks add a slice of orange peel for flavor.

Modern shortcuts: Pills or tinctures list doses of 500–1,000 mg, taken two or three times a day with meals.

Why dosing matters: Dan Shen can gently thin blood. That's good for flow, but if you're already on prescription blood thinners, doubling up can be risky. Doctors usually limit total daily raw herb to 15 grams.

Synergy star: TCM pairs Dan Shen with Dang Gui in a famous duo called **"Blood-Mover & Blood-Builder."** One keeps traffic moving, the other nourishes fresh red cells—like clearing the road and then sending a fuel truck.

"If there is free flow, there is no pain; if there is pain, there is lack of free flow." – Huang Di Nei Jing

9.1.2: QI, YIN, AND YANG EXPLAINED BRIEFLY
QI (Vital Energy)

Imagine your body is like a bustling city, where roads and highways carry food, water, and electricity to every building. In Traditional Chinese Medicine (TCM), **Qi** is like the steady flow of electricity that powers the entire city. When your Qi is balanced, you have enough energy to do your favorite activities, think clearly in school, and fight off sickness. But if the flow gets blocked or runs low, it's like having a blackout—your "city" can't function well, and you might feel tired, stressed, or sick more easily.

"Yin and yang, male and female, strong and weak, rigid and tender, heaven and earth, light and darkness, thunder and lightning, cold and warmth, good and evil... the interplay of opposite principles constitutes the universe." – Confucius

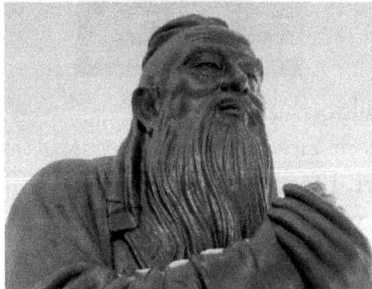

Confucius
Credit – Erika Wittlieb / Pixabay / Creative Commons 1.0 Universal Public Domain License

YIN (Cooling, Nourishing Energy)

Think of **Yin** as a calm, refreshing lake in the middle of a hot summer day. It represents coolness, moisture, and rest. Yin helps keep your body and mind from overheating, both physically—like preventing a fever—and emotionally—like stopping you from feeling too restless or anxious. When Yin is balanced, you feel relaxed and comfortable, and your body can heal and rebuild itself. If you don't have enough Yin, it's like a lake drying up in the sun—you might feel overheated, restless, or even dehydrated.

YANG (Warming, Active Energy)

Now, picture **Yang** as a campfire on a chilly night. It brings warmth, light, and energy to stay alert and strong. Yang helps your body move, digest food, and motivate you. When Yang is in balance, you have the drive to play sports, do your homework, or go out with friends, and your body stays warm and active. If Yang is too low, it's like trying to cook over a tiny flame—you'll feel tired and cold. But if Yang is too high, you might feel too hot or irritable, almost like standing too close to a big bonfire.

HOW THESE HERBS FIT IN

• Dang Gui feeds the river (blood) so Qi has something to push.
• Huang Qin pours ice into the lake when Yin is drying up.
• Dan Shen fans the campfire just enough to keep traffic flowing without overheating the system.

A seasoned TCM practitioner looks at your tongue, checks your pulse, and decides which teammate needs coaching. Then they build a custom "tea roster," mixing warming, cooling, or moving herbs so the trio stays balanced.

SAFETY TIPS WRAPPED IN COMMON SENSE

Buy clean herbs – Choose brands that lab-test for heavy metals and pesticides. Look for GMP or third-party certificates.

Start small, listen hard – Begin with the low end of any dose range. Note how you sleep, digest, and feel for a week before increasing.

Tell your doctor – Especially if you're on heart meds, diabetes drugs, or blood thinners. Herbs are powerful; mixing without guidance is like wiring extra lights into a house without checking the fuse box.

Respect tradition – These plants earned their reputations over centuries. Treat them as allies, not quick fixes, and pair them with good food, movement, and sleep.

Used this way, TCM herbs become quiet partners—helping the garden grow, cooling the system when it overheats, and clearing traffic so life's energy can roll on without jams.

KOBE BRYANT

Through my dear friend, *L.A. Lakers* coach **Frank Hamblen**, I was blessed to meet and share the same stage with legendary *NBA* Hall-of-Famer **Kobe Bryant** before his tragic passing. Late in his career, **Kobe Bryant** felt worn out from back-to-back games and a painful ankle sprain. Lakers nutritionist **Dr. Cate Shanahan** introduced him to a **Chinese medicinal bone-broth recipe** simmered with herbs that boost Qi and rebuild "essence." **Kobe** drank a steaming mug before practices. Reporters noticed he bounced back in just two missed games, and **Kobe** called the brew his Stone-Age secret for fresh legs and steadier energy through the season.

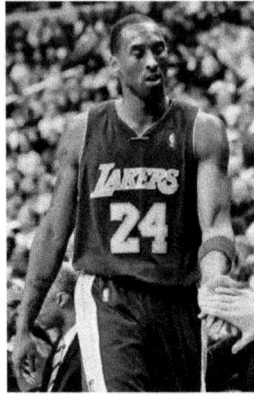

Kobe Bryant
Credit – Wikimedia Commons

9.1.3: KEY TCM FORMULAS (XAIO YAO SAN, LIU WEI DI HUANG WAN) AND LONGEVITY HERBS (JIAOGULAN)

XIAO YAO SAN ("Free & Easy Wanderer Powder")

Think of carrying an over-stuffed backpack all day—books, laptop, half-eaten snacks. Your shoulders ache and your mood sours. Xiao Yao San is the friend who takes half the load, lets you roll your shoulders, and says, *"Breathe! You've got this."*

Why TCM uses it

• Smooths stuck Qi that shows up as tension headaches, PMS cramps, or that cranky "don't-talk-to-me" feeling.

• Calms a jumpy stomach when stress makes digestion gurgle or stall.

Typical dose & taste

Two to three little tea-pills, three times a day, equal about 6 grams of powdered herbs. In loose powder, stir a rounded teaspoon into warm water; it tastes mildly sweet and earthy—like chamomile with a hint of licorice.

When to be careful

If you already run super-tired or very cold, ask a practitioner to tweak the mix (they'll often add a warming herb so you don't feel drained). Serious depression or sharp, stabbing pain needs medical evaluation first; this formula is gentle, not a stand-alone for big red-flag symptoms.

LIU WEI DI HUANG WAN ("Six-Ingredient Pill with Rehmannia")
Garden-roots for your body's battery

Picture your body as a tall oak tree. The leaves are your energy; the roots are your deep reserves (kidneys in TCM talk). Overwork, late nights, or aging can dry out the roots. This six-herb combo is like a slow-release fertilizer that soaks down and feeds the root system so the whole tree perks up.

Core benefits

• Recharges deep fatigue—the "I slept eight hours but still feel empty" kind.
• Moistens dryness: achy lower back, ringing ears, night sweats, dry eyes.

How people take it

Classic honeyed pills: 8–10 tiny pellets, twice a day. Modern capsules: about 1 gram of extract, two or three times daily. Because it's nourishing (and a bit heavy), people often swallow it after meals, not on an empty stomach.

Caution flags

Very damp digestion—think thick tongue coating, loose stools—may need a lighter version. If you're on prescription diuretics or thyroid meds, share the formula with your doctor so dosing can be spaced safely.

CASE STUDY

Meet **Eugenia**, a college student who felt "on edge" all the time—snappy with friends, irritable at small things, and frequently battling stomach cramps near her monthly cycle. After starting Xiao Yao San under the guidance of her TCM practitioner, **Eugenia** noticed her mood evened out within a few weeks. She felt calmer, her stomach aches reduced, and she was more patient during group projects. *"It's like my emotional backpack isn't so heavy anymore,"* she said. Xiao Yao San can be a gentle, natural option for supporting emotional balance, especially when stress and mild digestive issues go hand-in-hand.

LONGEVITY HERBS LIKE JIAOGULAN
Meet the mountain vine

In remote Chinese villages, elders sip a leafy tea called jiaogulan every morning. Locals joke that it keeps the grand-grand-grandparents working the rice fields. Scientists later found gypenosides—plant cousins to the ginsenosides in ginseng—that may support heart health, blood sugar, and stress resilience.

How to brew

Drop three or four dried leaves into hot (not boiling) water; steep five minutes. The flavor is mildly sweet, like green tea with a hint of licorice. Two cups a day is a common folk dose. Capsules run 200–400 mg once or twice daily.

Safety notes

Side-effects are rare but large amounts can loosen stools or lower blood pressure a little. Start with one cup and see how you feel. Pregnant women should wait—no solid safety data yet.

"If you ask what is the most single important key to longevity, I would have to say it is avoiding worry, stress, and tension. And if you didn't ask me, I'd still have to say it." — George Burns

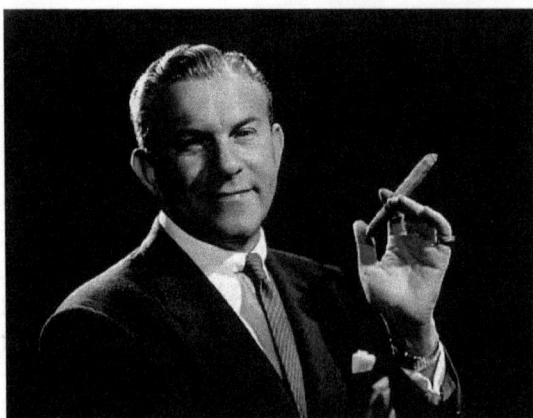

George Burns
Credit – Flickr / creativecommons.org / 2.0

SECTION TWO:
AYURVEDA AND OTHER GLOBAL TRADITIONS
9.2.1: AYURVEDIC STAPLES (AMLA, NEEM, GUDUCHI, GOTU KOLA)

AMLA IS RICH IN VITAMIN C, REVERED FOR REJUVENATION

Imagine you have a magic lemon that never seems to lose its sour power and bursts with vitamins. **Amla**, or Indian gooseberry, is like that—it's a small, green fruit incredibly high in vitamin C and antioxidants. In Ayurveda, people believe eating amla regularly can help you stay strong, keep your hair shiny, and protect you from getting sick, almost like a superhero shield for your body.

DIETARY SOURCES AND FORMS:

FRESH AMLA FRUIT: Eat raw or pickled. It can be pretty sour, so many people enjoy it with salt or spices.

AMLA POWDER: Used in smoothies, juices, or stirred into warm water.

AMLA OIL (HAIR & SKIN): Applied externally for hair nourishment or as a skin conditioner.

SUGGESTED DAILY DOSAGE AND MAXIMUM DOSAGE:
POWDER: 1–3 grams daily (about ½ to 1 teaspoon). Some traditional Ayurvedic regimens may go higher, up to 5 grams, but too much can cause stomach upset.
JUICE: 10–20 ml (about 2–4 teaspoons) diluted in water once or twice daily. Always follow product labels or a practitioner's guidance, as it's possible to experience **mild acidity or heartburn** if over-consumed.

SOLUBILITY: Amla's vitamin C is **water-soluble**, meaning it dissolves in liquids (like water or juice). Amla oil is used more for external applications (hair and scalp).

SYNERGY WITH OTHER SUBSTANCES: Consuming amla with honey or warm water can help balance the sour taste and make it easier on the stomach. In Ayurveda, it's often combined in poly-herbal formulas (e.g., Triphala).

OVERDOSE POTENTIAL: Amla is generally safe, but **excessive** intake may cause digestive discomfort or a drop in blood sugar for those on diabetic medications. Moderation is key.

NEEM FOR SKIN HEALTH, ANTIBACTERIAL PROPERTIES
Think of **Neem** as a super "cleaning" tree. Its leaves, bark, and oil taste bitter, but that bitterness is powerful. It helps fight germs on your skin, in your mouth, and even in your gut. Neem is so famous for its germ-fighting abilities that people in India have used its twigs as toothbrushes for centuries. Using Neem is like having a team of tiny, tough soldiers defending you against bad bacteria.

DIETARY SOURCES AND FORMS:
NEEM LEAVES: Consumed fresh (though very bitter!) or dried/powdered in capsules.
NEEM OIL: Applied to the skin or used as a natural pesticide in gardening.
NEEM TOOTHPASTE OR MOUTHWASH: Popular for oral hygiene.

SUGGESTED DAILY DOSAGE AND MAXIMUM DOSAGE:
CAPSULES (POWDERED NEEM): 500 mg to 1 gram daily is a standard range.
NEEM OIL (EXTERNAL USE): A few drops on problem skin areas or mixed with a carrier oil. Pure neem oil is very potent and can irritate skin if used in large amounts. Internal use of Neem should be monitored; very high doses can affect liver function.

SOLUBILITY: The **active compounds** in Neem (like azadirachtin) are more **oil-soluble**, which is why neem oil is so potent. Powdered neem leaves can be steeped in water as a tea, but the bitter compounds may not dissolve entirely.

SYNERGY WITH OTHER SUBSTANCES: Neem is extremely **bitter**, so many people prefer it in capsules or mixed with a sweetener (like honey) for teas. Pairing Neem with turmeric or aloe can help soothe skin, but be mindful not to overdo it (too many potent herbs together can upset the stomach).

OVERDOSE POTENTIAL: Neem in moderate amounts is safe, but **high doses** or consuming concentrated neem oil internally can be toxic (especially for children, pregnant women, or those with existing liver/kidney issues). Always follow guidelines.

GUDUCHI (Tinospora cordifolia)

Picture a climbing vine that can survive in challenging places and stay fresh and green—that's **Guduchi**. In Ayurveda, it's called "Amrit," meaning "divine nectar," because it's believed to boost your immune system, help your body recover faster from illnesses, and keep you energized. Think of it like a trusted hiking rope that supports you when scaling the mountains of everyday life—helping you stay steady and safe.

DIETARY SOURCES AND FORMS:

Powdered Guduchi: Commonly sold as a fine powder made from dried stems or leaves. It can be mixed into warm water, smoothies, or taken in capsules.

Guduchi Decoction (Kadha): Traditional Ayurvedic practice: boiling cut stem pieces in water to extract active compounds. Often consumed as a tea or mixed with other herbs.

Capsules or Tablets are convenient for standardized dosage. Make sure to choose high-quality brands that test for purity and potency.

Guduchi Satva (Starch/Extract): A more concentrated form of guduchi; looks like a fine, white powder. It is used traditionally to help with issues like acid reflux or to cool the body.

SUGGESTED DAILY DOSAGE AND MAXIMUM DOSAGE:

General Range: 300–500 mg of standardized extract **once or twice daily** is typical for adult supplementation.

Powder Form: Around 1–3 grams daily, split into 2–3 doses.

Decoction: 1–2 cups daily (using roughly 3–6 grams of dried stem).

Maximum Dosage: Some practitioners may go higher (up to 5–6 grams of powder daily) for short periods, but it's best done under professional guidance.

Important: Individuals with chronic medical conditions (like autoimmune diseases or diabetes) should seek advice from a healthcare professional before taking higher doses.

SOLUBILITY: The beneficial compounds in guduchi (polysaccharides and some alkaloids) extract well in water, teas, or decoctions.

Alcohol-based tinctures may also be used for a higher concentration of certain constituents. Most constituents have minimal oil solubility, **so Guduchi is not commonly prepared as an oil infusion (unlike herbs such as Neem or ashwagandha).**

SYNERGY WITH OTHER SUBSTANCES

Combined with Other Ayurvedic Herbs: Often paired with **amla, turmeric,** or **ashwagandha** to amplify immune-support benefits and rejuvenation.

Dietary Pairings: Consuming guduchi with **warm water** or **warm milk** (depending on your constitution) can help carry its active ingredients throughout the body. Honey is sometimes added to offset bitterness in powder form.

OVERDOSE POTENTIAL: Guduchi is well-tolerated when used in moderate amounts.

Potential Side Effects: Large doses or prolonged high intake could lead to digestive upset (e.g., nausea, diarrhea). There's limited evidence of severe toxicity, but it's wise to stick to recommended dosages.

Caution for Certain Health Conditions: If you have an autoimmune condition (e.g., rheumatoid arthritis, lupus), be cautious with immune-stimulating herbs like guduchi. Always consult a qualified professional, especially if you're taking medications affecting blood sugar levels or the immune system.

GOTU KOLA FOR HEALING PROPERTIES

Imagine your body is like a busy town with roads, bridges, and buildings that sometimes get worn out or damaged. **Gotu Kola** is like the friendly repair team that helps patch these roads and ensure the bridges stay strong. It supports healing on the outside (helping with scars and skin health) and works on the inside by improving blood flow and allowing you to stay focused and calm. Think of it as a handy helper that goes around your body, fixing cracks, boosting your "mental power," and keeping everything running smoothly.

Healing & Circulation: Gotu kola is known for promoting wound healing, improving skin health, and supporting blood flow to the brain (memory). It's often used in creams for scars or varicose veins and in teas for mental clarity.

SUGGESTED DAILY DOSAGE AND MAXIMUM DOSAGE:

TEA OR DECOCTION: 1–2 cups daily (about 2–5 grams of dried leaves).
CAPSULES: Typically 300–500 mg twice daily.
Overuse might cause headaches, dizziness, or sedation—stay within recommended limits.

SOLUBILITY: **For higher potency,** Gotu Kola's active compounds (like triterpenoids) **can be extracted in water** via teas or alcohol-based tinctures.

SYNERGY WITH OTHER SUBSTANCES: Often combined with other herbs that support circulation and relaxation, such as ashwagandha or holy basil, but best to consult an Ayurvedic practitioner.

OVERDOSE POTENTIAL: Excessive amounts can lead to **drowsiness** or stomach upset. Use responsibly.

A FAMILY IN INDIA

Each morning, the **Desai** family in India gathers around their courtyard tree—an old **neem**. **Grandpa Desai** snips a twig for each family member, and they chew the end until it becomes a natural toothbrush. They say it helps keep their teeth strong and gums healthy. While the children scrunch up their faces at the bitter taste at first, they then smile knowing they've grown used to it, knowing it's been a family tradition passed down through generations.

Neem is deeply ingrained in daily life in India for oral care and overall hygiene, reflecting the broader Ayurvedic concept that nature provides the tools we need for health.

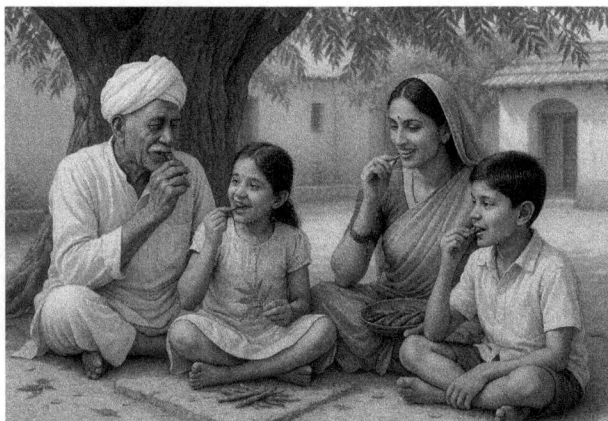

SOME AYURVEDIC REMEDIES HAVE ROBUST SCIENTIFIC BACKING, OTHERS LESS SO

Scientific Studies: Dozens of studies support the benefits of herbs like **Turmeric, Ashwagandha**, and **Ginger**. Promising research exists for amla, Neem, and gotu kola, but **more large-scale clinical trials** are often needed.

Use Evidence Wisely: Some claims (like Neem's antibacterial effect on skin) have decent scientific backing, while others (like specific "miraculous cures") may be more anecdotal.

Ask Questions: When you see an Ayurvedic product with grand promises, look for scientific references or third-party testing to confirm its quality and efficacy.

QUALITY CAN VARY; CHECK FOR CONTAMINANTS LIKE HEAVY METALS

Contamination Concerns: Poorly sourced Ayurvedic products can contain heavy metals (lead, arsenic, mercury) due to environmental pollution or improper manufacturing.

WHAT TO LOOK FOR::

REPUTABLE BRANDS: Choose products tested for purity (look for GMP or ISO certifications).

TRANSPARENT LABELS: Brands that list herb sourcing and lab testing are more reliable.

Avoid Cheap Unknowns: Super-cheap, unlabeled powders or oils are risky. Heavy metals can be very harmful, especially if taken over time.

"Because we cannot scrub our inner body we need to learn a few skills to help cleanse our tissues, organs, and mind. This is the art of Ayurveda."
-Sebastian Pole

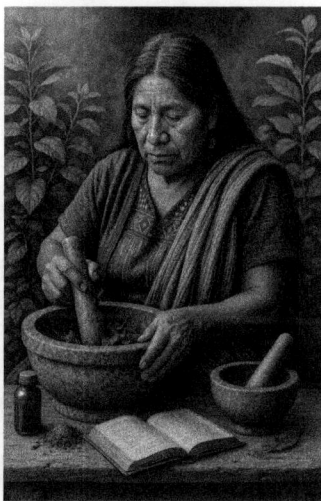

9.2.2: LATIN AMERICAN AND INDIGENOUS REMEDIES (GRAVIOLA, YERBA MATE)

GRAVIOLA (Soursop) – A FRIENDLY BODY GUARD DOG

Imagine a loyal guard dog standing outside your house, ready to bark and warn you of potential trouble. Some people believe that Graviola, also called soursop, acts like this for our bodies by helping our immune system stay on alert. It comes from a prickly green fruit that tastes sweet and tangy, often found in tropical places. While scientists are still studying how well it works, many people have used soursop leaves and fruits in traditional remedies to help keep their bodies strong.

Graviola is believed to support immune function, though research is inconclusive. It is commonly enjoyed as fruit or tea, but dosages aren't well-defined. Caution is advised for people on certain medications.

DIETARY SOURCES:
Primary Source: The fruit of the Annona muricata tree (soursop). It can be eaten fresh or used to make juices, smoothies, and desserts.
Leaves and Extracts: In some traditional practices, the leaves are brewed into teas or used to make supplements.

SUGGESTED DAILY DOSAGE AND MAXIMUM DOSAGE: There is **no widely established official dosage** for graviola in medical guidelines. Traditional use might involve **one cup of leaf tea daily** or small amounts of fruit. As a supplement, follow the **manufacturer's instructions** (e.g., 500 mg extract once or twice daily), but **always consult a healthcare provider** because research is limited.

SOLUBILITY AND BEST WAYS TO INGEST:
Main Active Compounds: Acetogenins and other phytochemicals can be extracted from water (teas) or sometimes alcohol-based tinctures. There's **no substantial evidence** that they need to be taken with fats or oils for better absorption; most people consume them in teas or juices.

OVERDOSE POTENTIAL:
Possible Neurotoxicity: Some studies suggest that large or frequent doses of Graviola might affect nerve cells. High amounts might **upset the stomach** or cause other side effects. Because there's not enough solid data, it's best to use graviola in **moderation** and not as a sole treatment for serious illnesses.
Lack of Large Human Trials: While test-tube and animal studies show interesting immune and cellular effects, we still lack conclusive evidence from large-scale clinical trials in humans.
Traditional and Cultural Use: Many communities use the leaves and fruit for various remedies, but practices vary significantly from region to region.

YERBA MATE - THE SOCIAL SPARK PLUG
Think of yerba mate as the spark plug in a car's engine—it helps get things going when you feel slow or tired. Yerba mate is a plant whose leaves make a tea-like drink that can boost energy. In many Latin American cultures, drinking yerba mate isn't just about feeling awake; it's also a social tradition. Friends share a hollow gourd with a metal straw, passing it around in a circle to chat, laugh, and stay connected.

Yerba Mate provides a natural caffeine boost and is a social drink in many Latin American cultures. Moderate use (1–2 cups daily) is generally safe but watch for too much caffeine.

DIETARY SOURCES:

Primary Source: Yerba mate leaves, which are dried, crushed, and used to make hot or cold beverages (often called "mate").

Common Forms: Loose-leaf tea, tea bags, bottled or canned beverages, and sometimes blended with other herbs.

SUGGESTED DAILY DOSAGE AND MAXIMUM DOSAGE: A typical serving might be 1–2 teaspoons of loose yerba mate leaves (about 2–4 grams) brewed in hot (but not boiling) water.

Maximum: Many guidelines suggest limiting total caffeine to around 300–400 mg daily for healthy adults. Since yerba mate can vary in caffeine content, it's wise to **start small** (1 cup) and see how you feel before increasing. Overconsumption of caffeine can lead to jitteriness, rapid heartbeat, or trouble sleeping.

SOLUBILITY AND BEST WAYS TO INGEST:

Water-Soluble Components: Yerba mate's key compounds (caffeine and antioxidants) dissolve in water. You don't need oil or fat for absorption. Some people add lemon juice or sweeteners, but it's not necessary for its effects. Because of the caffeine, it's **wise to avoid** taking it late in the day if you're sensitive to sleep disturbances.

OVERDOSE POTENTIAL: You can get too much caffeine, leading to anxiety or increased heart rate. Drinking very hot yerba mate has been studied for potential links to specific health issues; allowing it to cool slightly before drinking is recommended.

Social and Cultural Importance: Sharing mate is a big part of South American culture, symbolizing friendship and connection.

Health Benefits: It contains antioxidants and may boost mental alertness, but due to its caffeine content, it's best enjoyed in moderation.

COMMUNITY EXAMPLE

In the small rainforest village of **San Selva**, the elders pass down a recipe for "healing tea" made from sun-dried graviola leaves. They collect the freshest leaves early in the morning, wash them carefully, and set them out to dry. When a family member feels run-down, the mother brews the leaves in water, lets it cool, and serves it with local honey. They believe this warm, soothing drink helps the body fight off minor illnesses and keeps the spirit calm.

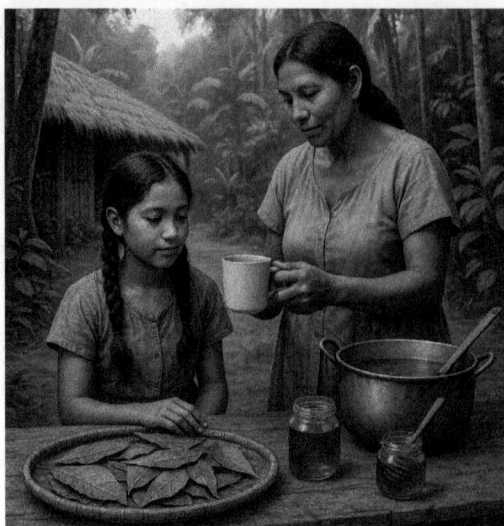

POTENTIAL INTERACTIONS WITH BLOOD PRESSURE MEDS OR ANTIDEPRESSANTS

Yerba Mate: Contains caffeine, which can **raise heart rate and blood pressure**. People on **blood pressure medication** should watch for changes in blood pressure. Caffeine can also interact with certain antidepressants that affect the body's breakdown of caffeine (leading to more potent side effects).

Graviola: Some preliminary data suggests it may **lower blood pressure** slightly. Combined with blood pressure meds, it might lead to overly low blood pressure. It may also **increase sedation** when combined with certain antidepressants or other medications. Always consult a healthcare professional if you're taking medication; these plants can have additive or unexpected effects.

ETHICAL SOURCING IS IMPORTANT –
PROTECTING BIODIVERSITY

Biodiversity: Both graviola and yerba mate grow in regions with delicate ecosystems. Overharvesting or poor farming practices can **harm local wildlife** and **reduce plant diversity**.

Fair Trade and Sustainable Practices: Look for **fair trade** or **organic** certifications that ensure farmers are paid fairly and that the environment is respected. Ethical sourcing often means that the people who've grown and used these plants for generations **benefit** economically and culturally.

> *"Mate keeps you awake ... and even regulates your digestion. It is antioxidant, perhaps even diuretic. And a lot more. It is a miraculous beverage. It has more virtues than we know. It's also a good companion. It includes iron, magnesium, vitamin B6, and caffeine. It's complete."*
> *- Andrés Calamaro*

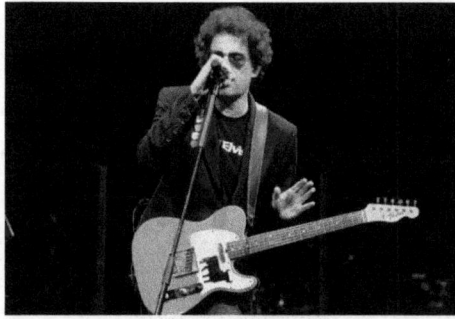

Andrés Calamaro

9.2.3: AFRICAN AND MIDDLE EASTERN HERBS (CINNAMON, FENUGREEK, FRANKINCENSE)

BLOOD SUGAR CONTROL AND LACTATION SUPPORT

Fenugreek seeds are small but mighty, like tiny superheroes with special powers. These tiny seeds can help balance blood sugar levels, vital for giving us a steady flow of energy instead of a sudden burst and crash—think of them as little traffic controllers for our blood sugar. Mothers who are breastfeeding sometimes use fenugreek to help produce more milk, making these seeds like caring helpers for both mom and baby. Fenugreek has a unique, slightly sweet taste that people often add to dishes or brew as tea. Whether sprinkled on food or taken as a supplement, fenugreek can quietly support our bodies in multiple ways.

Fenugreek seeds contain compounds that help regulate blood sugar by slowing the way our bodies absorb carbohydrates and improving insulin function. They are also traditionally used to support milk production in breastfeeding mothers, likely due to their phytoestrogen content.

DIETARY SOURCES: Fenugreek is commonly used in Indian, North African, and Middle Eastern cooking. The seeds can be soaked and eaten, ground into a spice blend, or brewed into tea. Supplements are available in capsule and powder form.

SUGGESTED DAILY DOSAGE:
For General Wellness/Blood Sugar Support: 1–3 grams of fenugreek seed powder or capsules daily.
For Lactation Support: Some sources recommend 3–6 grams per day in capsule form (often divided into two or three doses).

MAXIMUM DOSAGE AND OVERDOSE POTENTIAL: Clinical studies sometimes use up to 10 grams daily for short periods. Excessive amounts can cause gastrointestinal discomfort (bloating, diarrhea) and, in very high amounts, may interfere with certain medications (especially those for diabetes or blood clotting).

SOLUBILITY: Fenugreek contains water-soluble fibers; brewing it as a tea or soaking the seeds helps release these beneficial components. Taking fenugreek with meals can enhance its blood-sugar-balancing effects.

SYNERGY WITH COMPLEMENTARY SUBSTANCES: Fenugreek may work synergistically with other herbs that support metabolic health, such as cinnamon or ginger. Start low and increase slowly to gauge tolerance; consult a healthcare provider, especially if you are on blood-sugar-regulating medications or are pregnant or breastfeeding.

FRANKINCENSE FOR ANTI-INFLAMMATORY EFFECTS

Frankincense (Boswellia) might remind you of something magical because it's been used in places of worship and special ceremonies for centuries, like a fragrant gift from ancient times. It must be pretty cool if the three wise men brought it as a gift! It comes from tree sap, which hardens into a resin that can be burned for its soothing scent. Frankincense acts like a shield inside the body, helping reduce inflammation or swelling and protecting us from aches and pains. Some people describe its smell as woodsy or slightly sweet, and it has been cherished for its pleasant aroma and potential healing benefits. Think of frankincense as a calm, wise older friend who helps keep your body feeling its best.

Frankincense resin (from the Boswellia tree) is valued for its boswellic acids, which can reduce inflammatory markers in the body. This may help with osteoarthritis, rheumatoid arthritis, or other inflammatory issues.

DIETARY SOURCES: Frankincense is not typically eaten as a food; instead, you'll find it as:
Resin or Incense: Burned for its aromatic properties.
Capsules/Extracts: Standardized boswellic acid content for health benefits.
Essential Oil: Essential oils are used topically or in aromatherapy, though oral use is less common and requires caution.

SUGGESTED DAILY DOSAGE: For standardized Boswellia extract, 300–500 mg two to three times daily is commonly cited in research.

MAXIMUM DOSAGE AND OVERDOSE POTENTIAL: Some studies go up to around 1,200–1,500 mg daily in divided doses. Higher doses may cause digestive upset but rarely serious toxicity.

SOLUBILITY: Boswellic acids are more fat-soluble, so taking Frankincense capsules with a meal containing healthy fats may improve absorption.

SYNERGY WITH COMPLEMENTARY SUBSTANCES: Often paired with turmeric (curcumin) or ginger for enhanced anti-inflammatory effects.

USAGE IN RELIGIOUS CEREMONIES

Frankincense has a long history in spiritual and religious contexts, particularly in the Middle East and parts of Africa where Boswellia trees grow. Ancient Egyptians used frankincense in embalming and religious rituals. In Christian tradition, it was one of the gifts presented to the baby Jesus, symbolizing holiness and purification. Throughout the centuries, burning frankincense resin in temples, churches, and other sacred spaces was believed to cleanse the air and bring prayers closer to the divine. This deep-rooted cultural practice highlights frankincense's pleasant aroma and underscores its revered status as a precious and powerful substance.

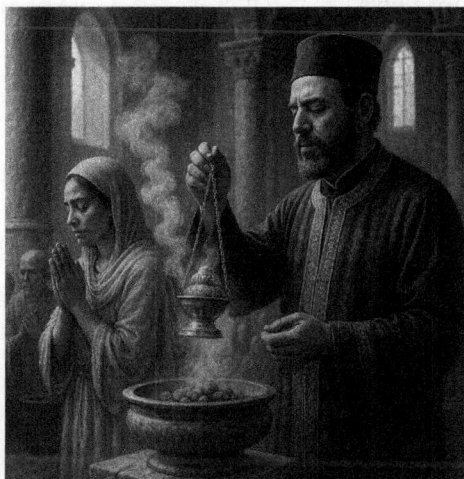

CINNAMON

Imagine coming home on a chilly day and smelling something sweet and spicy baking in the oven—that's how comforting Ceylon cinnamon can be. This type of cinnamon, often called "true" cinnamon, is known to help keep our blood sugar levels steady, a bit like a friendly traffic light that prevents sugar from zooming around too fast in our blood. Many people enjoy it in their tea or sprinkled on toast because it makes food taste warm and cozy. Ceylon cinnamon can also help protect our bodies by fighting inflammation, which is how we deal with tiny injuries. In short, Ceylon cinnamon is like a delicious, gentle helper that works quietly in the background to keep us healthy.

CINNAMON'S VARIETY: CASSIA VS. CEYLON, COUMARIN TOXICITY RISK IN HIGH DOSES

Cassia Cinnamon: The most common type found in grocery stores. Stronger flavor, darker color, and higher coumarin content.

Ceylon Cinnamon ("True Cinnamon"): Milder flavor, lighter color, and significantly lower coumarin content. Often preferred for regular or higher-volume consumption.

Coumarin Toxicity: Coumarin is a naturally occurring compound that, in large amounts, may stress the liver or pose other health risks. If you enjoy moderate quantities of cinnamon daily, choosing Ceylon cinnamon is safer to avoid excessive coumarin.

SUGGESTED DAILY DOSAGE: Most guidelines suggest 1–2 teaspoons (2–4 grams) of cinnamon powder daily as a general supportive amount. If using cassia cinnamon regularly, keep it to lower daily doses to reduce the risk of coumarin-related toxicity.

SOLUBILITY: Cinnamon's beneficial polyphenols are partially water-soluble; they can be steeped in teas or sprinkled on foods. For supplements, look for standardized extracts if specific dosing is required.

SYNERGY WITH COMPLEMENTARY SUBSTANCES: Cinnamon is often combined with other blood-sugar-supportive ingredients, like chromium or fenugreek, for synergistic effects.

MAXIMUM DOSAGE AND OVERDOSE POTENTIAL: Very high doses of cinnamon (particularly cassia) can lead to liver damage over time. Use caution and check with a healthcare professional if you plan to take large amounts as a supplement.

For those who love the flavor and use cinnamon liberally, switching to Ceylon cinnamon is an excellent choice.

UNDERSTANDING CULTURAL CONTEXTS HELPS US APPRECIATE THE VALUE OF THESE HERBS

Global Traditions & Wisdom: Each of these herbs—fenugreek, frankincense, and cinnamon—has been used for thousands of years in different cultures, whether in cooking, healing, or sacred rituals. Recognizing their origins and how they have been revered helps us grasp their therapeutic potential and show respect to the communities that perfected their use over centuries. When we learn about the roles these herbs play in various cultural diets, medicines, and ceremonies, we gain a richer appreciation for holistic health approaches. This can guide us to use these herbs more thoughtfully, blending modern scientific findings with ancestral wisdom.

"I can't tell you enough about cinnamon. Cinnamon is an awesome spice to use and it goes great with something like apples in the morning or in a mixture of fruit or in your oatmeal or even in your cereal."
– Emeril Lagasse

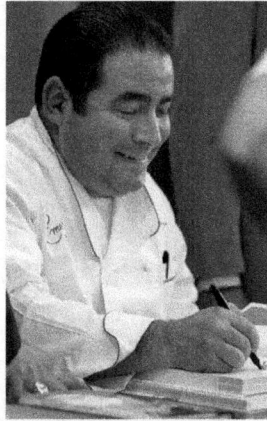

Emeril Lagasse
Credit – Picryl – Creativecommons.org

9.2.4: AFRICAN AND NATIVE AMERICAN TRADITIONS

When I was a teenager, my older sister **Judy** was in a terrible automobile accident on a cross-country trip in Albuquerque, New Mexico. She was airlifted to a hospital in Santa Fe, where she spend several months recuperating. Many of the nurses in the hospital were Native American, and my sister began a long journey into learning about the culture. She married a Native American and had a son. When I was fourteen, she took me to the Sundance in Wyoming. Only Native Americans are allowed, but since I was her brother I was considered part of their family. It was like taking a trip back 1,000 years, experiencing deer hunting and skinning, peyote meetings, dance rituals, and mostly wonderful, down-to-earth people who loved the land and loved each other with ferocity. It opened my eyes to a whole new world.

African and Native American cultures offer rich traditions for promoting health and longevity, blending herbal remedies, dietary practices, and holistic rituals. These approaches emphasize balance between body, mind, and spirit, providing insights for modern wellness.

AFRICAN TRADITIONAL MEDICINE

African traditional medicine, practiced for centuries, integrates herbalism, spiritual healing, and community care, often led by healers like sangomas or inyangas. These practices aim to enhance vitality and longevity through natural and holistic means.

Moringa oleifera: Known as the "miracle tree," moringa is packed with vitamins, minerals, and antioxidants. Used across Africa for nutrition, it supports energy, immunity, and metabolic health. Add moringa powder to smoothies or teas.

Sutherlandia frutescens (Cancer Bush): Traditionally used for immune support and inflammation, this herb is valued in South African medicine. Early studies suggest antiviral and anti-inflammatory properties.

Holistic Practices: Spiritual healing, bone setting, and community rituals foster mental and emotional well-being, reducing stress and promoting a balanced life, key to longevity.

NATIVE AMERICAN TRADITIONAL MEDICINE

Native American health practices, varying by tribe, focus on harmony among physical, mental, and spiritual health. These traditions use plants and rituals to support long-term wellness.

Echinacea: Widely used by Plains tribes for immune support, echinacea may reduce cold symptoms, though evidence is mixed. Available as teas or supplements.

Sage (Salvia apiana): Used in smudging for purification, sage has antimicrobial properties, supporting infection prevention. Burn sage or use it in cooking.

Sweat Lodges and Vision Quests: These rituals promote detoxification and mental clarity. A 2024 study notes improved circulation and stress reduction from sweat lodges, potentially aiding longevity.

These traditions highlight the value of community, nature, and balance, offering lessons for modern longevity practices.

SECTION THREE: INTEGRATING HISTORICAL WISDOM WITH MODERN SCIENCE
9.3.1: RESEARCH CHALLENGES

TRADITIONAL PRACTICES OFTEN LACK LARGE-SCALE CLINICAL TRIALS

Herbal systems like Ayurveda or TCM were built on what healers saw working over hundreds of years, not on lab trials. Running a modern clinical study with hundreds of volunteers costs millions of dollars, so only a handful of herbs ever get tested that way. Doctors who rely on strict data may hesitate to recommend a plant if no large study backs it up.

Hard to make every batch identical: A drug pill is made in a factory and is the same every time. A plant's strength changes with soil, weather, and harvest time. Researchers must spend extra effort to grind, extract, and measure each batch so every test dose matches—otherwise the results won't line up.

A small example of teamwork: A U.S. clinic tried an old TCM mix—ginger, licorice, and peony—for mild joint pain. They tracked both TCM signs (tongue and pulse) *and* Western numbers (pain scores, blood-inflammation tests). After eight weeks, patients hurt a little less and inflammation markers dipped. It was only a pilot study, but it showed how traditional know-how and lab tools can work together.

Money problems: Drug companies fund huge trials because they can patent and sell the final pill. No one can patent ginger or mint, so big investors stay away. Government or charity grants help, but their budgets are small compared with pharmaceutical cash.

Stories vs. strict experiments: Personal success stories (anecdotes) can point to useful herbs—but they might also be placebo or coincidence. Randomized controlled trials (RCTs) remove bias but take lots of time and money. The best plan is to start with good observations, then run well-designed RCTs, all while respecting local healers who know the plants best.

In short, traditional remedies may work, but proving *how well* and *how safe* they are takes careful, costly science—and that process is still catching up.

So, how do we know that herbal remedies work? Anecdotal evidence mixed with actual use gives us our answers depending upon how well they work for us.

9.3.2: RESPECTING AND PRESERVING CULTURAL KNOWLEDGE

MANY INDIGENOUS REMEDIES AT RISK OF DISAPPEARING

Many recipes live only in elders' memories. When people move to cities or forests are cut down, both the healers **and** the plants disappear. Every lost remedy could have been the clue to a new medicine. If we don't record and protect this knowledge now, it may be gone forever.

ETHICAL SOURCING TO SUPPORT LOCAL COMMUNITIES

Ethical sourcing means pay local pickers fairly and harvest without wrecking the forest. Fair-trade deals can fund village clinics, schools, and re-planting projects. Clear labels and third-party seals (Fair Trade, Rainforest Alliance) let shoppers know they're supporting the community, not exploiting it.

COOPERATIVES COULD HELP

In a growers' co-op in the Amazon, villagers set strict "only take what regrows" rules. They plant new seedlings for every root they dig. Universities test the plants and publish safety data. These practices promote healthier forests, steady income for families, and solid research that helps everyone.

COLLABORATIONS WITH UNIVERSITIES CAN VALIDATE TRADITIONAL MEDICINE

Scientists bring lab tools; healers bring centuries of know-how. Together they run proper studies to prove which plants work, at what dose, and why. Healers keep ownership of their recipes, and governments are more likely to approve proven herbs for wider use.

CULTURAL EXCHANGE FOSTERS BETTER GLOBAL HEALTH UNDERSTANDING

When Ayurvedic doctors, Indigenous shamans, TCM experts, and Western physicians swap ideas, each system fills the other's gaps. Good cross-cultural talks can make effective treatments available to more people and cut health-care inequality. Conferences and exchange programs build respect: modern science and traditional knowledge don't have to compete—they can cooperate. Protect the forests, pay local harvesters fairly, study the plants with modern science, and share the results. That's how we keep priceless healing traditions alive—and maybe find tomorrow's life-saving medicine.

The idea is for us all to get together to make a difference, working with people who think like us as well as others who don't. It all starts within us. My friend, **Congressman Scott Peters** said:

> *"I'm just not a purist. You set goals and you have to work with everyone to figure out how to get what you can."*

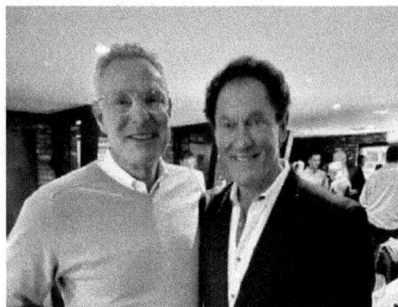

Congressman Scott Peters and Tad Sisler
Source – Sisler Private Collection

9.3.3: PERSONALIZED, HOLISTIC APPROACHES

BLENDING ANCIENT WISDOM WITH MODERN SCIENCE CAN YIELD COMPREHENSIVE HEALING

Systems like **Ayurveda** and **Traditional Chinese Medicine (TCM)** look at the *whole* person—body, mind, and spirit. Modern doctors rely on lab tests and clinical studies. When you combine the two—time-tested herbs and diets **plus** scientific safety checks—you can tackle both the *cause* of a problem and the painful symptoms. The result is a treatment plan that feels custom-made and usually leaves patients happier.

WORK YOUR DIET, ENVIRONMENT, MENTAL WELL-BEING, AND SUPPLEMENTS IN TANDEM

Holistic health approaches view these factors as interdependent: imbalances in one area can affect others. For instance, stress (mental well-being) can reduce nutrient absorption (diet), while poor-quality sleep (environmental factor) can disrupt hormonal balance and hinder the effectiveness of supplements.

Personalized plans might include tailored meal guidelines, mindfulness or meditation practices, targeted supplements, and modifications to one's living space.

INTEGRATIVE CLINICS COULD HELP

When I was a teenager, my parents divorced. My father was a medical doctor, and in a rebound relationship, my mother briefly married a chiropractor. During that period, most doctors considered chiropractors "quacks," although my father was open to the profession. My mother's second husband, **Bart**, imagined a world where modern, traditional, and progressive medical practitioners worked together for the common good.

Imagine walking into one office and meeting:
• a Western M.D. for scans and blood tests
• an Ayurvedic coach for meal plans and spices
• a TCM herbalist for energy-balancing tea

They compare notes, adjust dosages, and watch your progress as a team.
 This mix of viewpoints can solve tough, long-running health issues better than any one system alone.

EACH PERSON'S BODY AND CULTURAL BACKGROUND CAN INFLUENCE SUPPLEMENT CHOICES

Your genes, culture, and everyday foods change how you react to herbs or pills. A root that's common in India might upset a stomach in Norway. Good practitioners listen to your background first, then choose or tweak supplements so they suit **you**.

LONGEVITY IS MULTIFACTORIAL; NO SINGLE TRADITION HOLDS ALL THE ANSWERS

No single tradition has every answer. A real longevity plan blends balanced meals, regular movement, strong friendships, calm mind habits, and smart use of both ancient herbs **and** modern nutrients. Staying open-minded—and willing to borrow the best from each system—gives you the strongest roadmap to a long, healthy life.

"Healing is a matter of time, but it is sometimes also a matter of opportunity." – Hippocrates

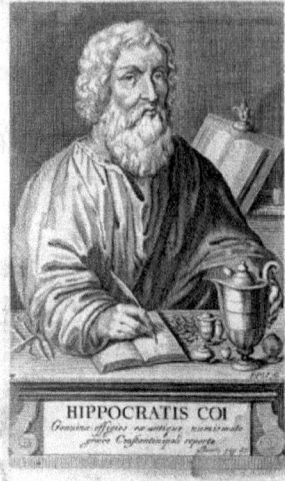

Hippocrates
Credit – Wikimedia Commons

9.3.4: VALIDATION OF HISTORICAL USES

Modern science is increasingly validating African and Native American health practices, confirming their benefits while respecting their cultural roots. This integration bridges traditional wisdom with contemporary health strategies.

VALIDATION OF AFRICAN TRADITIONAL MEDICINE

Moringa oleifera: A 2025 *Journal of Ethnopharmacology* study confirms moringa's high nutrient content and anti-diabetic effects, supporting its use for metabolic health. Clinical trials show improved blood sugar control in type 2 diabetes patients.

Hypoxis hemerocallidea (African Potato): Used for inflammation and immune support, a 2025 study found it reduces inflammatory markers in animal models, validating traditional claims.

Artemisia afra: Traditionally used for respiratory issues, 2024 research confirms its antimicrobial and anti-inflammatory properties, effective against bronchitis.

VALIDATION OF NATIVE AMERICAN TRADITIONAL MEDICINE

Echinacea: A 2024 *Cochrane Database* review found mixed results, with some trials showing reduced cold duration, supporting its immune-boosting use. Further studies are needed for consistency.

Sage: A 2025 *Journal of Ethnopharmacology* study confirms antimicrobial activity against pathogens, validating its use in purification rituals.

Sweat Lodges: A 2024 study reports physiological benefits like improved circulation and stress reduction, supporting mental and physical health.

CHALLENGES AND FUTURE DIRECTIONS

Standardizing herbal preparations and conducting large-scale clinical trials remain challenges due to variability in plant compounds and cultural practices. Ethical concerns include respecting indigenous intellectual property and ensuring communities benefit from commercialized remedies. A 2025 WHO report calls for collaborative research with traditional healers to preserve knowledge and advance science. Future studies should focus on rigorous testing while honoring cultural contexts.

PRACTICAL STEPS

Incorporate Herbs: Add moringa to your diet or try echinacea supplements, consulting a doctor for safety.

Explore Rituals: Engage in community wellness practices inspired by these traditions, like meditation or group activities.

Support Ethical Research: Advocate for studies that respect cultural knowledge.

SECTION FOUR:
NUTRITION FROM LIVING ORGANISMS
9.4.1: COMMON STAPLES

MILK (e.g., from cows, goats, buffalo)

Milk is a powerhouse drink.

• It packs **protein** for muscles, **calcium** for strong bones, and key vitamins like **B-12** and **D**.

• Some people choose goat or buffalo milk instead of cow's milk because the nutrients differ a little and may suit their bodies better.

• For centuries, many cultures have relied on milk as a symbol of comfort and good nutrition.

That said, some people can't handle lactose or are allergic to dairy, so they need other options. If your body tolerates it, milk can be an easy way to boost overall health and help you stay strong as you age.

EGGS (e.g., from chickens, ducks)

Eggs are nutrition all-stars.

• They give you top-notch **protein** for muscles.

• They carry **choline** for a sharp brain and healthy liver, plus **selenium** to help your body fight damage.

• Few foods have natural **vitamin D**, but eggs do—good for bones and immunity.

• The **yolk** supplies healthy fats and extra vitamins; the **white** is pure, lean protein. Boiled, scrambled, or baked into recipes, eggs are a staple food around the world.

HONEY (produced by bees)

Bees turn flower nectar into this thick, golden syrup. Besides tasting sweet, honey carries tiny bits of vitamins, minerals, and antioxidants. Clover, manuka, and wildflower honeys all taste a little different and may offer slightly different perks. People have long used honey to calm sore throats and help small cuts because it can slow the growth of germs. Remember, it's still sugar, so enjoy it in small amounts.

Propolis is a resinous mixture collected by bees from tree buds and sap to seal and protect their hives. When bees need "glue" to seal cracks in the hive, they mix tree sap with wax and make propolis. This sticky stuff is loaded with plant chemicals that fight germs and swelling. Many cultures turn propolis into throat sprays, salves, or tinctures to boost immunity and speed up healing. Buy it from trusted beekeepers to be sure it's pure.

Royal Jelly: Worker bees create a milky food called royal jelly for one special bee—the queen. Thanks to this super-food, the queen grows bigger and lives much longer than the rest. Royal jelly contains protein, vitamins, and minerals, so some people take it in capsules or tonics hoping for extra energy and immune support. Scientists are still studying exactly how it works, but it has been part of traditional medicine for centuries.

FISH OIL (e.g., from salmon, cod, or anchovies)

We've already touched on the benefits of fish oil in other chapters. Fish oil is prized for its high levels of omega-3 fatty acids, in particular EPA and DHA, which support cardiovascular health by helping to reduce inflammation and maintain healthy triglyceride levels, playing a critical role in brain function, and possibly aiding cognition and mood regulation. Cultures with traditionally high fish intake often display lower rates of certain chronic diseases. Taking a supplement makes it easier for people who do not consume fish regularly to meet their omega-3 needs. Even still, sustainability and purity (i.e., low mercury levels) are key considerations when selecting fish oil products.

COLLAGEN AND GELATIN

Collagen and gelatin are the "glue" proteins in animal skin, bones, and cartilage.
Why people take them:
• Keep skin stretchy and smooth
• Lubricate joints for easier movement
• Soothe the stomach lining
• Strengthen hair and nails

Where you see them:
- **Collagen powder** stirred into coffee or smoothies
- **Gelatin** in bone broths, gummies, and Jell-O-style desserts

CHEESE (fermented dairy product)

Cheese is a long-lasting dairy food packed with good stuff:

Nutrients: lots of calcium for bones, solid protein, healthy fats, plus vitamins B-12 and riboflavin.

Probiotics: some cheeses (especially the aged or fermented kinds) add friendly gut bacteria.

Variety: from soft ricotta to sharp cheddar and nutty gouda, every culture has its own style and flavor. Because some cheeses are high in salt and saturated fat, it's best to enjoy them in sensible portions. Eaten wisely, cheese can be a tasty, nutrient-dense part of your diet.

MAPLE SYRUP (from sap of maple trees)

Maple syrup is a North-American tree sap boiled into a thick, earthy-tasting syrup.
- It offers a little manganese, zinc, and antioxidants—nutrients plain white sugar lacks.
- Light syrup tastes mild; darker syrup is stronger and richer.
- It's still mostly sugar, so use small pours to keep your diet balanced. Enjoy it for flavor, but don't overdo it.

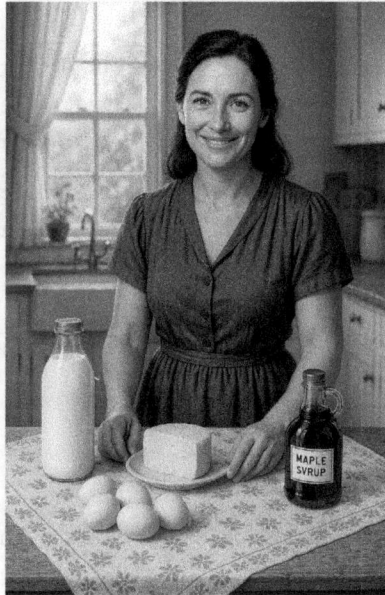

GLUTATHIONE (from bacteria, animals, fungi, and plants)

Glutathione is your body's built-in "clean-up crew."

- It's made from three amino acids and acts as a **master antioxidant**, mopping up harmful free radicals.
- It also recharges other defenders like vitamins C and E so they keep working.
- Aging, junk food, and pollution can drain your glutathione supply. Eating colorful fruits and veggies, getting enough sleep, and (if needed) taking targeted supplements can help keep your glutathione levels strong.

9.4.2: ORGANIC DETOX AND CLEANSING AGENTS

MILK THISTLE (Supports Liver Detoxification)

Milk thistle is an herb best known for **silymarin**, a compound that acts like a shield for your liver.
- Helps the liver break down toxins and repair itself.
- Used in traditional tonics for centuries; scientists are still studying exactly how well it works.
- Usually safe, but check with your doctor before adding any new supplement.

ACTIVATED CHARCOAL (Used for Binding Toxins in Digestion)

When wood or coconut shells are super-heated, they turn into a black powder full of tiny holes. Those holes act like sponges, grabbing onto chemicals in your stomach so they can't get into your blood.

People sometimes use it for:
- **Minor stomach troubles** like gas or bloating
- **Emergencies** after swallowing something harmful (only under medical care)

But be careful:
- It can also soak up medicines and nutrients if you take them at the same time.
- Taking too much can be harmful. So always check with a healthcare professional and watch your timing if you decide to use it.

CHLORELLA AND SPIRULINA (Algae for Heavy Metal Detoxification)

- They're tiny blue-green algae packed with protein, vitamins, minerals, and antioxidants.
- These algae can latch onto some heavy metals in the body, which is why people use them for gentle "detox."
- You'll usually find them as green powders or tablets to mix into smoothies or take with water.

Because they're strong concentrates, check with a doctor first—especially if you have any health issues or take other medicines.

What if you have a specific disease or illness? What other options do you have? Let's look at specific remedies that can help.

CHAPTER TEN
DISEASE AND ILLNESS PREVENTION

SECTION ONE: MAJOR DISEASES
10.1.1: THE GREATEST KILLERS

U nintentional injuries account for approximately 200,000 deaths per year in the USA, according to injuryfacts.nsc.org. Although this is listed among the ten greatest killers, our only remedy is to be as careful as possible, hoping that life will become safer as new advancements and inventions come into fruition. The following supplements may help in prevention, slowing the onset, or assisting in treatment of their corresponding illnesses.

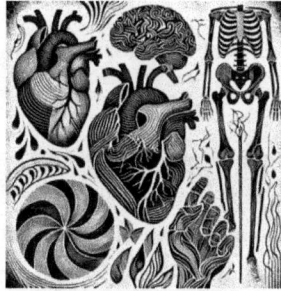

HEART DISEASE

Approximately 680,909 deaths per year in USA. (Source, New York Post)

Key Concerns: High cholesterol, inflammation, atherosclerosis, blood pressure.

VITAMINS AND MINERALS

Vitamin D3: Linked with cardiovascular health; deficiencies may contribute to higher heart disease risk.

Vitamin K2 (MK-7): Helps direct calcium to bones rather than arteries, potentially reducing plaque buildup.

Magnesium: Supports healthy blood pressure and normal heart rhythms.

B Vitamins (especially B6, B9, B12): Essential for homocysteine metabolism; elevated homocysteine can harm cardiovascular health.

SUPPLEMENTS

Omega-3 Fatty Acids (Fish Oil, Algal Oil): May reduce triglycerides, support healthy blood pressure, and help modulate inflammation.

Coenzyme Q10 (CoQ10): Vital for energy production in heart cells; may benefit patients on statin therapy.

Red Yeast Rice: Used traditionally for cholesterol management (though must be monitored for liver function and interactions).

HERBS

Garlic (Allium sativum): May help support healthy blood pressure and cholesterol levels.

Hawthorn (Crataegus spp.): Historically used to support heart function and circulation.

CANCER

Approximately 600,000 deaths per year in USA (Source – healthline.com)

Key Concerns: Oxidative stress, chronic inflammation, abnormal cell growth. Some supplements are listed twice as we also address effects of chemo and radiation.

VITAMINS AND MINERALS

Vitamin D3: Emerging evidence suggests a role in immune regulation and possibly cancer prevention.

Vitamin C (Ascorbic Acid): Powerful antioxidant; supports immune health and collagen synthesis.

Selenium: An antioxidant mineral that may help protect cells from oxidative damage.

SUPPLEMENTS

Curcumin (from Turmeric): Potent anti-inflammatory and antioxidant properties; studied extensively in cancer research.

Green Tea Extract (EGCG): Contains polyphenols that may inhibit tumor cell proliferation and promote detoxification.

Resveratrol (from Grapes or Japanese Knotweed): Antioxidant and anti-inflammatory effects; some promising lab studies.

HERBS

Turmeric (Curcuma longa): Source of curcumin, supports healthy inflammation response.

Milk Thistle (Silybum marianum): May support liver function, helping the body detoxify.

CHEMOTHERAPY AND RADIATION EFFECTS

I am not a medical professional, and the information provided here is for general educational purposes only. Always make sure you consult with a qualified healthcare provider before adding any supplements or herbs to your regimen, especially during chemotherapy or radiation. Individual needs can vary greatly depending on specific type of cancer, your treatment plan, and overall health status.

CONSULT YOUR ONCOLOGIST

Certain supplements, particularly antioxidants, may interfere with chemotherapy or radiation by reducing the treatments' effectiveness.

Your oncologist or a registered dietitian specializing in oncology can offer guidance tailored to your situation.

QUALITY AND SAFETY

Many herbal and supplement products are not strictly regulated. If you decide to use them, choose reputable, third-party-tested brands for purity and safety.

TIMING OF SUPPLEMENTATION

The timing of when you take certain supplements can be critical. In some cases, it might be recommended to avoid high doses of specific vitamins on treatment days, but they may be permissible in moderate amounts at other times.

COMMON SUPPLEMENTS AND NUTRIENTS

Below are some nutrients and herbs people commonly explore to help manage side effects or support overall health during cancer therapy. **Again, please discuss these with your medical team before taking them.**

VITAMINS

Vitamin D • Vital for bone health, immune function, and mood support. • Chemotherapy and radiation can sometimes contribute to vitamin D deficiencies. • Your doctor will measure your vitamin D level (25-hydroxyvitamin D test) and recommend supplementation if needed.

Vitamin B Complex (B12, B6, Folate, etc.) • Helps support energy production, function of your nerves, and red blood cell formation. • Certain chemotherapy drugs can lead to deficiencies or increase the need for B vitamins. • High doses should be monitored by a professional to avoid interactions or masking other conditions.

Vitamin C is an antioxidant that may support immune function.
Caution: High-dose vitamin C is controversial during active treatment because it could potentially reduce the effectiveness of certain chemo or radiation therapies. Moderate dietary intake is generally considered safe, but supplemental use should be cleared by your oncologist.

Vitamin E is another antioxidant that helps protect cells from damage.
Caution: As with vitamin C, high-dose vitamin E has similar concerns regarding treatment interference.

MINERALS

Zinc • Important for wound healing, immune support, and taste perception (which can be affected by chemotherapy). • High doses can cause nausea or potentially interfere with copper absorption, so balanced supplementation is key.

Magnesium • Supports muscle and nerve function. • Some chemo drugs can deplete magnesium levels. A doctor may recommend supplements if your levels are low.

HERBS AND BOTANICALS

Ginger • Often used to help manage nausea and vomiting, common side effects of chemotherapy. • Fresh ginger tea, ginger candies, or standardized supplements can be considered, but check dosage guidelines.

Turmeric/Curcumin • Known for its anti-inflammatory properties. • There is ongoing research into its potential benefits for cancer patients, but high doses can interact with certain medications, and not all forms are well absorbed.

Astragalus • Used in Traditional Chinese Medicine to support the immune system and general vitality. • Some studies suggest it may help reduce certain side effects of chemotherapy; however, more research is needed. Must be supervised by a knowledgeable practitioner.

Milk Thistle • Commonly used to support liver function. • Research is mixed regarding benefits during cancer therapy; discuss with your healthcare provider to avoid possible drug interactions.

PROBIOTICS (e.g., Lactobacillus, Bifidobacterium)
May help with gut health, especially if chemotherapy leads to digestive issues or if antibiotics are prescribed. The safety of probiotics can vary based on your immune status; in some situations (like very low white blood cell counts), they might not be recommended.

PRACTICAL TIPS FOR SUPPORTING RECOVERY
Balanced Diet: Focus on whole, minimally processed foods: vegetables, fruits, whole grains, legumes, and lean proteins rich in vitamins, minerals, and antioxidants, supporting overall health

Stay Hydrated: Adequate water intake can help flush out toxins and support kidney function, especially if you're experiencing diarrhea or vomiting.

Manage Nausea and Appetite: Small, frequent meals and gentle, bland foods can reduce nausea. Consider ginger tea or peppermint tea to settle the stomach, with your doctor's approval.

Monitor Blood Counts and Lab Work: Regular blood tests can highlight deficiencies (e.g., low magnesium, calcium, iron). Your healthcare provider can then recommend targeted supplementation.

Rest and Gentle Exercise: Quality sleep supports healing. Light activities like short walks or gentle yoga can help reduce fatigue and maintain muscle tone, but always follow your doctor's guidance regarding exercise.

Stress Management: Stress can weaken the immune response. Consider techniques like meditation, breathing exercises, or counseling to help cope with the emotional side of treatment.

There is no one-size-fits-all supplement strategy during chemotherapy or radiation, and in some cases, certain vitamins or herbs could interfere with treatment. Always talk with your oncologist or a registered dietitian specialized in cancer care to develop a safe, personalized plan. This individualized approach ensures you get the potential benefits of supportive supplements without reducing the effectiveness of your life-saving treatments.

PARKINSON'S DISEASE

Approximately 35,000 deaths per year in USA according to ajmc.com

Key Concerns: Dopamine depletion, oxidative stress, mitochondrial dysfunction.

VITAMINS AND MINERALS

Vitamin D3: Low levels have been associated with worse motor symptoms in Parkinson's; helps with bone density and immune health.

B Vitamins (especially B6, B9, B12): May support brain health and proper nerve function.

SUPPLEMENTS

CoQ10 (Ubiquinol): Supports mitochondrial function; some preliminary studies suggest benefits in Parkinson's.

N-Acetylcysteine (NAC): May help replenish glutathione, the brain's master antioxidant.

Omega-3 Fatty Acids: Anti-inflammatory; some evidence suggests they may support overall neurological health.

HERBS

Mucuna Pruriens: Natural source of L-DOPA, used in traditional medicine for Parkinsonian symptoms.

ALZHEIMER'S DISEASE

Approximately 120,000 deaths per year in USA according to healthline.com

Key Concerns: Beta-amyloid plaque buildup, neuroinflammation, cognitive decline.

VITAMINS AND MINERALS

Vitamin B12, Folate (B9), B6: Vital for homocysteine control; high homocysteine is linked to cognitive decline.

Vitamin D3: May play a role in cognitive function and immune regulation in the brain.

Vitamin E (Mixed Tocopherols/Tocotrienols): Antioxidant that may help protect neurons from oxidative stress.

SUPPLEMENTS

Omega-3 Fatty Acids (DHA/EPA): Essential for neuronal membrane integrity; some studies suggest cognitive benefits.

Curcumin: Anti-inflammatory properties; may reduce amyloid plaque aggregation in lab studies.

Phosphatidylserine (PS): Component of neuronal membranes, potentially supportive of cognition and memory.

HERBS

Ginkgo Biloba: Traditionally used to support cognitive function and circulation to the brain.

Ashwagandha (Withania somnifera): Adaptogen with potential neuroprotective effects.

TYPE 2 DIABETES

Approximately 100,000 deaths per year in USA according to healthline.com

Key Concerns: Insulin resistance, high blood sugar, metabolic syndrome.

VITAMINS AND MINERALS

Vitamin D3: Low levels are linked with reduced insulin sensitivity.

Magnesium: Deficiency correlates with increased insulin resistance and risk of diabetes.

Chromium: May enhance insulin action and improve glucose metabolism in some individuals.

SUPPLEMENTS

Alpha-Lipoic Acid (ALA): Antioxidant that may help reduce diabetic neuropathy and support glucose metabolism.

Berberine: Found in plants like barberry and goldenseal; research shows it may help improve insulin sensitivity.

Probiotics: Supporting gut health can positively impact glucose metabolism and overall metabolic function.

HERBS

Cinnamon (Cinnamomum verum/C. cassia): Some evidence suggests it can help lower fasting blood glucose.

Fenugreek (Trigonella foenum-graecum): May help modulate blood sugar levels when taken in seed or supplement form.

Please be advised that changes in diet may help immensely as well.

OSTEOPOROSIS

While osteoporosis itself is not typically listed as the direct cause of death, fractures leading to serious complications resulting in death are high. In the USA, approximately 31,000 deaths occur annually within six months following a hip fracture, according to pmc.ncbi.nlm.hih.gov

Key Concerns: Low bone density, risk of fractures, calcium and mineral deficiency.

VITAMINS AND MINERALS

Vitamin D3 + Calcium: Classic duo for bone health, with D3 enhancing calcium absorption.

Vitamin K2 (MK-7): Guides calcium to bones; may reduce risk of arterial calcification.

Magnesium: Works synergistically with calcium and vitamin D to maintain bone density.

SUPPLEMENTS

Collagen Peptides: May help support bone matrix and overall bone strength.

Strontium Ranelate (in some regions): Shown in some studies to help increase bone mass.

HERBS

Horsetail (Equisetum arvense): Traditionally used for silica content to support bone health.

Red Clover (Trifolium pratense): Contains phytoestrogens that may help support bone density in menopausal women (though more research is needed).

ARTHRITIS (Osteoarthritis & Rheumatoid)

Arthritis deaths primarily occur due to associated comorbidities such as cardiovascular disease, particularly in individuals with Rheumatoid Arthritis.

Key Concerns: Joint inflammation, cartilage breakdown, pain management.

VITAMINS AND MINERALS

Vitamin D3: Adequate levels help maintain joint and bone health.

Vitamin C: Needed for collagen synthesis, which supports cartilage and connective tissues.

SUPPLEMENTS

Glucosamine & Chondroitin: Commonly used to support cartilage repair and reduce joint stiffness.

Omega-3 Fatty Acids (Fish Oil): Anti-inflammatory properties, may help ease joint pain.

MSM (Methylsulfonylmethane): May help reduce inflammation and support collagen production.

HERBS

Boswellia Serrata (Frankincense): Anti-inflammatory properties that may help reduce arthritic pain.

Turmeric/Curcumin: Potent anti-inflammatory; used widely for joint health support.

DEPRESSION AND ANXIETY

While not purely "diseases," mood disorders have a strong impact on longevity and quality of life. Mental health disorders are linked to an increased risk of mortality, both from natural causes and suicide. In addition to our suggestions, prescription medication may be strongly advised, so check with your medical professional.

VITAMINS AND MINERALS

B Vitamins (especially B12, Folate): Essential for neurotransmitter production and mood regulation.

Magnesium: Involved in stress response and relaxation pathways.

SUPPLEMENTS

Omega-3 Fatty Acids: EPA in particular has shown some benefit for depressive symptoms.

Probiotics: Growing research links gut health with mental health ("gut-brain axis").

SAM-e (S-Adenosylmethionine): May support neurotransmitter balance and mood in some individuals.

HERBS

St. John's Wort (Hypericum perforatum): Traditionally used for mild to moderate depression (must watch for drug interactions).

Ashwagandha (Withania somnifera): Adaptogen that may help modulate stress and anxiety.

STROKE PREVENTION (Cerebrovascular Disease)

Approximately 162,639 deaths per year in USA – Source-New York Post

Key Concerns: Hypertension, atherosclerosis, blood clot risk, inflammation.

VITAMINS AND MINERALS

Vitamin D3: Low levels correlate with increased risk of hypertension and stroke.

Vitamin B12, Folate, B6: Help manage homocysteine levels, which can affect stroke risk.

Potassium: Helps regulate blood pressure when consumed at adequate levels (typically via diet but sometimes supplemented).

SUPPLEMENTS

Omega-3 Fatty Acids: Can support healthy blood pressure and reduce inflammation.

CoQ10: Helps maintain healthy blood pressure levels in some studies, supports cardiovascular function.

HERBS

Garlic (Allium sativum): May reduce platelet aggregation and help keep blood pressure in check.

Ginkgo Biloba: Some evidence suggests it may help improve circulation, though its role in stroke prevention is still being researched.

CHRONIC LOWER RESPIRATORY DISEASES [Including Chronic Obstructive Pulmonary Disease (COPD)]

Approximately 150,000 deaths per year in USA, according to healthline.com

Key Concerns: Lung function, inflammation, oxidative stress, immune support.

VITAMINS AND MINERALS

Vitamin D3: Low levels often found in patients with chronic respiratory issues; may support immune health.

Vitamin C & E: Antioxidants that can help reduce oxidative stress in lung tissues.

SUPPLEMENTS

N-Acetylcysteine (NAC): Helps replenish glutathione in the lungs, supports mucous clearance.

Omega-3 Fatty Acids: May help modulate inflammation and support respiratory function.

HERBS

Ginger (Zingiber officinale): Anti-inflammatory and antioxidant properties; may help ease inflammation in airways.

Mullein (Verbascum thapsus): Traditionally used to soothe respiratory tract irritation (often in teas or tinctures).

KIDNEY DISEASE (Nephritis, Nephrotic Syndrome, and Nephrosis):

Approximately 50,000 deaths per year occur in the USA from Kidney Disease, according to healthline.com

Key Concerns: Impaired filtration of waste and toxins, Fluid and electrolyte imbalances, High blood pressure and cardiovascular risks, Protein loss in urine (in nephrotic syndrome).

VITAMINS AND MINERALS

Vitamin D (supports bone health, often deficient in kidney disease)

B vitamins (help with energy production and red blood cell formation)

Iron (for anemia, common in kidney disease)

Magnesium and Potassium (need to be monitored, as imbalances can be harmful)

SUPPLEMENTS

Omega-3 fatty acids (reduce inflammation and cardiovascular risk)

Coenzyme Q10 (CoQ10) (supports mitochondrial function and reduces oxidative stress)

L-Carnitine (can help with muscle weakness in kidney disease)

HERBS

Astragalus (may support kidney function and immunity)

Dandelion root (acts as a natural diuretic, helping with fluid balance)

Nettle leaf (rich in nutrients, may help reduce inflammation)

CHRONIC LIVER DISEASE AND CIRRHOSIS

Approximately 50,000 deaths per year occur in the USA from Chronic Liver Disease and Cirrhosis, according to healthline.com

Key Concerns: Liver scarring and reduced detoxification ability, Poor protein metabolism and risk of ammonia buildup, Increased risk of fatty liver and liver cancer, Vitamin and mineral deficiencies due to malabsorption.

VITAMINS AND MINERALS

Vitamin E (antioxidant that may protect liver cells)

Vitamin D (often deficient in liver disease)

Zinc (supports liver function and helps with ammonia detoxification)

Selenium (important for liver enzyme function and detoxification)

SUPPLEMENTS

Milk thistle (silymarin) (supports liver cell regeneration)

N-Acetylcysteine (NAC) (helps replenish glutathione, a key antioxidant for liver detox)

Lipoic acid (reduces oxidative stress and supports liver metabolism)

HERBS

Turmeric (curcumin) (anti-inflammatory and supports liver repair)

Dandelion root (may help with bile production and liver detoxification)

Schisandra berry (traditionally used to protect liver cells and improve liver function)

These recommendations should be personalized based on individual health status and under medical supervision.

"Advances in technology and in our understanding of illness and disease together with an expanded workforce and greater resources will allow us to provide more services to a higher quality." – John Hutton

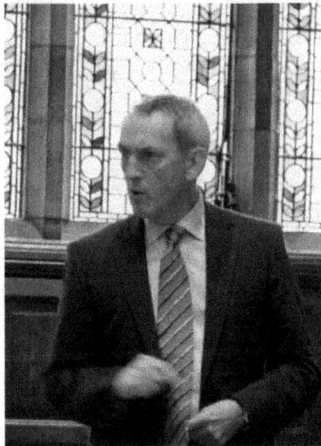

John Hutton
Credit – Wikimedia Commons

10.1.2: MINOR ILLNESSES

Below is a high-level overview of vitamins, supplements, and herbs that are frequently referenced for **ten common or "minor" ailments**—from colds and flu to everyday aches. Keep in mind that "minor" doesn't mean trivial; these conditions can still impact quality of life. As always, this is **not medical advice**—consult a qualified healthcare provider before making any changes to your health regimen.

COMMON COLDS AND FLU

Key Concerns: Immune support, viral load, inflammation, symptom relief.

VITAMINS AND MINERALS:

Vitamin C (Ascorbic Acid): Supports immune function; high doses may reduce cold duration.

Vitamin D3: Low levels are linked to increased susceptibility to infections; helps modulate immune response.

Zinc: Essential for immune cell function; may help shorten cold duration when taken at onset.

SUPPLEMENTS:

Elderberry (Sambucus nigra): Traditionally used to reduce the severity and duration of colds and flu.

Echinacea: May support immune cell activity and strengthen defenses against common pathogens.

Probiotics: A healthy gut microbiome can bolster overall immunity.

HERBS – REMEDIES:

Ginger (Zingiber officinale): Anti-inflammatory and warming, can ease congestion and soothe sore throats.

Garlic (Allium sativum): Known for antimicrobial properties; can be consumed fresh or in capsule form.

SEASONAL ALLERGIES (HAY FEVER)

Key Concerns: Histamine response, nasal congestion, watery eyes, sneezing.

VITAMINS AND MINERALS:

Vitamin C: Natural antihistamine effects, may reduce inflammatory responses in allergic reactions.

Quercetin (technically a flavonoid): Often taken with vitamin C; may inhibit histamine release.

SUPPLEMENTS:

Butterbur (Petasites hybridus): Some clinical studies show it helps alleviate allergic rhinitis symptoms.

Stinging Nettle (Urtica dioica): Traditional remedy for reducing nasal inflammation and congestion.

Probiotics: Gut health can influence immune and allergic responses.

HERBS – REMEDIES:

Nettle & Peppermint Teas: Can soothe irritated nasal passages and provide mild decongestant effects.

Local Raw Honey (anecdotal): Some people believe it helps build tolerance to local pollen (research is mixed).

MILD PULMONARY COMPLAINTS
(Simple Bronchitis, Mild Asthma Flare-ups)

Key Concerns: Airway inflammation, mucus clearance, breathing ease.

VITAMINS AND MINERALS:

Vitamin D3: Adequate levels can support lung health and immune modulation.

Magnesium: May help with smooth muscle relaxation in the airways, sometimes beneficial for mild asthma.

SUPPLEMENTS:

N-Acetylcysteine (NAC): Supports mucus thinning and clearance, replenishes glutathione in lung tissue.

Omega-3 Fatty Acids: Anti-inflammatory properties that may help with respiratory function.

HERBS – REMEDIES:

Mullein (Verbascum thapsus): Traditionally used to soothe the respiratory tract and reduce irritation.

Licorice Root (Glycyrrhiza glabra): In herbal medicine, used for soothing inflamed tissues, but caution in hypertension.

MILD DIGESTIVE DISTURBANCES
(Indigestion, Bloating, Occasional Constipation)

Key Concerns: Gut motility, healthy gut flora, inflammation in the GI tract.

VITAMINS AND MINERALS:

Magnesium (Citrate form): Can help loosen stool and support regular bowel movements.

B Vitamins (especially B1, B2, B3): Important for overall digestive enzyme function and energy metabolism.

SUPPLEMENTS:

Probiotics: Helps rebalance gut flora, alleviate bloating, and improve bowel regularity.

Digestive Enzymes: Aid in the breakdown of proteins, fats, and carbs—useful for overeating or mild malabsorption issues.

Peppermint Oil Capsules: May soothe gas and bloating, especially in IBS-like symptoms.

HERBS – REMEDIES:

Ginger: Stimulates digestion and alleviates nausea.

Chamomile: Calming effect on the GI tract; helps reduce mild inflammation and spasms.

TENSION HEADACHES AND MILD MIGRANES

Key Concerns: Vascular health, muscular tension, possible nutrient deficiencies.

VITAMINS AND MINERALS:

Magnesium (Glycinate or Citrate): Often low in migraine sufferers; can relax blood vessels and muscles.

B2 (Riboflavin): Clinical research suggests high-dose riboflavin may reduce migraine frequency.

SUPPLEMENTS:

CoQ10: Plays a role in mitochondrial energy production; some evidence supports migraine prevention.

5-HTP (5-Hydroxytryptophan): May help support serotonin levels, which can affect migraine onset (consult healthcare provider).

HERBS – REMEDIES:

Feverfew (Tanacetum parthenium): Traditionally used to reduce migraine frequency and severity.

Butterbur (Petasites hybridus): Another herbal option studied for migraine prevention (make sure it's a PA-free extract).

MILD SKIN IRRITATIONS (Exzema, Mild Acne)

Key Concerns: Inflammation, dryness, bacterial overgrowth, immune response.

VITAMINS AND MINERALS:

Vitamin D3: May help modulate immune response in skin conditions like eczema.

Zinc: Important for skin repair and sebum regulation, often used for acne support.

Vitamin C: Supports collagen formation and skin healing.

SUPPLEMENTS:

Omega-3 Fatty Acids: Reduce inflammation, can improve skin barrier function.

Probiotics: Research shows a gut-skin connection; balancing gut flora can alleviate some skin issues.

HERBS – REMEDIES:

Aloe Vera (topical or oral juice): Soothes irritated skin and supports healing.

Calendula (topical): Mild anti-inflammatory and antimicrobial properties, used for eczema or minor wounds.

URINARY TRACT DISCOMFORT
(Minor UTIs, Mild Irritation)

Key Concerns: Bacterial overgrowth, urinary pH, inflammation of the urinary tract.

VITAMINS AND MINERALS:

Vitamin C: Acidifies urine, which can inhibit bacterial growth.

Zinc: Supports immune function and may help the body fight infections.

SUPPLEMENTS:

Cranberry Extract (Vaccinium macrocarpon): Contains proanthocyanidins that may prevent bacteria from adhering to the urinary tract.

D-Mannose: A sugar shown to help flush out bacteria (especially E. coli) from the bladder.

Probiotics: Particularly Lactobacillus strains for urogenital health.

HERBS – REMEDIES:

Uva Ursi (Arctostaphylos uva-ursi): Traditionally used for mild UTIs; contains arbutin (use caution with long-term or high doses).

Horsetail (Equisetum arvense): Mild diuretic properties; sometimes used to help flush the urinary tract.

MILD EYE STRAIN AND DRYNESS

Key Concerns: Computer eye strain, lack of tear production, oxidative stress.

VITAMINS AND MINERALS:

Vitamin A: Essential for healthy vision, night vision, and corneal health.

Omega-3 Fatty Acids: Particularly EPA/DHA for tear production and reducing inflammation.

SUPPLEMENTS:

Lutein & Zeaxanthin: Carotenoids concentrated in the retina; may help filter blue light and protect eye tissues.

Astaxanthin: Antioxidant that supports eye health and may reduce eye fatigue.

HERBS – REMEDIES:

Bilberry (Vaccinium myrtillus): Traditionally used to support night vision and reduce eye fatigue.

Eyebright (Euphrasia officinalis): Historically used in herbal eye washes for irritation (use caution and sterile solutions).

MILD JOINT AND MUSCLE PAIN
(Everyday Aches, Overuse)

Key Concerns: Inflammation, collagen synthesis, stiffness, minor injury recovery.

VITAMINS AND MINERALS:

Vitamin C: Necessary for collagen formation, helps with repair of cartilage and connective tissue.

Vitamin D3 & Magnesium: Work synergistically for muscle and bone support.
SUPPLEMENTS:
Collagen Peptides: Can support cartilage health and improve joint comfort.
Glucosamine & Chondroitin: Commonly used for joint lubrication and mild osteoarthritis.
MSM (Methylsulfonylmethane): May help reduce inflammation and support connective tissue repair.
HERBS – REMEDIES:
Turmeric/Curcumin: Potent anti-inflammatory; helps alleviate minor joint pain.
Boswellia Serrata (Frankincense): Supports a healthy inflammatory response in joints.

MILD SLEEP DISTURBANCES
(Trouble Falling Asleep, Light Insomnia)
Key Concerns: Relaxation, circadian rhythm, stress management.
VITAMINS AND MINERALS:
Magnesium (Glycinate): Often called the "relaxation mineral," can help calm nerves and support better sleep.
Vitamin B6 (Pyridoxine): Helps produce neurotransmitters like serotonin and melatonin, important for sleep quality.

SUPPLEMENTS:
Melatonin: Directly regulates the sleep-wake cycle; helpful for short-term circadian rhythm adjustments.
5-HTP: May boost serotonin levels, thereby improving sleep onset (consult healthcare provider for proper dosing).
L-Theanine (from Green Tea): Promotes relaxation without sedation.
HERBS – REMEDIES:
Valerian Root (Valeriana officinalis): Traditional sedative herb to reduce sleep latency.
Chamomile (Matricaria chamomilla): Mildly sedative herb that calms the nervous system.

Individual Variation: Nutrient needs and responses to supplements vary greatly based on genetics, lifestyle, age, and existing health conditions. Everyone's biochemistry is different—what works for one person may not work for another
Quality & Dosage Matters: Seek out reputable brands that provide **third-party testing** and **transparent labeling** to ensure purity and potency.
Professional Guidance: Certain supplements can interact with medications or exacerbate health conditions. Always discuss any new supplement or herb with

a qualified healthcare provider, especially if you have a diagnosed condition or take prescription drugs.

Lifestyle Integration: Supplements are most effective when combined with a nutrient-dense diet, regular exercise, stress management, and adequate sleep.

"In terms of flu prevention, for my son I'll do a quick smoothie, usually with spinach, avocado or broccoli. And then throw in strawberries and blueberries to hide the greens." – Tia Mowry

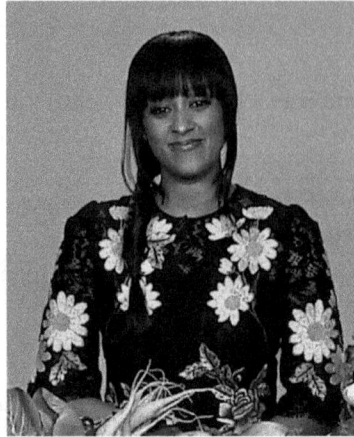

Tia Mowry
Credit – Wikimedia Commons

10.1.3: LIFESTYLE FACTORS BEYOND SUPPLEMENTS

Supplements can support health, but lifestyle factors like diet, exercise, sleep, stress management, and social connections are critical for preventing chronic diseases and promoting longevity. These habits work together to reduce inflammation, enhance immunity, and improve overall well-being.

DIET

A nutrient-rich diet is key to preventing diseases like heart disease, diabetes, and cancer. The Mediterranean diet, rich in fruits, vegetables, whole grains, lean proteins, and olive oil, is linked to a 25% lower risk of cardiovascular events (*Nature Aging*). The DASH diet, focusing on low sodium and high potassium, effectively lowers blood pressure. A 2025 study found plant-based diets reduce inflammatory markers by 15%, supporting longevity (*Nature Aging*). For more information on this and every other diet in the last century, get my book **The Ultimate AI Diet - Consolidating the Best Diets Over the Last 100 Years: Achieve Fast, Lasting Weight Management with a Personalized, Modern Approach Backed by a Century of Proven Success.**

240

EXERCISE

Regular physical activity strengthens the heart, muscles, and bones while boosting mental health. The American Heart Association recommends 150 minutes of moderate aerobic exercise or 75 minutes of vigorous exercise weekly, plus strength training. A 2025 meta-analysis showed a 30% lower all-cause mortality risk for active individuals compared to sedentary ones (*The Lancet*).

SLEEP

Quality sleep (7–9 hours nightly) supports tissue repair, hormone regulation, and cognitive health. Poor sleep increases risks of obesity, diabetes, and cognitive decline. A 2025 study linked consistent sleep to lower inflammation and better immune function (*Sleep Medicine Reviews*).

STRESS MANAGEMENT

Chronic stress raises cortisol, contributing to hypertension and mental health issues. Mindfulness, yoga, and deep breathing can lower stress. A 2025 study found regular mindfulness practice reduced cortisol by 20% and improved immunity (*Psychosomatic Medicine*).

SOCIAL CONNECTIONS

Strong social ties reduce depression and mortality risks. A 2025 study showed individuals with robust social networks have a 50% lower risk of premature death (*PLOS Medicine*). Community activities and relationships foster mental and physical health.

PRACTICAL TIPS

Eat more fruits, vegetables, and whole grains, aiming for a Mediterranean-style diet.
Walk, cycle, or lift weights regularly to meet exercise guidelines.
Prioritize 7–9 hours of sleep with a consistent schedule.
Practice 10 minutes of mindfulness or yoga daily.
Join community groups or maintain close relationships to stay connected.

10.1.4: PERSONALIZED MEDICINE AND GENETICS

Personalized medicine tailors prevention and treatment to your genetic profile, lifestyle, and environment, offering precise strategies to reduce disease risk.

GENETIC TESTING

Genetic tests identify predispositions to diseases like breast cancer (BRCA1/2 mutations) or heart disease. Direct-to-consumer kits like 23andMe provide health risk insights, but interpretation requires professional guidance. A 2025 study found genetic testing increased preventive actions in 60% of users (*Genetics in Medicine*).

PHARMACOGENOMICS

Pharmacogenomics studies how genes affect drug responses, ensuring safer and more effective treatments. For example, variations in the CYP2CI9 gene influence responses to antidepressants. A 2025 review showed pharmacogenomic testing improved outcomes for depression and cardiovascular treatments (*Clinical Pharmacology & Therapeutics*).

NUTRIGENOMICS

Nutrigenomics explores how genes interact with nutrients to influence health. For instance, MTHFR gene variants may require higher folate intake to reduce cardiovascular risk. A 2025 study found personalized nutrition based on genetics improved metabolic health by 20% compared to standard diets (*Nutrients*).

PRACTICAL STEPS

Consider genetic testing through reputable providers like 23andMe (*23andMe*) and consult a genetic counselor.

Ask your doctor about pharmacogenomic testing if on multiple medications.

Use nutrigenomic insights to adjust your diet, focusing on foods that match your genetic needs.

Work with a healthcare provider to interpret genetic data and create a prevention plan.

By combining lifestyle changes with personalized medicine, you can proactively prevent disease and enhance longevity.

SECTION TWO: MODERN CHALLENGES

Many of the **infectious diseases** (Plague, Diphtheria, Tetanus, TB, Malaria) we outline in **Sections 2 and 3** require **urgent medical treatment** with **pharmaceuticals** (antibiotics, antitoxins, or antiparasitics). Vitamins, supplements, and herbs can be **complementary** but **do not** replace standard care.

Autoimmune and chronic conditions often need prescription therapies (immunosuppressants, biologics, etc.). Supplements, vitamins, and herbs can sometimes help manage symptoms or support overall health but should be integrated under professional supervision.

Dosages of the supplements and herbs mentioned vary widely based on individual circumstances (age, weight, comorbidities). Always **consult a qualified healthcare provider** before starting any new regimen. Nutritional interventions work best as part of a comprehensive approach, including **dietary changes, exercise, stress management**, and other **lifestyle factors**.

This information is for **educational** purposes only and does not constitute medical advice. Each person's situation is unique. If you suspect or are diagnosed with any of these conditions, please work closely with a healthcare professional.

10.2.1: MODERN CHRONIC CONDITIONS

ASTHMA

Key Concerns: Airway hyperresponsiveness, inflammation, mucus overproduction, restricted breathing.

VITAMINS AND MINERALS:

Vitamin D3: Low levels are often linked with worse respiratory outcomes; supports immune modulation in the lungs.

Magnesium: May help relax bronchial smooth muscles; low magnesium can exacerbate asthma symptoms.

SUPPLEMENTS:

Omega-3 Fatty Acids: Anti-inflammatory properties can help reduce airway inflammation.

N-Acetylcysteine (NAC): Helps thin mucus and replenish glutathione in lung tissue.

HERBS – REMEDIES:

Mullein (Verbascum thapsus): Traditionally used to soothe respiratory tract irritation and reduce coughing.

Licorice Root (Glycyrrhiza glabra): Has demulcent properties to coat and soothe airways; caution in hypertension.

Other Therapies: Inhaled bronchodilators, inhaled corticosteroids, leukotriene inhibitors (standard medical treatments).

"Hindered by asthma since I was six weeks old, I had begun experimenting with my diet and discovered a disquieting correlation. When I stopped eating the normal America diet of sugar, fats, alcohol, chemicals, and additives, I felt better. I could breathe freely. When I tried to sneak in a hamburger and a Coke, my body rebelled." – Paul Hawken

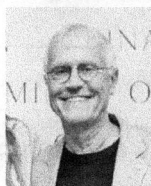

Paul Hawken
Credit – Wikimedia Commons

10.2.2: NEURODEVELOPMENTAL AND BEHAVIORAL CONDITIONS

AUTISM SPECTRUM DISORDER (ASD)

Key Concerns: Communication and social interaction challenges, sensory sensitivities, possible GI issues, nutrient imbalances.

VITAMINS AND MINERALS:

Vitamin D3: Some research suggests low levels may be linked with more severe autism traits; supports immune and brain function.

B Vitamins (B6, B9, B12): Important for neurotransmitter synthesis and methylation pathways; some clinicians use higher-dose B6 or methylated folate in certain cases.

Magnesium: May help with relaxation and reduce certain behaviors if deficiency is present.

SUPPLEMENTS:

Omega-3 Fatty Acids: May support brain development and help with inflammation linked to neurological function.

Probiotics: GI symptoms are common in autism; rebalancing gut flora can sometimes improve discomfort and behavior.

HERBS – REMEDIES:

Chamomile (Matricaria chamomilla): Gentle calming effect; can help with mild anxiety or restlessness.

Lemon Balm (Melissa officinalis): Traditionally used for calming; sometimes used in children with hyperactivity or insomnia.

Other Therapies: Behavioral therapy, occupational therapy, speech therapy, specialized diets (e.g., gluten-free/casein-free) may be recommended.

ADD & ADHD

Key Concerns: Attention span, impulsivity, possible dopamine/norepinephrine dysregulation, stress and anxiety co-morbidities.

VITAMINS AND MINERALS:

Iron & Zinc: Low levels have been associated with reduced attention and cognitive function.

Magnesium & B6: Often used together to support neurotransmitter balance and calm hyperactivity.

SUPPLEMENTS:

Omega-3 Fatty Acids (EPA/DHA): Some studies show improved attention and mood regulation in children and adults with ADHD.

Phosphatidylserine (PS): May support cognitive function, memory, and attention.

HERBS – REMEDIES:

Ginkgo Biloba: May improve circulation to the brain and support focus in some individuals.

Bacopa Monnieri: Traditionally used in Ayurvedic medicine for cognition and memory.

Standard Treatments: Stimulant medications (e.g., methylphenidate, amphetamines) or non-stimulants (atomoxetine) often prescribed.

Remember, with ADHD, we must always highlight the potential creative strengths associated with the condition. **Albert Einstein's** famous quote below connects the potential for high creativity with the introspective nature that can sometimes accompany ADHD:

"The monotony and solitude of a quiet life stimulates the creative mind."

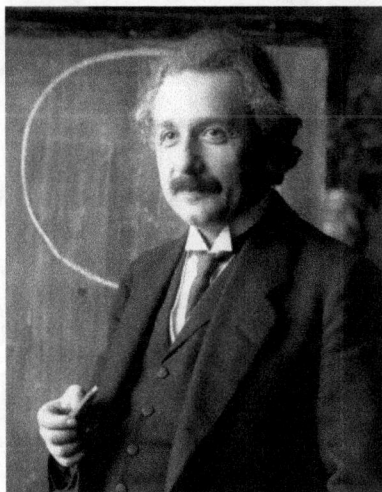

Albert Einstein
Credit – PICRYL / creativecommons.org

Many parents of children with ADHD or autism spectrum disorder (ASD) are caught between a rock and a hard place: standard prescription medications can calm restlessness and improve focus, but they often come with side-effects like poor sleep, appetite loss, or a "flat" mood. That has created a growing demand for gentler, more natural approaches—especially ones that don't require juggling several different pills every day. Enter *Regencell Bioscience (RGC)*, a Hong Kong company that's modernizing a traditional Chinese multi-herb liquid formula and testing it as a single, ready-to-drink treatment.

Early results are encouraging, but they're still just a first step. In RGC's second small study, seven school-age children took the herbal blend for three months and showed an average 37 percent drop in overall ADHD/ASD symptoms. That sounds impressive, yet it's important to remember two big caveats: the study group was tiny, and everyone knew they were taking the treatment (there was no placebo for comparison). Because expectations alone can influence how kids behave and how parents rate progress, researchers need larger, blinded trials before anyone can call this a proven breakthrough.

If you've already read about single-compound "brain boosters" like caffeine, L-theanine, or citicoline in earlier chapters, RGC's approach may feel very different. Those nootropics isolate one active ingredient and aim it at a specific pathway—say, boosting dopamine or sharpening alertness for a few hours. By contrast, the RGC formula keeps the herbs together as they've been used for centuries, hoping the mix of plant chemicals works in harmony to smooth mood, calm the mind, and support attention over the long haul. That holistic philosophy could offer a broader, gentler effect, but it also makes it harder to pin down exactly how (or why) the remedy works—another reason robust, placebo-controlled studies are so crucial before parents and clinicians can fully trust the results.

10.2.3: AUTOIMMUNE CONDITIONS

These are chronic diseases in which the immune system attacks the body's own tissues. Below are three examples:

PSORIASIS

Key Concerns: Overactive immune response leading to rapid skin cell turnover, inflammation, scaly patches.

VITAMINS AND MINERALS:

Vitamin D3: Topical and oral forms may help modulate immune activity in the skin.

Omega-3 Fatty Acids (while not a vitamin or mineral, it's often used similarly): Can reduce systemic inflammation.

Zinc: Important for skin integrity and immune modulation.

SUPPLEMENTS:

Probiotics: The gut-skin axis suggests a balanced microbiome may reduce autoimmune flare-ups.

Turmeric/Curcumin: Potent anti-inflammatory properties; may reduce plaque severity in some individuals.

HERBS – REMEDIES:

Aloe Vera (topical): Cooling, may reduce itching and inflammation on the skin.

Milk Thistle (Silybum marianum): Liver support may indirectly help manage inflammation.

Other Therapies: Topical corticosteroids, phototherapy, immune-modulating drugs (e.g., methotrexate, biologics).

> *"Autoimmunity is probably the next frontier. The majority of cases of autoimmune disease result from a complex genetic problem that has environmental influences. It is a colossal task for the immune system to*

maintain tolerance of self and yet be ready to react to everything in the world around us." – Bruce Beutler

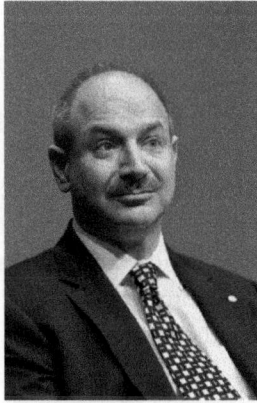

Bruce Beutler
Credit – Wikimedia Commons

MULTIPLE SCLEROSIS (MS)

Key Concerns: Demyelination in the central nervous system, inflammation, autoimmune attack on neurons.

VITAMINS AND MINERALS:

Vitamin D3: Low levels linked with increased MS risk and relapse; essential for immune regulation.

B Vitamins: Support nerve function (B12 particularly important for myelin health).

Magnesium: Muscle and nerve function support; helps reduce spasms and cramps.

SUPPLEMENTS:

Omega-3 Fatty Acids: Anti-inflammatory effects may help slow progression and reduce flare-ups.

N-Acetylcysteine (NAC): Antioxidant support for potentially reduced oxidative damage.

CoQ10: Mitochondrial support, may aid in energy production in neurons.

HERBS – REMEDIES:

Turmeric/Curcumin: Anti-inflammatory and neuroprotective in some studies.

Ginkgo Biloba: Some MS patients report improvements in cognitive function and fatigue.

Other Therapies: Disease-modifying medications (e.g., interferons, monoclonal antibodies), physical therapy.

INFLAMMATORY BOWEL DISEASE (IBD)
(Includes Crohn's Disease and Ulcerative Colitis)

Key Concerns: Chronic inflammation of the GI tract, malabsorption, potential for nutrient deficiencies, immune dysregulation.

VITAMINS AND MINERALS:

Vitamin D3: May help modulate immune response in the gut; often low in IBD patients.

Iron & B12: Deficiencies common due to malabsorption and chronic GI blood loss.

Magnesium & Calcium: Chronic diarrhea can deplete electrolytes.

SUPPLEMENTS:

Probiotics (e.g., Lactobacillus, Bifidobacterium strains): May help restore healthy gut flora and reduce inflammation.

Omega-3 Fatty Acids: Anti-inflammatory; some evidence for reduced flare frequency.

L-Glutamine: Can support intestinal lining repair.

HERBS – REMEDIES:

Aloe Vera (oral juice): Some anecdotal evidence for soothing gut mucosa; use caution (may cause diarrhea).

Boswellia Serrata: Anti-inflammatory resin that may help reduce GI inflammation.

Other Therapies: Immunosuppressants (e.g., corticosteroids), 5-ASA drugs, biologics (anti-TNF agents).

SECTION THREE: MEDIEVAL, HISTORIC, THIRD-WORLD AND ENVIRONMENTAL INFECTIOUS DISEASES

10.3.1: MEDIEVAL AND HISTORIC INFECTIOUS DISEASES

Unfortunately, some diseases have survived for hundreds or thousands of years, only to emerge again. The good news is that we have made incredible strides to abolish or lessen the effects of these diseases that killed millions.

PLAGUE (Yersinia pestis)

Key Concerns: Highly infectious bacterial disease (bubonic, pneumonic forms), can be fatal if untreated, fever, swollen lymph nodes.

STANDARD MEDICAL TREATMENT:

Antibiotics: Aminoglycosides (e.g., streptomycin) or fluoroquinolones (e.g., ciprofloxacin) are first-line. **Rapid treatment is critical.**

VITAMINS AND MINERALS: (as adjuncts, not primary treatment)

Vitamin C: Supports immune function and tissue repair.

Zinc: May help immune response, but must be careful with dosing.

SUPPLEMENTS:

Elderberry: Immune-modulating properties; historically used for infections (adjunct only).

Garlic: Traditional antimicrobial supportive; again, only a supportive measure.

HERBS/REMEDIES:

Echinacea: Some use for immune support.

Goldenseal (Hydrastis canadensis): Historically used for bacterial infections (berberine content).

Note: Plague is a medical emergency—seek immediate professional medical intervention.

DIPHTHERIA (Corynebacterium diphtheriae)

Key Concerns: Bacterial toxin-producing infection affecting throat/nose; can lead to severe breathing issues, heart failure, nerve damage.

STANDARD MEDICAL TREATMENT:

Diphtheria Antitoxin and **Antibiotics** (e.g., penicillin or erythromycin).

Vaccination is key for prevention (DPT or Tdap).

VITAMINS AND MINERALS: (as adjuncts)

Vitamin C: May support recovery and immune response.

Zinc: Essential for immune function.

SUPPLEMENTS:

Probiotics: Support general immune function and gut flora during/after antibiotic use.

HERBS/REMEDIES:

Licorice Root: Historically used to soothe throat inflammation (adjunct only).

Sage (Salvia officinalis): Traditional antiseptic gargle; mild support.

Note: Medical intervention is critical; herbs and supplements are only complementary.

TETANUS (Clostridium tetani)

Key Concerns: Toxin-mediated muscle spasms ("lockjaw"), can be fatal if untreated.

STANDARD MEDICAL TREATMENT:

Tetanus Immunoglobulin (TIG), **Wound debridement**, and **Antibiotics** (metronidazole, penicillin).

Tetanus Vaccine is highly effective in prevention.

VITAMINS AND MINERALS:

Magnesium: May help reduce muscle spasms, but must be carefully monitored.

SUPPLEMENTS/HERBS:

Generally supportive for immune health only (vitamin C, mild adaptogens).

Chamomile or **Valerian** might help with mild sedation, but in a clinical setting sedation is more complex.

Note: Tetanus is an emergency; immediate professional care is essential.

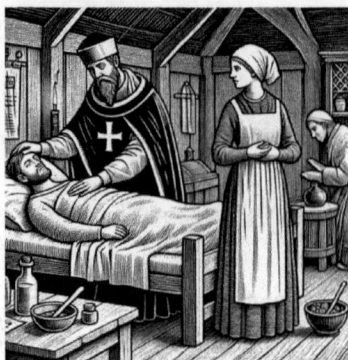

10.3.2: THIRD-WORLD INFECTIOUS DISEASES

TUBERCULOSIS (TB) (Mycobacterium tuberculosis)

Key Concerns: Chronic lung infection, can affect other organs, spread via airborne droplets, potential for antibiotic resistance.

STANDARD MEDICAL TREATMENT:

RIPE Therapy (Rifampin, Isoniazid, Pyrazinamide, Ethambutol) for active TB. **Treatment is lengthy (6+ months).**

VITAMINS AND MINERALS:

Vitamin D3: Historical link between vitamin D deficiency and increased TB susceptibility.

B Vitamins: Isoniazid can deplete B6 (pyridoxine); supplementation often recommended.

Iron: Monitor levels; chronic infection can cause anemia, but excess iron can also feed bacteria—balance is key.

SUPPLEMENTS:

Probiotics: May help with gut flora balance during prolonged antibiotic use.

N-Acetylcysteine (NAC): Antioxidant, can support lung health.

HERBS/REMEDIES:

Garlic (Allium sativum): Traditional antimicrobial; mild adjunct only.

Echinacea: May support immune function; no direct TB-specific evidence.

Note: TB requires strict medical supervision; herbal remedies are only complementary.

MALARIA (Plasmodium spp.)

Key Concerns: Parasitic infection spread by mosquitoes; fever, chills, organ damage if severe.

STANDARD MEDICAL TREATMENT:

Antimalarial Medications: Chloroquine, artemisinin-based combination therapies (ACTs), mefloquine, etc.

Prevention: Mosquito nets, repellents, prophylactic meds when traveling.

VITAMINS AND MINERALS: (adjunctive)

Vitamin A & D: General immune support in regions with deficiencies.

Iron: Caution—some forms of malaria can worsen with iron supplementation in certain populations; assess case by case.

SUPPLEMENTS:

Probiotics: Supports overall gut health, especially when taking antimalarial drugs that may affect microbiome.

Antioxidants (like vitamin C or NAC) to reduce oxidative stress.

HERBS/REMEDIES:

Artemisia annua (Sweet Wormwood): Source of artemisinin, used in standard malaria treatments (ACT).

Neem (Azadirachta indica): Traditional use for fever management, though more research needed.

Note: Immediate medical intervention is vital if malaria is suspected; herbal usage is supportive and does not replace standard therapy.

CHOLERA

Key Concerns: Cholera is caused by the bacterium *Vibrio cholerae*, typically transmitted through contaminated water or food. It is characterized by acute watery diarrhea, which can quickly lead to severe dehydration if untreated.

STANDARD MEDICAL TREATMENT:

Rehydration Therapy/Oral Rehydration Solution (ORS): The mainstay treatment; standard WHO-ORS packets contain a precise balance of glucose and electrolytes.

Intravenous (IV) Fluids: Required if the patient is unable to drink or is severely dehydrated.

Antibiotics like **doxycycline** or **azithromycin** can reduce the duration and volume of diarrhea. Antibiotics are typically used in moderate to severe cases or to reduce transmission, but they are secondary to rehydration therapy.

Zinc Supplementation (for Children): The WHO recommends zinc for children with diarrhea (including cholera) to shorten the duration and reduce the severity.

VITAMINS AND MINERALS:

While rehydration and proper antibiotic therapy are the cornerstones of cholera treatment, the following vitamins, minerals, and supplements may offer **support** to the immune system and assist in recovery:

Zinc: Proven to reduce the duration and severity of diarrheal illnesses, especially in children. WHO recommends 10–20 mg of zinc per day for 10–14 days in children with diarrhea.

Vitamin C: Supports immune function and may help decrease oxidative stress. **Sources:** Citrus fruits, tomatoes, bell peppers (or in supplement form if local produce is unavailable).

Vitamin A: Critical for maintaining healthy mucosal surfaces and immune defenses. In areas where Vitamin A deficiency is common, supplementation is often recommended, especially in children.

B-Complex Vitamins: Important for energy metabolism, especially helpful if the patient has poor nutritional intake. **Sources:** Whole grains, legumes, or a balanced multi-vitamin if available.

Electrolytes: Dehydration from cholera leads to massive losses of sodium, potassium, and chloride. **ORS:** Contains these critical electrolytes. Additional potassium (e.g., from bananas or coconut water) can be supportive if accessible.

Probiotics: May help restore healthy gut flora after or during severe diarrheal episodes. **Potential Sources:** Fermented foods (yogurt, kefir, certain fermented vegetables) or probiotic supplements if available.

SUPPLEMENTS/HERBS: (Supportive Measures)

No herb or natural remedy can replace medical treatment for cholera (i.e., rehydration and antibiotics). However, certain herbs and home remedies may provide **support** by helping with mild antimicrobial properties, soothing the digestive tract, or adding nutritional value. Keep in mind that evidence for these is limited, and they should be used only as **complementary** measures alongside proper medical care.

Ginger: May help reduce nausea and vomiting, mild anti-inflammatory properties. **Use:** Ginger tea or grated ginger in warm water.

Garlic: Traditionally considered to have broad-spectrum antimicrobial properties; may support overall immunity. **Use:** Incorporate into meals or, if tolerable, consume raw in small amounts.

Turmeric (Curcumin): Anti-inflammatory properties; some studies suggest it may help gut health. **Use:** Can be added to soups or teas.

Holy Basil (Tulsi): Traditionally valued in some cultures for its antibacterial properties and immune support. **Use:** As a tea or added to warm water, if accessible.

Lemon/Lime Juice: Has mild antimicrobial effects against some waterborne pathogens; can improve taste and encourage fluid intake. **Use:** Add to safe, purified water (but do **not** rely on it alone to purify unsafe water).

Coconut Water: Natural source of some electrolytes, can be helpful to maintain hydration. **Caution:** Not a complete replacement for ORS, as it lacks the precise balance of electrolytes in standard rehydration solutions.

Immediate Rehydration Is Crucial

The most life-threatening aspect of cholera is fluid and electrolyte loss. Oral Rehydration Solution (ORS) or IV fluids are the top priority.

Seek Medical Help Early

Even mild cases can progress rapidly. Antibiotics can be important, but **they do not replace** the absolute need for rapid rehydration.

Nutritional and Herbal Support

Supplements (zinc, vitamins) and certain herbs can **support** overall health and recovery but **cannot** replace medical treatments.

Prevention

Access to safe water, proper sanitation, and community education significantly reduce the risk of outbreaks.

"The rewards for biotechnology are tremendous – to solve disease, eliminate poverty, age gracefully. It sounds so much cooler than Facebook." – George M. Church

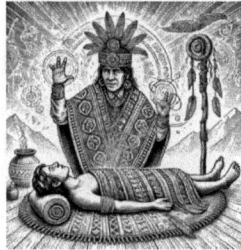

10.3.3: TOXIC MATERIAL ABSORPTION AND ENVIRONMENTAL POISONING

(**Examples: Heavy metals like lead/mercury, industrial chemicals, pollutants.**)

Key Concerns: Accumulation of toxins, oxidative stress, organ damage (liver, kidneys, brain), neurological deficits.

STANDARD MEDICAL TREATMENT:

Chelation Therapy (EDTA, DMSA, DMPS) for significant heavy metal poisoning; must be medically supervised.

VITAMINS AND MINERALS:

Vitamin C: Supports antioxidant defenses and may assist with detox pathways.

Selenium: Supports glutathione peroxidase, helps protect cells from oxidative damage.

Zinc: Helps maintain healthy metabolism; can sometimes displace more toxic metals.

SUPPLEMENTS:

N-Acetylcysteine (NAC): Helps replenish glutathione, crucial for detoxification.

Alpha-Lipoic Acid (ALA): Chelating properties and antioxidant support.

Chlorella/Spirulina: Some evidence suggests they can bind heavy metals in the gut, though data vary.

HERBS/REMEDIES:
Milk Thistle (Silybum marianum): Liver support for detox processes.
Cilantro (Coriandrum sativum): Folk remedy for heavy metal chelation; evidence is mixed.

SECTION FOUR: HOW VITAMINS AND SUPPLEMENTS AFFECT EACH OF YOUR ORGANS

How can we maintain each of our organs with maximum efficiency? Recently, I took a blood test, and in my lab results, my creatinine levels were somewhat high. I wanted to research what I may be taking that would be affecting my kidneys, and as a result, I cut back on my Vitamin C and Calcium supplements. Much of this information is dispersed throughout the book, but this section should be helpful if you're concerned about any one of your major organs.

HEART
Positive: Supplements like omega-3 fatty acids (found in fish oil) help your heart by lowering inflammation, cholesterol, and triglycerides. Magnesium and potassium can keep your blood pressure steady, helping reduce stress on the heart. Coenzyme Q10 (CoQ10) is also great for heart health, improving the heart's energy and potentially reducing symptoms in heart failure patients.
Negative: However, too much calcium from supplements might actually raise the risk of heart problems by causing calcium buildup in your arteries. High-dose vitamin E has been linked to a greater risk of heart failure in some studies, so moderation is key.

BRAIN
Positive: Omega-3 fatty acids, particularly DHA, are amazing for your brain. They help maintain clear thinking, memory, and may even lower the risk of dementia. Vitamin B12 and folate also keep your brain healthy by supporting nerve function and preventing mental fatigue. Supplements like ginkgo biloba might improve blood flow to the brain, boosting memory and concentration.
Negative: High doses of certain supplements, like iron or copper, can harm brain cells or increase dementia risks. Excess vitamin B6 intake over a long period can even cause nerve damage or confusion, showing how balance is crucial.

LIVER
Positive: Milk thistle and turmeric (curcumin) can protect your liver by reducing inflammation and helping it detoxify harmful substances. Vitamin E can support the liver, particularly if you have fatty liver disease.
Negative: High doses of vitamin A, niacin, and certain herbal supplements (such as kava and green tea extracts) can seriously harm your liver. It's essential not to exceed recommended doses of these supplements to avoid liver damage.

KIDNEYS

Positive: Vitamin D is good for kidney function, especially if you're deficient. It helps manage calcium and phosphorus levels in your blood, protecting kidney health.

Negative: Taking too much vitamin D, vitamin C, or calcium can put a strain on your kidneys. High doses can increase your risk of kidney stones or kidney damage, so always follow recommended amounts.

LUNGS

Positive: Vitamin C, vitamin E, and antioxidants like selenium can protect your lungs by reducing inflammation and damage from pollutants or smoke.

Negative: Surprisingly, some studies suggest high doses of beta-carotene supplements (a type of vitamin A) may actually increase lung cancer risk, especially among smokers. So, be cautious with high-dose antioxidant supplements.

STOMACH AND DIGESTIVE SYSTEM

Positive: Probiotics (beneficial bacteria supplements) help your digestive system run smoothly by improving gut health and nutrient absorption. Ginger and peppermint supplements ease digestive discomfort and nausea.

Negative: Too much iron, zinc, or magnesium can upset your stomach, causing nausea, diarrhea, or constipation. Overuse of fiber supplements without enough water can lead to bloating or digestive blockages.

BONES

Positive: Vitamin D, calcium, magnesium, and vitamin K are essential for strong bones. They help prevent osteoporosis by building bone density and keeping your bones healthy as you age.

Negative: Excessive vitamin A intake can actually weaken your bones, increasing fracture risk. Also, too much calcium without balanced magnesium and vitamin D may cause calcium deposits in the wrong places, like your arteries.

SKIN

Positive: Vitamins C, E, and A (especially retinol) can keep your skin looking youthful by fighting off damage from sunlight and pollution. Collagen supplements might help reduce wrinkles and improve elasticity.

Negative: Overdosing on vitamin A supplements can lead to dry, peeling skin, and too much niacin can cause severe flushing, redness, or itching.

EYES

Positive: Vitamin A, lutein, zeaxanthin, and omega-3 fatty acids help your eyes by protecting them from age-related macular degeneration and cataracts.

Negative: High-dose beta-carotene (vitamin A) supplements, particularly in smokers, may harm rather than protect eyes, potentially increasing health risks.

PANCREAS
Positive: Chromium supplements can help your pancreas regulate insulin better, which might improve blood sugar control in people with diabetes.
Negative: Taking excessive chromium or herbal supplements like bitter melon without medical supervision could negatively affect your blood sugar, causing unexpected spikes or drops.

IMMUNE SYSTEM
Positive: Vitamin C, zinc, vitamin D, and echinacea help your immune system, pushing your body to fight off illnesses faster or reducing how often you get sick.
Negative: Overusing zinc supplements (especially for longer than recommended) can actually weaken your immune system over time, making infections harder to fight off.

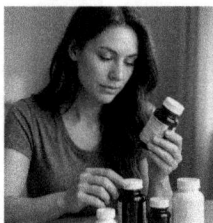

Vitamins and supplements can offer powerful benefits if used thoughtfully, but too much or improper use can lead to significant risks. Always check with a professional before adding high-dose supplements or new products to your routine to make sure you're staying safe and truly supporting your health.

Our final chapter will guide you in creating a customized, sustainable plan — combining the best of everything we've explored.

I WANT TO OFFER YOU A FREE GIFT
I hope you're loving this book so far. In my **HEALTH AND LONGEVITY SERIES,** I address slowing aging, vitamins and supplements for longevity (this book), an excellent AI diet and weight management plan, how positive thinking can add years to your life, and the power of your mind and body. Before we get into crafting your own personalized longevity blueprint, I've also created a **TWELVE-STEP ACTION PLAN FOR LONGEVITY AND HEALTHSPAN**, a roadmap for health and longevity encompassing elements from **all** my books, and I want to share it with you.

If you want a free copy of my plan, email us at...
<<   modernrenaissancepublishing@gmail.com   >>

with the subject line **12-STEP ACTION PLAN FOR LONGEVITY,** and I'll email you back a free copy at no obligation whatsoever to you as a heartfelt thanks for reading this book. Or you can access it through our website at https://www.modernrenaissancepublishing.com.

CHAPTER ELEVEN
CRAFTING YOUR PERSONALIZED HEALTH AND LONGEVITY BLUEPRINT

The Chinese philosopher **Lao Tzu** said, *"The journey of a thousand miles begins with a single step."* It's never too late to reverse the terrible health decisions we all made when we were young and carefree. My old friend, famous **Moody Blues** and **Paul McCartney & Wings** guitarist **Denny Laine** said:

"You can't get tied into your past. It's not fun for me.
You can't just keep doing the same material forever.
Some people just play the hits, and it's the same show every night.
They're happy to do that. I personally am not."

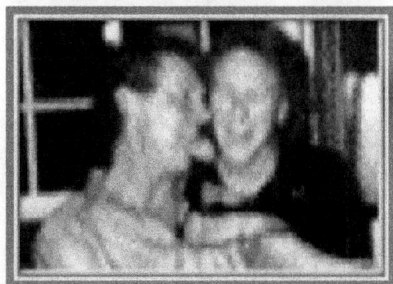

Tad Sisler singing with Denny Laine
Source – Sisler Private Collection

What if you could start now, designing a daily regimen – aligned with your body's unique needs – that keeps you energized, resilient, and focused on living life to the fullest?

SECTION ONE
ASSESSING YOUR INDIVIDUAL NEEDS
11.1.1: HEALTH STATUS AND GOALS

BEGIN WITH A COMPREHENSIVE CHECKUP (BLOODWORK, LIFESTYLE, FAMILY HISTORY).

Start with a thorough health assessment to get a clear baseline for your wellness plan. Start with standard blood tests (like a complete blood count, metabolic panel, and nutrient levels) and a careful review of your personal and family medical history. Combine these findings with insights into your daily habits—

like diet, sleep, and exercise—to pinpoint areas that need improvement and lay the groundwork for a more targeted vitamin and supplement strategy. The whole idea is to take care of yourself. *Pretty Little Liars* actress **Lucy Hale** got so caught up in her work that she lost her priorities briefly and became ill. **Lucy** said:

"I've never really talked about this, but I would go days without eating. Or maybe I'd have some fruit and then go to the gym for three hours. I knew I had a problem... It was a gradual process but I changed myself."

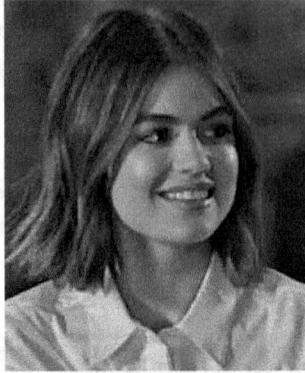

Lucy Hale
Credit – Wikimedia Commons

CLARIFY TOP PRIORITIES: IMMUNITY, ENERGY, JOINT HEALTH, ETC.

Before exploring specific supplements, you need to know what you want to achieve. Whether you want to boost immune function, increase daily energy, improve joint and bone health, or address other specific concerns, identifying these core objectives will shape your choices. Tackle the problems most relevant to your current lifestyle and long-term well-being.

ALIGN YOUR GOALS WITH REALISTIC, TIME-BOUND STEPS

Set achievable milestones to transform your ambitions into practical action plans. For instance, if you want to boost your vitamin D levels, pick a specific dose, schedule follow-up blood work in three months, and track changes in your energy or mood. Break down your objectives into smaller steps with clear deadlines to maintain momentum and measure your progress effectively.

DIFFERENTIATE BETWEEN SHORT-TERM FIXES VS. LONG-TERM STRATEGY

While short bursts of supplemental support—like high-dose vitamin C when you feel a cold coming on—can help address immediate concerns, they don't replace a consistent, well-rounded regimen designed for longevity. Strike a balance between quick interventions and a sustained plan to make sure you're not simply "patching" issues but working on lasting change in your health. The goal is to prevent nutrient imbalances and support better vitality and resilience over the long haul.

"When you have a system, you kind of get in a routine of what's important. And then you spend a lot more time on thinking of things that would make it better." – Nick Saban

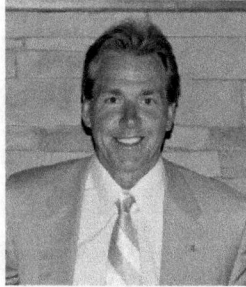

Nick Saban
Credit – Wikimedia Commons

11.1.2: LIFESTYLE AUDIT (DIET, SLEEP, STRESS)

SUPPLEMENTS CAN NOT COMPENSATE FOR CHRONIC STRESS OR POOR SLEEP

While vitamins and herbs are great, they can't undo the effects of persistent stress or a chronic lack of rest. High cortisol levels and insufficient sleep can suppress your immunity, disrupt your digestion, and reverse the benefits of a healthy diet or targeted supplements. Work on your stress levels by practicing mindfulness, relaxation techniques, or counseling and prioritizing quality sleep to really see a meaningful, lasting health transformation.

IDENTIFY DAILY DIET PATTERNS - WHERE ARE THE GAPS?

Before supplementing, take a good look at what you eat each day. Are you consistently short on nutrient-dense fruits and vegetables, or do you rely heavily on processed foods? Start by recognizing any dietary gaps you have, and this will help you decide which vitamins, minerals, or herbs to emphasize. It also paves the way for informed changes, like adding more leafy greens for magnesium or incorporating fish for essential fatty acids, rather than guessing or over-supplementing.

LENNY KRAVITZ

Lenny Kravitz is known for his revolutionary music and his eccentric style, In a recent story on the New Beauty website, he talked about how he maintains his cool composure inside and out. Despite his A-list status, **Kravitz's** self-care routine is pretty low-key as he relies on a few simple products to keep his mind and body in shape.

One of the few wellness-products he swears by is Magnesium Gummies. "I tend to get very creative at night and sometimes need a little help relaxing," **Lenny** says, "this dose of magnesium starts to wind me down, and it comes in a gummy form, so it's like I'm just eating candy." **Kravitz** mentions that these stress-relieving gummies are a perfect addition to his nightly ritual that includes *"turning off all my devices, taking a bath, eating some of these gummies, and then, hopefully, falling asleep easier."*

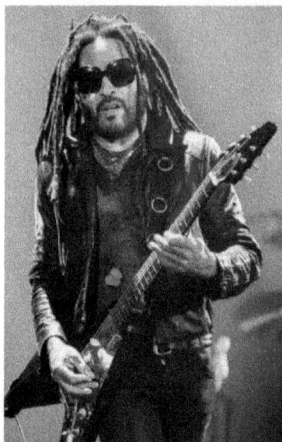

Lenny Kravitz
Credit – Wikimedia Commons

EVALUATE TIME CONSTRAINTS – REALISTIC CHANGES MATTER

It's hard to adopt healthy habits if your schedule is already packed. It's important to be realistic: Commit to simple, sustainable changes. Doing this can be more powerful than taking on an all-or-nothing approach that collapses under day-to-day pressure. If you only have fifteen minutes for a quick home workout or meal prep, use that window effectively—small, consistent adjustments over time can yield significant, long-lasting benefits.

SLEEP HYGIENE IS PIVOTAL FOR NUTRIENT ASSIMILATION AND HORMONE REGULATION

It's great to get enough rest, but sleep is much more than just that. Good, deep sleep is when your body performs critical tasks like tissue repair, hormone balance, and cellular cleanup. Adequate, uninterrupted sleep enhances how well your body absorbs and utilizes nutrients. Even the most carefully selected supplements won't deliver their full benefits without restorative sleep. Cultivate good sleep habits—like minimizing screen time and creating a consistent bedtime routine—and you will support your body's capacity for healing and rejuvenation.

"Sleep is the best meditation." – Dalai Lama

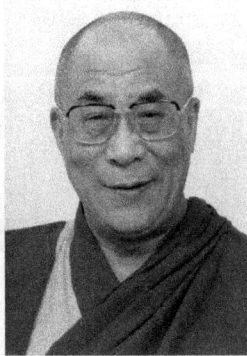

Dalai Lama
Credit – Wikimedia Commons

II.I.3: NAVIGATING INFORMATION OVERLOAD AND UTILIZING AI FOR GENERAL HEALTH

THE INTERNET IS FLOODED WITH CONFLICTING DATA - ALWAYS USE PEER-REVIEWED SOURCES

With endless blogs, articles, and social media posts claiming to offer the "best" health advice, it's easy to be overwhelmed. When researching vitamins, supplements, and herbs, prioritize reputable, peer-reviewed journals and verified medical organizations. These sources use rigorous review processes and scientific data, making sure that the information you rely on for your health decisions is accurate and current.

GET ADVICE FROM HEALTH PROFESSIONALS

Learning on your own is great, but it can only take you so far. Talking with experts like nutritionists, dietitians, or doctors trained in holistic and integrative medicine can make a huge difference. They can help you pick the best supplements based on your unique body and health goals, instead of just guessing.

KEEP A HEALTH JOURNAL TO SEE WHAT WORKS

Keeping a daily diary of what you eat, how well you sleep, your stress levels, and any supplements you try can teach you a lot. For instance, you might notice more energy after starting a B-vitamin complex or better sleep after adding magnesium. Writing things down also helps your healthcare provider make smart adjustments to your plan.

KAMILA VALIEVA

Kamila Valieva, a talented teenage figure skater from Russia, was given a mix of 56 different supplements and medications by her team to enhance her performance. One of these substances was banned, leading to her suspension from competitions. Even though it wasn't technically her fault, she paid the price. There can be a danger in taking numerous supplements without proper oversight, especially for young athletes.

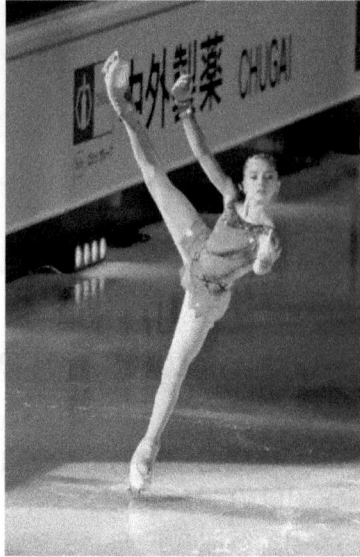

Kamila Valieva
Credit – Wikimedia Commons

MAKE SMALL, STEADY CHANGES INSTEAD OF BIG ONES

Trying to change everything overnight often leads to frustration and giving up. It's better to focus on small steps, like adding just one new supplement at a time and paying attention to how it affects you, or slowly improving your diet. Little changes are easier to stick with and can lead to bigger, lasting improvements in your overall health.

II.1.4: TOOLS FOR TRACKING PROGRESS

Various tools can monitor diet, exercise, sleep, supplement intake, and overall well-being, helping you optimize your regimen. Here is your one-stop breakdown, including some we've already mentioned in the book:

HEALTH AND FITNESS APPS

Nutrition Tracking: Apps like MyFitnessPal or Cronometer track food intake, nutrients, and supplement schedules, ensuring you meet dietary goals. A 2025 study found app users improved nutrient intake by 15%.

Exercise Tracking: Strava or Fitbit apps log physical activity, setting goals for steps or workouts.

Sleep and Mood Tracking: Sleep Cycle or Headspace monitor sleep quality and mental well-being, linking habits to health outcomes.

Supplement Management: Medisafe reminds you to take supplements and tracks adherence.

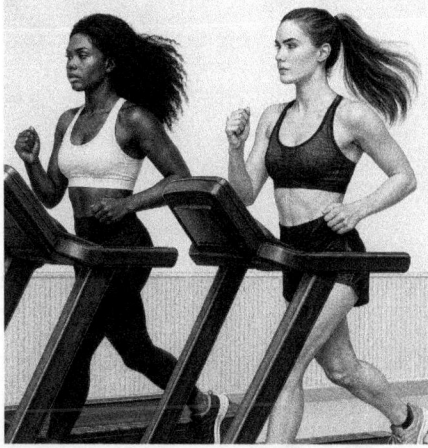

WEARABLE DEVICES

Fitness Trackers: Fitbit or Garmin devices measure steps, heart rate, and calories burned, providing real-time activity data.

Smartwatches: Apple Watch or Samsung Galaxy Watch offer advanced features like ECG and blood oxygen monitoring, useful for tracking cardiovascular health.

Sleep Trackers: Oura Ring provides detailed sleep stage analysis and recovery scores, aiding in lifestyle adjustments.

JOURNALING

Physical Journals: Log daily habits, moods, and supplement effects in a notebook to identify patterns.

Digital Journals: Apps like Day One or Notion organize entries for easy review and trend analysis.

BIOMETRIC TESTING

Blood Tests: Regular tests for cholesterol, blood sugar, or nutrient levels (e.g., vitamin D, B12) provide objective health data. A 2025 study showed testing guided supplement use in 70% of users.

At-Home Kits: Tests for hormones, gut health, or genetic markers are increasingly accessible, offering insights into personalized needs.

TELEHEALTH PLATFORMS

Virtual Consultations: Platforms like Teladoc or Amwell allow you to share tracking data with doctors or nutritionists for tailored advice.

Data Integration: Some platforms sync with wearables or apps, enhancing personalized recommendations.

COMMUNITY SUPPORT

Online Forums: Join communities on X (@TadSislerOne) or Reddit to share experiences and gain insights.

Local Groups: Health clubs or support groups provide motivation and accountability.

PRACTICAL TIPS

Choose tools that match your goals (e.g., nutrition apps for diet, wearables for activity).

Use consistent tracking to spot trends and measure progress.

Consult a healthcare provider to interpret biometric data and adjust your plan.

Combine tools (e.g., app with journal) for a comprehensive view of your health.

CUTTING-EDGE AI TOOLS, APPS, AND PROCESSES FOR VITAMINS, SUPPLEMENTS, AND GENERAL HEALTH

Here's a more complete breakdown of some of the more popular and effective tools:

InsideTracker uses a combination of advanced blood analysis, DNA insights, and AI-driven algorithms to provide customized health recommendations. By examining biomarkers like vitamin D, cholesterol, and inflammation markers, InsideTracker creates a data-backed action plan, suggesting dietary tweaks and supplementation strategies to optimize health over time.

Baze offers an at-home blood testing kit that measures key nutrient levels. Its AI-powered platform interprets your results and curates a monthly personalized vitamin subscription. The service regularly re-tests your blood to track progress and refine supplement choices, ensuring you only take what you truly need.

Care/of starts with an interactive online quiz that gathers information about your goals, diet, and lifestyle. Its AI system then recommends a custom vitamin and supplement plan delivered in daily packs. The platform refines its suggestions by asking follow-up questions over time, helping you stay on track with evolving health needs.

Persona Nutrition, similar to Care/of, employs an AI-driven quiz to pinpoint individual nutrient gaps, allergy concerns, and health objectives. It then crafts a precise regimen of vitamins, minerals, and herbs. Users also have access to nutritionists for extra guidance, ensuring they can continually tweak their plans as their lifestyles change.

Viome analyzes your gut microbiome through a stool sample, using AI to interpret trillions of microbial data points. The platform suggests specific foods to include or avoid and may recommend targeted supplements for better digestion, immune function, and overall health. Regular testing allows you to monitor how changes in diet or supplements affect your microbiome.

Cronometer is a robust nutrient-tracking app with data analytics and AI-driven insights to help you understand your daily macro and micronutrient intake. Logging your meals and supplements reveals patterns and identifies nutrient shortfalls, making it easier to determine if your current regimen meets your health goals.

Lumen is a breath-analysis device connected to an AI-driven app that measures your metabolism in real-time. Analyzing CO_2 levels in your breath determines whether you're burning carbs or fat. This immediate feedback helps tailor your supplement and dietary choices to optimize energy levels, weight management, and overall metabolic health.

MyFitnessPal: While primarily known as a calorie tracker, MyFitnessPal leverages machine learning and AI features to provide personalized tips on meal composition, nutrient balance, and progress trends. By logging supplements, meals, and exercise, users can visualize how each factor affects their overall health goals, making it more straightforward to identify where small changes can have significant impacts.

MyGeneFood focuses on genetic testing to guide dietary and supplement choices. The AI platform analyzes genetic markers linked to nutrient metabolism, potential sensitivities, and various health risks. It then recommends a personalized diet plan and supplement protocol tailored to your genetic blueprint, aiming for a customized path to better health.

Nutrient Optimiser syncs with your dietary data—often pulled from trackers like Cronometer—and uses an AI-based algorithm to pinpoint which foods and supplements can help you reach your nutrient targets. By focusing on maximizing nutrient density and suggesting incremental dietary changes, this tool allows you continually improve your micronutrient profile.

"He who has health, has hope; and he who has hope, has everything."
— Thomas Carlyle

SECTION TWO
BUILDING A TARGETED SUPPLEMENT STACK
11.2.1: CORE ESSENTIALS
(MULTIVITAMIN, FISH OIL, PROBIOTIC)

Truly, the minimum you might do to begin a targeted regimen is to just include a multivitamin, fish oil, and probiotic into your daily routine.

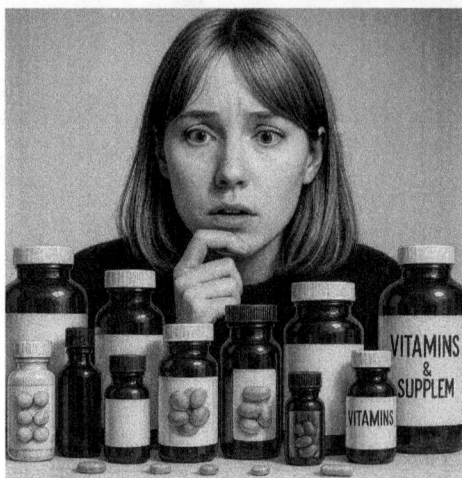

START WITH A GOOD DAILY MULTIVITAMIN

Think of a high-quality multivitamin as your nutritional safety net. Even if you eat well, it's easy to miss some nutrients here and there. A good multivitamin provides all the essential vitamins and minerals your body needs daily, helping with energy, keeping your cells healthy, and supporting overall wellness. Look for multivitamins that use easily absorbed forms of nutrients for better results.

CHOOSE OMEGA-3 FROM FISH OIL OR ALGAE TO FIGHT INFLAMMATION

Omega-3 fatty acids—especially EPA and DHA—are great for your heart and brain and help lower inflammation throughout your body. Fish oil is a popular choice, but if you're vegetarian or vegan, algae-based omega-3s offer the same benefits. Just be sure to pick products that are high-quality and tested for contaminants like heavy metals.

SAMPLE DAILY SUPPLEMENT ROUTINE

A simple daily routine might look like this: Take your multivitamin in the morning with a healthy breakfast to improve absorption. At lunch, have your omega-3 supplement (either fish oil or algae-based) to support your brain and fight inflammation. Then, if your digestion feels calm in the evening, take a probiotic to help healthy bacteria grow in your gut. Feel free to adjust these times based on what feels best for your digestion and convenience.

BOOST YOUR GUT HEALTH WITH PROBIOTICS

Your gut health affects your immune system, digestion, and even your mood. Probiotics—either from supplements or fermented foods like yogurt, kefir, kimchi, or sauerkraut—help fill your gut with friendly bacteria. These helpful microbes can make digestion easier, reduce bloating, and keep your digestive system balanced and healthy.

CHECK BRAND QUALITY AND TESTING RESULTS

Before buying supplements, take a moment to research the brands. Good brands are transparent about where they get their ingredients and how they make their products. They also usually have third-party testing to confirm their supplements are pure, safe, and effective. Choosing trusted brands means you can be confident you're getting exactly what's promised on the label.

"I believe that you can, by taking some simple and inexpensive measures, lead a longer life and extend your years of well-being. My most important recommendation is that you take vitamins every day in optimum amounts to supplement the vitamins that you receive in your food." – Linus Pauling

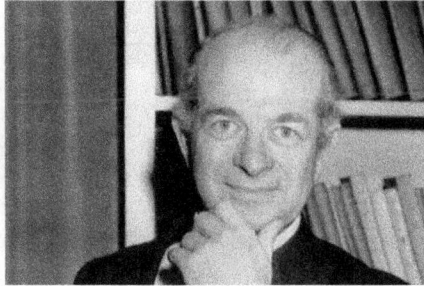

Linus Pauling

Credit – PICKRL - https://creativecommons.org/publicdomain/mark/1.0/

11.2.2: SPECIALTY ADD-ONS (ADAPTOGENS, NOOTROPICS, TARGETED MINERALS)

IF YOU FEEL STRESSED, TRY ADAPTOGENS LIKE ASHWAGANDHA

Adaptogens are special herbs that help your body handle stress and feel balanced. Ashwagandha, in particular, is popular because it helps lower stress hormones like cortisol and promotes a calmer mood. Over time, adaptogens can also give you more energy and help you bounce back faster from everyday stress.

FOR BETTER MEMORY OR FOCUS, CONSIDER NOOTROPICS

Nootropics, often called "brain boosters," are supplements designed to sharpen your memory and focus. Bacopa monnieri has been used for centuries to improve learning and concentration. Lion's Mane, a type of mushroom, may also help your brain grow new nerve connections and keep existing ones healthy. Combined with good daily habits, these supplements can help your mind feel clearer and sharper.

THE POWER OF COMBINING SUPPLEMENTS

Using adaptogenic herbs alongside basic supplements like a multivitamin and enough protein can boost their effectiveness. Your body needs a variety of vitamins and minerals to function at its best, while adaptogens help you manage stress more effectively. Together, these supplements create a solid foundation, helping your body and mind stay strong and balanced.

IF BLOOD TESTS SHOW YOU NEED IT, ADD SPECIFIC MINERALS LIKE IRON OR MAGNESIUM

I found out I had low white blood cells, so I added iron supplements (I chose comfort iron tablets). I don't take them every day because too much iron isn't healthy either, but now my white blood cell count is back to normal. Before adding specialized supplements, it's smart to check your mineral levels. Iron, magnesium, and other minerals affect your energy, muscles, and nerves. Correcting any deficiencies first ensures your body is ready to make the most of other supplements.

ADD NEW SUPPLEMENTS ONE AT A TIME TO SEE HOW THEY AFFECT YOU

When you start taking new supplements, add them slowly, one at a time. This helps you clearly see how each supplement affects you—good or bad. This careful approach makes it easy to figure out what's working best, what you should avoid, and how to build a supplement plan that perfectly suits your body and health goals.

"Observational studies show that exercise, nutritional supplements and reducing psychological stress can help. Chronic high stress and smoking can lead to accelerated telomere shortening." – Elizabeth Blackburn

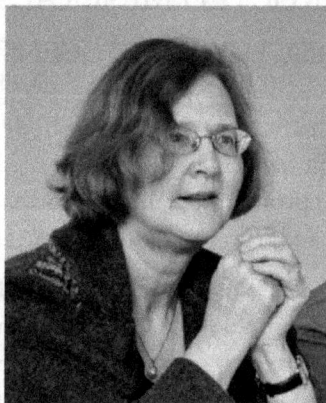

Elizabeth Blackburn
Credit – Wikimedia Commons

11.2.3: CYCLING AND PERIODIC ADJUSTMENTS

USE SOME SUPPLEMENTS IN CYCLES (LIKE SENOLYTICS OR STRONG ANTIOXIDANTS)

Some powerful supplements—like senolytics (which remove old, worn-out cells) or high-dose antioxidants—work better and are safer when taken in cycles, rather than continuously. Taking breaks between cycles can prevent side effects, keep the supplements effective, and give your body a chance to reset. This way, you'll get all the benefits without accidentally interfering with your body's natural processes.

CHECK YOUR LEVELS REGULARLY TO AVOID TAKING TOO MUCH

Regular lab tests or home-testing kits help you make sure you're getting just enough of each supplement—not too little, and not too much. This is especially important for vitamins and minerals that can build up in your body over time, like vitamin D or iron. Regular checks help you adjust your supplements as needed, saving money and keeping you healthy.

FOLLOW A SIMPLE THREE-MONTH CHECK-IN SCHEDULE

Start by checking your nutrient levels and overall health to set your baseline. After about 6-8 weeks, do a quick check to see how things are going, so you can make early changes if needed. At three months, do a more detailed review to see how you've improved and decide if your supplements still match your needs. This approach helps you stay consistent while making smart adjustments along the way.

PAY ATTENTION TO YOUR BODY: ENERGY, DIGESTION, AND SLEEP

Besides tests, your body gives you important clues about whether your supplements are helping or hurting. Notice how energized you feel in the morning, your mood during the day, and how comfortable your digestion is. Feeling tired, cranky, or bloated could mean something needs adjustment. Good energy and restful sleep usually indicate you're on the right track. Listening to these signals helps you fine-tune your plan.

UPDATE YOUR PLAN DURING BIG LIFE CHANGES

Major life events—like pregnancy, getting older, or starting a stressful new job—can change your body's nutritional needs dramatically. Hormones, stress levels, and lifestyle changes can all affect how your body uses nutrients. Updating your supplements to match your current life situation helps ensure your plan stays effective and supports your long-term health. Check 11.2.4 for more information.

If we set our sights on becoming the best version of ourselves, we can achieve anything. Single-mindedness will help you accomplish the wellness goal or anything you put your mind to. My friend, legendary actor **Gene Barry**, exemplified single-mindedness when he said:

"My earliest dreams were of acting, and I have never considered anything else."

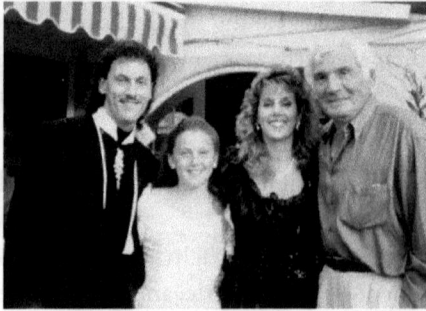

Tad, Rachel and Stephanie Sisler with Gene Barry
Source – Sisler Private Collection

11.2.4: ADJUSTING REGIMENS FOR LIFE STAGES

Your health needs evolve through life stages, requiring tailored supplement and lifestyle adjustments to optimize vitality and longevity. Below is a guide to adapting your regimen for key stages, with professional guidance recommended.

GENERAL APPROACH

Identify Health Goals: Focus on stage-specific priorities, like growth in youth or disease prevention in adulthood.

Consult Healthcare Providers: Regular check-ups and tests pinpoint needs or deficiencies.

Tailor Supplements: Adjust types and dosages based on age-related requirements.

Modify Lifestyle: Adapt diet, exercise, and stress management to suit each stage.

Track and Adjust: Use tools from 11.1.4 to monitor progress and refine your plan.

LIFE STAGES AND ADJUSTMENTS

CHILDHOOD AND ADOLESCENCE

Goals: Support growth, brain development, and immune health.

Supplements: Multivitamins, calcium, vitamin D for bone growth, omega-3s for cognitive health. A 2025 study emphasizes calcium's role in adolescent bone density.

Lifestyle: Balanced diet with fruits and vegetables, 60 minutes of daily physical activity, 8–10 hours of sleep, limited screen time.

ADULTHOOD

Goals: Prevent chronic diseases, maintain energy and mental clarity.

Supplements: Omega-3s, probiotics, vitamin D, magnesium to support heart and gut health. Antioxidants like vitamin C reduce oxidative stress.

Lifestyle: 150 minutes of moderate exercise weekly, stress management (e.g., meditation), Mediterranean diet, social engagement.

PREGNANCY

Goals: Support fetal development, maintain maternal health.

Supplements: Prenatal vitamins with folate (400–800 mcg), iron, calcium, DHA to prevent neural tube defects and support brain development. A 2025 study highlights folate's importance.

Lifestyle: Nutrient-rich diet, moderate exercise (e.g., walking), avoiding alcohol and smoking, regular prenatal care.

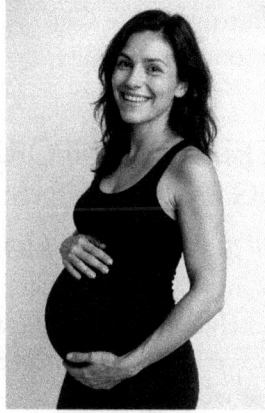

MENOPAUSE

Goals: Manage hormonal changes, protect bone and heart health.

Supplements: Calcium, vitamin D, magnesium for bone density, phytoestrogens (e.g., soy isoflavones) for symptom relief. Black cohosh may reduce hot flashes.

Lifestyle: Weight-bearing exercises, heart-healthy diet, stress reduction (e.g., yoga), regular health screenings.

AGING (60+)

Goals: Preserve muscle, cognitive function, and immunity.

Supplements: Vitamin B12 (absorption decreases with age), CoQ10, antioxidants, omega-3s to support energy and brain health. A 2025 study supports B12 for cognitive maintenance.

Lifestyle: Strength training, mental exercises (e.g., puzzles), social activities, balanced diet with adequate protein.

SPECIAL CONSIDERATIONS

Chronic Conditions: Adjust regimens for conditions like diabetes or arthritis with medical guidance.

Life Transitions: Events like retirement or loss may require emotional and physical support adjustments.

Genetic Factors: Use insights from genetic testing (see 10.1.4) to personalize supplement choices.

PRACTICAL TIPS

Work with a doctor or nutritionist to tailor supplements and lifestyle to your stage.

Use tracking tools to monitor how changes affect your health.

Adjust gradually to avoid overwhelming your routine.

Stay informed via trusted sources like X (@TadSislerOne) for updates on longevity science.

By adapting your health plan to your life stage, you can support your body's changing needs and promote long-term vitality.

SECTION THREE
STAYING MOTIVATED AND INFORMED
11.3.1: CELEBRATING SMALL WINS

KEEP AN EYE ON YOUR ENERGY, MOOD, AND LAB TESTS

Tracking your progress isn't just about lab results. How you feel each day—your morning energy, mood stability, and concentration—is just as important. Combine these everyday observations with periodic lab tests for a full picture of how your supplements are working. Using a simple notebook or app can help you notice trends, make changes as needed, and celebrate your real-life improvements.

REWARD YOURSELF FOR STICKING TO YOUR PLAN (BUT NOT WITH FOOD!)

Building and sticking to a supplement routine takes real commitment, so celebrate your successes! Reward yourself after milestones like a week of consistent supplement use or a month of feeling better. Pick non-food rewards—maybe a new book, a massage, or a short trip—to keep you motivated and make your new healthy habits fun and sustainable.

SHARE YOUR WINS WITH FRIENDS, FAMILY, OR GROUPS

Talking about your journey with supportive people—whether it's family, friends, or an online community—can help you stay motivated and accountable. It's also a great way to pick up new tips and ideas. Sharing your experiences helps everyone benefit from each other's successes and challenges, creating a supportive environment that keeps you moving forward.

BE REALISTIC—CHANGE TAKES TIME

Remember, real and lasting improvements don't usually happen overnight. It can take weeks or even months for your body to fully benefit from new nutrients, balance hormones, or rebuild its stores. Being patient and keeping your expectations realistic will help you avoid getting frustrated and stay focused on your long-term health goals.

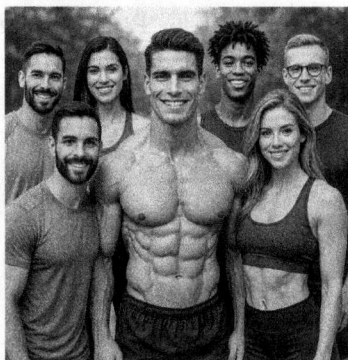

11.3.2: CONTINUOUS LEARNING AND ADAPTATION

CHECK RELIABLE HEALTH NEWS & USE SMART AI TOOLS

One of the easiest ways to stay on top of new health and longevity tips is to subscribe to trustworthy newsletters or medical journals. Add in AI tools (like the ones we talked about earlier), and you can quickly find what matters to you, skip the noise, and get the latest updates based on real science.

TALK TO YOUR DOCTOR ABOUT NEW INFO

Even the best research articles are more useful when you go over them with a healthcare pro. Try checking in with your doctor, naturopath, or dietitian every so often to talk about what you've read and see if it makes sense for your health goals.

Keep in mind: most doctors are trained to treat diseases and nutrient deficiencies—not necessarily to recommend supplements for prevention. That's changing, though. Integrative and functional medicine are becoming more popular, and more experts now see how vitamins and supplements can support overall wellness.

That said, doctors still vary in how they view supplements. Some are cautious and only suggest them when there's a proven need (like iron for anemia). Others are more proactive, recommending supplements based on lab work or your personal health history. The key is to work with a provider who keeps up with the latest science and gives advice tailored to you.

DON'T FALL FOR FAD SUPPLEMENTS—STICK TO THE SCIENCE

It's easy to get excited when a flashy headline or influencer claims a supplement will change your life—but most of those trends aren't backed by strong research. Before trying anything new, check if it's supported by real science or experts. Staying skeptical helps you avoid wasting time and money on things that don't work.

BE OPEN TO UPDATING YOUR PLAN AS SCIENCE EVOLVES

Health research is always moving forward, so your supplement plan might need to shift too. What works great for you today may be even better tomorrow with new evidence. Stay flexible, keep learning, and be open to trying new things—especially if they're backed by solid research. Being adaptable can lead to amazing improvements in how you feel and function, from better energy to sharper focus.

"Live as if you were to die tomorrow. Learn as if you were to live forever." –
Mahatma Gandhi

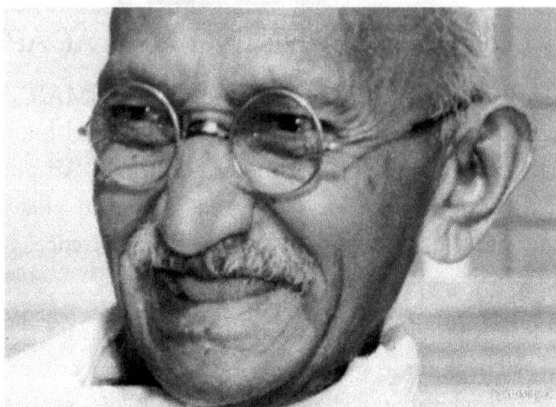

Mahatma Gandhi
Credit – PICRYL / creativecommons.org

II.3.3: BALANCING SUPPLEMENTS WITH OVERALL WELLNESS

SUPPLEMENTS HELP—BUT THEY'RE JUST ONE PIECE OF THE PUZZLE

Vitamins, herbs, and other supplements can help fill in the gaps, but they're not a magic fix. To really feel your best, you still need the basics: eating well, moving your body, and getting good sleep. Think of supplements like tools in your toolbox—they work best when you're already building a healthy lifestyle.

FEELING CONNECTED AND HAVING PURPOSE MATTERS FOR LONG LIFE

Studies show that strong relationships, a sense of community, and feeling like your life has meaning can make a big difference in your health. Whether it's through helping others, spending time with loved ones, or doing work you care about, emotional wellness plays a big role in how long and how well you live.

THE BLUE ZONES EXAMPLE

People in "Blue Zones"—places where people regularly live into their 90s and beyond—tend to have tight communities and shared purpose. They show us that staying socially connected can be just as powerful as any supplement or medication when it comes to living a longer, healthier life.

ADD STRESS-RELIEVING HABITS LIKE MEDITATION OR JOURNALING

Stress can undo a lot of your hard work. Even if you're eating well and taking great supplements, too much stress can throw your hormones off and weaken your immune system. That's why it helps to build in calming habits like meditation, deep breathing, or writing in a journal. Just a few quiet minutes each day can boost your focus, calm your mind, and support your overall health.

BALANCE YOUR MIND, BODY, AND SPIRIT

Real health isn't just about your body—it's also about how you think and feel. Take time to check in with yourself. Are your food choices, workouts, relationships, and daily routines all pointing you toward a life that feels meaningful? When everything is in sync, your supplements will work even better, and you'll be setting yourself up for a healthier, more fulfilling life.

"Wellness is the complete integration of body, mind, and spirit – the realization that everything we do, think, feel, and believe has an effet on our state of well-being." – Greg Anderson

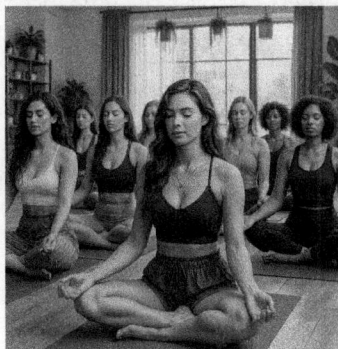

Now that you've constructed your personalized blueprint, let's review the key takeaways and inspire you to continue on this path to health and longevity.

CONCLUSION

As we wrap things up, I hope you feel more confident and inspired than ever. What you've learned here goes far beyond facts and charts—it's about giving yourself the tools to feel better, live stronger, and take charge of your health in a real, lasting way.

Together, we've explored vitamins, minerals, herbs, and cutting-edge research on how to stay energized, support your immune system, and age with strength and grace. But if there's one takeaway to carry with you, it's this: supplements work best as part of a bigger picture. Nothing beats the power of nourishing food, regular movement, good sleep, and taking care of your emotional health.

The real magic? It's in staying curious. Keep learning, stay open to new research, and don't be afraid to try what feels right for you—especially with the guidance of a trusted healthcare professional. Listen to your body, celebrate your wins (big or small), and trust that every step you take matters.

With each healthy choice you make—every deep breath, every morning walk, every mindful moment—you're building a life that's full of energy, clarity, and joy. Let your knowledge be your compass. Keep that spark alive. You have everything it takes to feel amazing and keep thriving—not just today, but for many vibrant years ahead.

Here's to your health, your happiness, and your journey. You've got this!

PLEASE LEAVE A REVIEW

Now that you have everything you need to **work towards a longer, healthier life**, it's time to share your newfound knowledge and show other readers where they can find the same support.

By leaving your honest opinion of this book on Amazon or wherever you purchased it, you'll help others discover the guidance they need to elevate their voices and share their passion for **a healthy, meaningful, long life.**

Thank you for your help. The **quest for answers** lives on when we pass on what we've learned, and you're helping **me** to do just that.

If you purchased my book on Amazon, please leave your review.

REFERENCES

I. License Link References
- Creative Commons. (n.d.). Attribution-ShareAlike 2.0 International (CC BY-SA 2.0) [License]. Retrieved from https://creativecommons.org/licenses/by/2.0/
- Creative Commons. (n.d.). Attribution-ShareAlike 4.0 International (CC BY-SA 4.0) [License]. Retrieved from https://creativecommons.org/licenses/by/4.0/

II. Quotes & Inspiration

- AZQuotes. (n.d.). Quotes on cinnamon. Retrieved from
https://www.azquotes.com/quotes/topics/cinnamon.html
- AZQuotes. (n.d.). Quotes on probiotics. Retrieved from
https://www.azquotes.com/quotes/topics/probiotics.html
- BrainyQuote. (n.d.). Various quotes by authors and thinkers. Retrieved from
https://www.brainyquote.com/
- Elevate ADK. (n.d.). Voices on cannabis: 11 insightful quotes by influential figures. Retrieved from
https://elevateadk.com/voices-on-cannabis-11-insightful-quotes-by-influential-figures/
- Goodreads. (n.d.). Therapeutic 2: Metformin – The "low-risk" wonder drug. Retrieved from
https://www.goodreads.com/quotes/11169440-therapeutic-2-metformin-the-low-risk-wonder-drug-
metformin-may-have-already
- Goodreads. (n.d.). Yin and yang quote. Retrieved from
https://www.goodreads.com/quotes/9045081-yin-and-yang-male-and-female-strong-and-weak-
rigid#:~:text=Sign%20Up%20Now-
,Yin%20and%20yang%2C%20male%20and%20female%2C%20strong%20and%20weak%2C,oppos
ite%20principles%20constitutes%20the%20universe
- Hathaway, A. (2014). Interview in Harper's Bazaar.
- IMDb. (n.d.). Quotes by [Name redacted]. Retrieved from
https://www.imdb.com/name/nm0058001/quotes/
- India Today. (2020, November 13). Inspirational quotes about Ayurveda and Ayurvedic lifestyle.
Retrieved from https://www.indiatoday.in/information/story/inspirational-quotes-about-ayurveda-
and-ayurvedic-lifestyle-1740776-2020-11-13
- Naidoo, U. (n.d.). Probiotics and prebiotics quote. In QuoteFancy. Retrieved from
https://quotefancy.com/quote/3434128/Uma-Naidoo-Probiotics-and-Prebiotics-If-you-re-suffering-
from-gut-induced-depression-how
- Paltrow, G. (2010). GOOP Newsletter. Retrieved from https://goop.com
- PeaceJoyAustin (Author). (n.d.). Top quotes: Lifespan — Why We Age and Why We Don't Have
To by David Sinclair. Retrieved from https://peacejoyaustin.medium.com/top-quotes-lifespan-why-
we-age-and-why-we-dont-have-to-david-sinclair-c8df323db153
- Quotio.com. (n.d.). Quotes by Mark Redman. Retrieved from https://quotio.com/by/Mark-
Redman
- coolsandiegosights.com. (2018, October 4). "There is no shortcut to true success." Retrieved from
https://coolsandiegosights.com/2018/10/04/there-is-no-shortcut-to-true-success/

III. Vitamins & Minerals

- BodyCarre. (n.d.). *Zinc*. Retrieved from https://bodycarre.com/food-nutrition/zinc/
- Consistent Reviews. (n.d.). *Vitamin C serum benefits uncovered: Your secret to glowing skin*.
Retrieved from https://www.consistentreviews.com/vitamin-c-serum-benefits/
- Elanza Wellness. (n.d.). *Does folic acid affect fertility? What the science says*. Retrieved from
https://www.elanzawellness.com/post/does-folic-acid-affect-fertility-what-the-science-says
- Elm & Rye. (n.d.). *A comprehensive guide to essential vitamins: What you need to know*. Retrieved
from https://elmandrye.com/blogs/news/a-comprehensive-guide-to-essential-vitamins-what-you-need-
to-know
- Gugi Health. (n.d.). *Zinc: The essential mineral for immune health and beyond*. Retrieved from
https://gugihealth.com/nutrition-supplements/6ovlmufnexuczaxkjxs1/
- Health Guide Info. (n.d.). *How much vitamin C is too much? Side effects of consuming excess
vitamin C*. Retrieved from https://www.healthguideinfo.com/vitamins-minerals/p82066/
- Health Views Online. (n.d.). *Complete info on Vitamin B9: Functions, RDA, deficiency & more*.
Retrieved from https://healthviewsonline.com/about-vitamin-b9-folic-functions-food-source-
recommended-amount-deficiency/
- Health and the City. (n.d.). *Vitamin B12 shots for B12 deficiency*. Retrieved from
https://healthandthecity.ca/b12-shots/
- Lakshmi, P. (2016). *Love, Loss, and What We Ate: A Memoir*. Ecco.

- Life Answers HQ. (n.d.). *Can you take multivitamins without food?* Retrieved from https://millerfortexas.com/can-you-take-multivitamins-without-food/
- Lindberg, J. S., Zobitz, M. M., Poindexter, J. R., & Pak, C. Y. (1990). Magnesium bioavailability from magnesium citrate and magnesium oxide. *Journal of the American College of Nutrition, 9*(1), 48–55.
- Media Express24. (n.d.). *Vitamins required for our body in winter*. Retrieved from https://mediaexpress24.com/health/vitamins-required-for-our-body-in-winter/
- NZ Nutrition Foundation. (n.d.). *Antioxidant supplementation*. Retrieved from https://nutritionfoundation.org.nz/antioxidant-supplementation/
- Nourishing Our Children. (2022, June 7). *Vitamin B12 can not be obtained from plant foods*. Retrieved from https://nourishingourchildren.org/2022/06/07/vitamin-b12/
- Oxygens.co.uk. (n.d.). *Combine vitamins with hyperbaric oxygen therapy*. Retrieved from https://oxygens.co.uk/combine-vitamins-with-hyperbaric-oxygen-therapy/
- Radcliffe, P. (2005). *Paula: My Story So Far*. Simon & Schuster.
- Rise of Kingdoms Answers. (n.d.). *Which of the following vitamins is most helpful for maintaining good vision?* Retrieved from https://rokanswers.com/which-of-the-following-vitamins-is-most-helpful-for-maintaining-good-vision/
- Spelling, T. (2013). *Spelling It Like It Is*. Gallery Books.
- We Train Phlebotomists. (n.d.). *Case studies of therapeutic phlebotomy in treating hemochromatosis*. Retrieved from https://wetrainphlebotomists.com/case-studies-of-therapeutic-phlebotomy-in-treating-hemochromatosis/

IV. Herbs & Natural Remedies
- 40 Aprons. (n.d.). *All about Ashwagandha*. Retrieved from https://40aprons.com/ashwagandha/
- Acupuncture Wellness Services. (n.d.). *Chinese herbal remedies: A holistic approach to health*. Retrieved from https://acupuncturewellnessservices.com/chinese-herbs-and-herbal-remedies/
- American Journal of Traditional Chinese Veterinary Medicine. (2021). Mai Wei Di Huang Wan. https://doi.org/10.59565/xyko4588
- Boshi Beauty. (n.d.). *Waterless Bōshi Beauty® nanofiber technology unlocks the full potential of antioxidants*. Retrieved from https://boshibeauty.com/ja/waterless-boshi-beauty-nanofiber-technology-unlocks-the-full-potential-of-antioxidants/
- Fleurance Nature. (n.d.). *Royal jelly in dispensers*. Retrieved from https://www.fleurancenature.com/en/p/royal-jelly-in-dispensers-03130.html
- Greenway Magazine. (2023, July 18). *Midwest Magic launches Midwest Magic Mushroom Gummies*. Retrieved from https://mogreenway.com/2023/07/18/midwest-magic-launches-new-thc-infused-gummies-adding-benefits-of-adaptogenic-mushrooms/
- Laviano, E., et al. (2020). Association between preoperative levels of 25-hydroxyvitamin D and hospital-acquired infections after hepatobiliary surgery. *PLOS ONE, 15*(3), e0230336.
- NootropicsPlanet. (n.d.). *The secret life of mushrooms: How they can boost immunity, support your gut, and even fight cancer*. Retrieved from https://nootropicsplanet.com/mushrooms-boost-immunity/
- ProcuRSS.eu. (n.d.). *What is oxidative stress & how does it affect the mind and body?* Retrieved from https://procurss.eu/what-is-oxidative-stress-how-does-it-affect-the-mind-and-body/
- Science News. (n.d.). Warming to a Cold War Herb. Line 40—quote by Georg Wikman on Valery Polyakov.
- Urdega. (n.d.). *Unveiling the science behind Testosil ingredients: Powering men's vitality*. Retrieved from https://urdega.com/unveiling-the-science-behind-testosil-ingredients-powering-mens-vitality/

V. Longevity & Advanced Research
Armitage, H. (2020, April 6). 'Smart toilet' monitors for signs of disease. *Stanford Medicine News Center*. Retrieved from https://med.stanford.edu/news/all-news/2020/04/smart-toilet-monitors-for-signs-of-disease.html
Fisetin Unveiled: 5 Surprising Health Benefits of This Mighty Flavonoid. (n.d.). *Piracetam.net*. Retrieved from https://piracetam.net/fisetin-health-benefits/

Gene Editing Opens Faster, Cheaper Way to Introduce New Crop Traits. (n.d.). *Grain Central*. Retrieved from https://www.graincentral.com/news/gene-editing-opens-faster-cheaper-way-to-introduce-new-crop-traits/

Navigating the World of Nootropics: Natural Brain Boosters. (n.d.). *No Ordinary Moments Nutrition*. Retrieved from https://www.noordinarymoments.co/blogs/news/navigating-the-world-of-nootropics-natural-brain-boosters

Ozfirat, Z., & Chowdhury, T. A. (2010). Vitamin D deficiency and type 2 diabetes. *Postgraduate Medical Journal*. https://doi.org/10.1136/pgmj.2009.078626

PMC. (n.d.). *Article on metformin*. Retrieved from https://pmc.ncbi.nlm.nih.gov/articles/PMC6814615/

S, D., S, A., V, S., G, S., & G, C. (2021). Carotenoids and cognitive outcomes: A meta-analysis of randomized intervention trials. *Antioxidants, 10*(2), 223. https://doi.org/10.3390/antiox10020223

Unveiling the Connection Between Vitamin D, Obesity, and Longevity. (n.d.). *PrimeMDPlus*. Retrieved from https://primemdplus.com/trending/unveiling-the-connection-between-vitamin-d-obesity-and-longevity/

What Is Gamma-linolenic Acid? High and Low Values | Lab Results Explained. (2021, June 14). *HealthMatters.io*. Retrieved from https://blog.healthmatters.io/2021/06/14/what-is-gamma-linolenic-acid-high-and-low-values-lab-results-explained/

VI. Additional Health & Lifestyle

10 Reasons Why You Need To Eat Your Greens! (n.d.). *Live Love Fruit*. Retrieved from https://livelovefruit.com/why-you-need-to-eat-your-greens/

About Black Seed Oil. (n.d.). Retrieved from https://aboutblackseedoil.com/black-seed-quotes/

AcuAtlanta – Supplements: Vitamin D & K. (n.d.). Retrieved from https://acuatlanta.net/vitamins/vitamin-d-k/

(Note: Overlaps with "Vitamins & Minerals," included here if discussing lifestyle integration.)

Ask The Doctor. (n.d.). *What Is Sensitive Gut and Irritable Bowel Syndrome?* NorthwestPharmacy.com. Retrieved from https://www.northwestpharmacy.com/askthedoctor/what-is-sensitive-gut-and-irritable-bowel-syndrome

Can Coffee Cause Anxiety or Depression? (n.d.). *SourceEC – Corporate Gift Information*. Retrieved from https://sourceec.com.sg/corporate-gift-knowledge-detail/can-coffee-cause-anxiety-or-depression/

Can You Take Too Much Metformin? (2023, September 2). *Porter Brothers Ltd*. Retrieved from https://porterbrothersltd.com/2023/09/02/can-you-take-too-much-metformin/

LiveWellMedicine.com. (n.d.). *If there is free flow, there is no pain*. Retrieved from https://www.livewellmedicine.com/if-there-is-free-flow-there-is-no-pain/

Mayo Clinic. (n.d.). *Fish oil (omega-3 fatty acids)*. Retrieved from https://www.mayoclinic.org/drugs-supplements-fish-oil/art-20364810#:~:text=There's%20strong%20evidence%20that%20omega

National Eczema Association. (n.d.). *Open letter to eczema*. Retrieved from https://nationaleczema.org/blog/open-letter-to-eczema/

ORBilu (n.d.). *Detailed reference*. Retrieved from https://orbilu.uni.lu/handle/10993/51650

The Issue. (n.d.). *The nutritional benefits of eating eggs every day*. Retrieved from https://theissue.co.uk/health-fitness/the-nutritional-benefits-of-eating-eggs-every-day/

Rizzo, N. (2024, February 5). BEETS: HEALTH BENEFITS AND NUTRITION. Today. **https://www.today.com/health/diet-fitness/beets-benefits-rcna135124**

Alba, J. (2013). *The Honest Life: Living Naturally and True to You*. Rodale Books.

VII. Reference Tools & Journals for Further Reading

Nature Portfolio. (n.d.). *Nature Aging*. https://www.nature.com/nataging

Elsevier. (n.d.). *The Lancet*. http://thelancet.com/

Oxford Academic. (n.d.). *Sleep*. https://www.sleep-journals.com/

Segerstrom, S. C. (2025, May). [Article page]. *Behavioral Sleep Medicine*. https://journals.lww.com/bsam/pages/default.aspx

Public Library of Science. (n.d.). *PLOS Medicine*. https://journals.plos.org/plosmedicine/

23andMe, Inc. (n.d.). *Personal genetic testing & ancestry service*. https://www.23andme.com/

American College of Medical Genetics and Genomics. (n.d.). *Genetics in Medicine.*
https://www.gimjournal.org/
Van der Graaf, P. H. (n.d.). [Editorial profile]. *CPT: Pharmacometrics & Systems Pharmacology.*
https://ascpt.onlinelibrary.wiley.com/journal/15326535
MDPI. (n.d.). *Nutrients.* https://www.mdpi.com/journal/nutrients

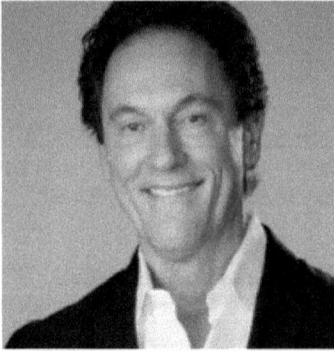

ABOUT THE AUTHOR

Tad Sisler is an American Composer, Author and Producer of feature films and music. More than a thousand of his original works are available through *iTunes, Amazon* and virtually every other major marketplace. Through the years, **Tad** created and released independent feature films and documentaries, television shows, developed a music store and vast collection of music for film and television usages, in addition to published screenplays and books.

Tad is a voting member of *The Academy of Recording Arts & Sciences.* **Tad** invented a wireless karaoke all-in-one microphone that became a best-seller on *Amazon.* A child prodigy, Tad was playing advanced piano pieces at the age of 8, and rating superior in Classical piano competitions at 12. Tad won his first scholarship for singing at 12, attending the Idyllwild School of Music and the Arts, then affiliated with the University of Southern California.

FEATURE FILMS

Tad produced, edited, and released "**The Ghosts of Brewer Town**", a mystery feature film, currently available on *YouTube.*

TELEVISION PROJECTS

Tad launched the **Journey To An Extraordinary Life-Legends Among Us** documentary series, which chronicles the lives and careers of legendary artists, actors, sports figures and heroes of medicine, in a feature-film format.

BOOKS

Books, Audio Books and Podcasts released by **Tad** include "**Reflections in the Key of Life-The Steve Madaio Story**", chronicling the life and times of America's most prolific trumpeter. This book garnered a **Readers' Favorite Book Award** for Tad.

"**Mafia Baby**" is a shocking true story of a woman raped by a Mafioso, who then raised his child alone. Tad's autobiography, "**It's a Long Climb to The Middle**" *is* available currently on *Amazon* and *Barnes & Noble.* Screenplays in development by Tad Sisler include "**The Incredible Spark of Franklin Benjamin**", and "**Please Don't Forget**". Tad's latest **Music Mastery** collection of books is designed to educate and inspire musicians to become masters. His **Health and Longevity Mastery** series of books is crafted to educate on longevity, age reversal, and general wellness.

MUSIC

Tad's production music catalog tripled in size with the addition of thousands of excellent production music tracks, as well as hundreds of sound-alike tracks for the DJ/Karaoke industry, now distributed on **iTunes, Amazon Marketplace, CD Baby, Spotify, Rdio, Xbox Music** and dozens of other outlets Worldwide.

Tad produced and released "The Barcelona Sessions" to 1000 radio stations Worldwide, with never-before-heard original performances by Miles Davis' bassist, Bill Evan's drummer, Frank Sinatra's saxophonist, Maynard Ferguson's guitarist, and Andrae Crouch' flutist/saxophonist, produced by Tad Sisler in his recording studio.

Tad Sisler composed the full score to "**The Encore Of Tony Duran**", an indie feature film starring **Elliott Gould, William Katt, Nicki Ziering and Cody Kasch**, along with his co- composer Andrew Fraga, Jr. After having the distinction of being the first film to sell-out at the prestigious *Palm Springs International Film Festival*, the film won the **Jury Award** for **Best Feature Film** at the *Las Vegas Film Festival* and the *Santa Fe Film Festival*, as well as the **Indie Spirit Award** at the *Fort Lauderdale Film Festival* and the **Audience Favorite Award** at *Tallgrass Film Festival*, in conjunction with a **Lifetime Achievement Award** for **Elliott Gould**. The film is available on *Amazon Prime*.

Tad completed the music and audio editing for the TV Series "**American M.C.**". The first 7 episodes are complete and in the process of distribution through **iTunes**. Tad scored the Main Title theme to **American M.C.** as well as underscore and providing Music Supervision and source music.

PRODUCTION

Tad Sisler has been a valuable member of the team of specialists and project developers for **Yamaha Corporation of America**, delivering hundreds of intricate projects to exact **Yamaha** specifications over a 10-year period.

Tad received accolades in 2011 after being given the honor and challenge of doing the "official" remake of the iconic "**Andy Griffith Theme**" for the estate of the composer **Earle Hagen** as a perfect sound-alike, along with his composing associate Andrew Fraga, Jr.

Following a stint composing for a series entitled "**Famous Families**" on **Foxstar** and working as assistant to composer Jeff Edwards on the television series "**Silk Stalkings**" and "**Renegade**" in the late 1990's, Tad Sisler and founded & developed a production music catalog, containing thousands of high-quality music tracks available for sync licenses in film, television and advertising in more than 150 genres.

In addition to handling Music Supervision on "**The Encore Of Tony Duran**", and on "**American M.C.**", "**The Ghosts of Brewer Town**", "**'Tis' The Season**", the "**Journey To an Extraordinary Life**" series, **Tad** placed his original music on **NBC, ABC/Disney, Warner Brothers Television**, **TNT**, US National Infomercial campaigns through **Guthy/Renker** and **Script To Screen**, as well as custom composing for the TV and Advertising industry.

Tad released contains hundreds of top-quality soundalike tracks produced by **Tad** and his associates, for DJ and Karaoke usages, currently on *ITunes, Amazon Marketplace, Spotify, Rdio, Xbox Music,* and many other outlets.

LIVE PRODUCTION

In the 1980's and 1990's, **Tad** and his team produced a series of live headliner events at multiple venues from the ground up, including sold-out performances by **Kenny Rogers, Earth, Wind & Fire, Los Lobos, Glen Campbell, The Righteous Brothers, Lou Rawls, Tito Puente,** the **Power Jam** featuring **Timmy T, Tara Kemp, Candyman, Soul To Soul** and more.

HISTORY

As a very young man, Tad Sisler worked as a performer for **Frank Sinatra**, studied music in choreography under world-famous Broadway Dancer/Choreographer **Jacque D'Amboise**, received superior ratings in classical piano performance in tough **Joanna Hodges** international competitions, and received private acting lessons from **Richard Burton**, a friend of his family.

Tad attended the prestigious **Idyllwild School of Music and the Arts** on vocal music scholarships during the period when it was affiliated with the **University of Southern California**. In High School, Tad was one of 100 statewide vocalists elected to the prestigious **All-State Choir** in Missouri.

During his storied career, Tad has also had the honor of performing with and working among such greats as **Gladys Knight, Rita Coolidge, B.B. King, Marilyn McCoo, Johnny Mathis, Kenny Rogers, Tito Puente, Sonny and Mary Bono, Gene Barry, Terry Cole-Whittaker, Shecky Greene, Peter Marshall, Mary Hart, Blackwell, Herb Jeffries, Trini Lopez, Glen Campbell, Jennifer Hudson** and other legends.

Tad Sisler's extensive experience, state of the art facility and history of delivering quality feature films and music <u>on time and on budget</u>, as well as the ability to draw from an extensive catalog of production music, allows his experienced team to offer complete services in custom film and television production as well as in music composition and production efficiently.

Tad is proud and humbled to be a voting member of the **Academy of Recording Arts & Sciences**, which allows him to have a voice to vote for great artists worthy of winning a **Grammy Award**. Many of Tad's works have been placed into Grammy consideration.

In 2023, Tad won a prestigious **Telly Award** for creative excellence in his *Journey to an Extraordinary Life* film series.

Modern Renaissance Publishing is at the forefront of a new intellectual awakening, dedicated to fostering a renaissance of ideas that resonate in today's world. Our mission is to bring cutting-edge concepts and timeless wisdom to the public through a diverse array of publishing formats, including books, eBooks, and audiobooks.

We are proud to launch our **Music Mastery** series, offering comprehensive guides and insights for musicians of all levels. Our **Health and Longevity Mastery** series highlights the latest discoveries and insights into extending the human healthspan and lifespan. In addition to our literary endeavors, we also publish original music, enriching the cultural landscape with creative expressions. Whether you're seeking to expand your knowledge, enhance your skills, or simply be inspired,

Modern Renaissance Publishing provides the resources and content to empower your journey. Join us as we bridge the rich heritage of the past with the innovative spirit of the present to shape a brighter, more enlightened future.

©2025 by Tad Sisler

Publisher: MODERN RENAISSANCE PUBLISHING

IN USA +1 (818) 845-6700

modernrenaissancepublishing.com

Email: modernrenaissancepublishing@gmail.com

ISBN# 978-1-966258-29-2

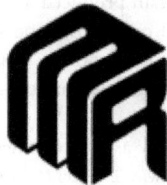

MODERN RENAISSANCE
PUBLISHING

www.ingramcontent.com/pod-product-compliance
Lightning Source LLC
Chambersburg PA
CBHW062120020426
42335CB00013B/1043